HANDBOOK FOR

BRUNNER AND SUDDARTH'S
TEXTBOOK OF MEDICAL–SURGICAL NURSING

HANDBOOK FOR

BRUNNER AND SUDDARTH'S
TEXTBOOK OF MEDICAL–SURGICAL NURSING

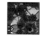 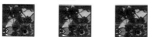

DIANE C. BAUGHMAN, EdD, RNCS
Professor
Weber State University
Nursing Program
Ogden, Utah

JoANN C. HACKLEY, MSNC, RN
Assistant Professor
Weber State University
Nursing Program
Ogden, Utah

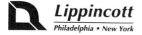 *Lippincott*
Philadelphia • New York

Acquisitions Editor: Lisa Stead
Sponsoring Editor: Brian MacDonald
Production: Berliner, Inc.
Production Manager: Janet Greenwood

Library of Congress Cataloging-in-Publication Data
Baughman, Diane C.
    Handbook for Brunner and Suddarth's textbook of medical–surgical nursing / Diane C. Baughman, JoAnn C. Hackley
        p.   cm.
    Handbook for: Brunner and Suddarth's textbook of medical–surgical nursing / [edited by] Suzanne C. Smeltzer, Brenda G. Bare. 8th ed. 1995.
    Includes index
    ISBN 0-397-55162-2.
    1. Nursing—Handbooks, manuals, etc.   2. Surgical nursing—Handbooks, manuals, etc.   I. Hackley, JoAnn C.   II. Brunner and Suddarth's textbook of medical–surgical nursing.   III. Title.
    [DNLM: 1. Nursing Care—handbooks.   2. Surgical Nursing—handbooks.   WY 49 B345h 1996]
    RT51.B38   1996
    610.73—dc20
    DNLM/DLC
    for Library of Congress   95-25922

The material contained in this volume was submitted as previously unpublished material, except in the instances in which credit has been given to the source from which some of the illustrative maaterial was derived.

Great care has been taken to maintain the accuracy of the information contained in the volume. However, neither Lippincott–Raven Publishers nor the editors can be held responsible for errors or for any consequences arising from the use of the information herein.

The authors and publisher have exerted every effort to ensure that drug selection and dosage set forth in this text are in accord with current recommendations and practice at the time of publication. However, in view of ongoing research, changes in government regulations, and the constant flow of information relating to drug therapy and drug reactions, the reader is urged to check the package insert for each drug for any change in indications and dosage and for added warnings and precautions. This is particularly important when the recommended agent is a new or infrequently employed drug.

Materials appearing in this book prepared by individuals as part of their official duties as U.S. Government employees are not covered by the above mentioned copyright.

9 8 7 6 5 4 3 2 1

PREFACE

This *Handbook for Brunner & Suddarth's Textbook of Medical–Surgical Nursing* is a comprehensive yet concise clinical reference designed for use by students and nurses. Perfect for both the hospital and community settings, it presents need-to-know information on the most commonly seen diseases and disorders in an easy-to-use outline format. Each entry is formatted consistently for quick access to vital information on:

A general overview of the disease process
Most common clinical manifestations
Main diagnostic evaluation methods
Medical management
Major nursing diagnoses and collaborative problems
Nursing interventions

For readers requiring more in-depth information, the *Handbook* is completely cross-referenced to *Brunner and Suddarth's Textbook of Medical–Surgical Nursing*, by Smeltzer and Bare, the leading comprehensive medical surgical textbook.

Special Features

Because of the revolution in health care and the increasing emphasis on home care, many entries include a separate section entitled "Patient Education and Health Maintenance: Care in the Home and Community." This section focuses on information vital to nurses in the home and community settings, who play an increasingly independent role as patient care providers. Patient and family teaching information is included in these sections.

"Gerontologic Considerations" provide an understanding of specific issues related to the care of older adults and help today's nurses and nursing students deal with this growing population.

"Clinical Alerts" call the reader's attention to priority care issues and highlight potential life-threatening situations.

The *Handbook*'s convenient pocket size and A to Z organization allow the user to reference pertinent information quickly and easily wherever care is being given.

We have written this text with an eye to providing content that as nurses we need to know. We hope it will provide a valuable guide to assist you in your education and nursing practice.

Diane C. Baughman, EdD, RNCS
JoAnn C. Hackley, MSNC, RN

Acknowledgments

We would like to thank Paul Streeter, Nursing Editor, at Lippincott–Raven for initiating this project and providing continuous support and guidance. Special thanks to Joanne De Carlo for her valuable transcription skills which helped this book come to completion; and Jeffrey L. Christensen for his phenomenal computer knowledge and patience in troubleshooting our computer glitches.

Contents

ABSCESS, BRAIN

See Brain Abscess

ABSCESS, LUNG

See Lung Abscess

ACNE VULGARIS

Acne vulgaris is a common follicular disorder affecting susceptible pilosebaceous follicles (hair follicles) most commonly found on the face, neck, and upper trunk. It is the most often encountered skin condition, becoming more marked at puberty and adolescence. The etiology of acne appears to stem from an interplay of genetic, hormonal, and bacterial factors. Diagnosis is most often made on signs and symptoms.

CLINICAL MANIFESTATIONS

1. Closed comedones (whiteheads).
2. Open comedones (blackheads).
3. Erythematous papules (inflammatory condition).
4. Inflammatory pustules.
5. Inflammatory cysts.

MANAGEMENT

The goals are to reduce bacterial colonies, decrease sebaceous gland activity, prevent the follicles from becoming plugged, reduce inflammation, combat secondary infection, minimize scarring, and eliminate factors that predispose the person to acne.

Dietary Therapy

Eliminate foods associated with acne flare-up, e.g., chocolate, colas, fried foods, and milk products.

Skin Hygiene

1. In mild cases: wash at least two times daily with cleansing soap; dislodge comedones with abrasive sponge (Buf-Puf).
2. Discourage use of oil-based cosmetics or creams.

Topical Pharmacotherapy

1. Benzoyl peroxide preparation.
2. Vitamin A acid (tretinoin).
3. Topical antibiotics, e.g., tetracycline, erythromycin.

Systemic Therapy

1. Systemic antibiotics, e.g., tetracycline, minocycline (Minocin).
2. Oral retinoids, e.g., vitamin A, isotretinoin (Accutane).
3. Hormone therapy, e.g., progesterone-estrogen preparations.

Surgical Treatment

1. Comedo extraction.
2. Injections of steroids into the inflamed lesions.
3. Incision and drainage.
4. Cryosurgery.
5. Dermabrasion.

NURSING PROCESS

Assessment

1. Observe and listen to how patient perceives skin condition.
2. Approach the adolescent with empathy and compassion.
3. Inspect lesions by gently stretching the skin. Closed comedones appear as slightly elevated small

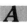

papules. Open comedones appear flat or slightly raised with a central follicular impaction.
4. Document the presence of inflammatory lesions.

Major Nursing Diagnosis

1. Ineffective management of therapeutic regimen related to insufficient knowledge about the condition and its causes, course, prevention, treatment, and skin care.
2. Body image disturbance related to embarrassment and frustration over appearance.

Collaborative Problems

1. Scarring.
2. Infection.

Planning and Implementation

The major goals may include understanding of the condition to enhance compliance with prescribed therapy, development of self-acceptance, and absence of complications.

Interventions

INCREASING TREATMENT COMPLIANCE AND UNDERSTANDING

1. Counsel and assure that problem is not related to uncleanliness, dietary indiscretions, masturbation, sexual activity, or other misconceptions.
2. Reinforce concept that acne arises from many factors.
3. Teach rationale for using oral and topical medications.
4. Explain actions and side effects of medications; encourage frequent blood tests.
5. Encourage consistent treatment every day.

PROMOTING SELF-ACCEPTANCE

1. Make patient a partner in therapy; take problems seriously; give understanding, reassurance, and support.
2. Consider all aspects of emotional factors.
3. Assist with stress reduction techniques as needed.

MONITORING AND MANAGING POTENTIAL COMPLICATIONS

1. Scarring: Caution against manipulation of lesions; inform patient of potential scarring from surgical intervention.
2. Infection: Advise to watch for signs and symptoms of oral or vaginal candidiasis when on long-term antibiotic therapy.

✎ **PATIENT EDUCATION AND HEALTH MAINTENANCE: CARE IN THE HOME AND COMMUNITY**

1. Instruct patient to wash face with mild soap and water twice a day; use of Buf-Puf may be helpful.
2. Advise patient to avoid all forms of friction and trauma to the face; to avoid cosmetics, shaving creams, and lotions; to follow a nutritious diet; and to keep hands away from the face and not to squeeze pimples or blackheads.
3. Counsel on need to be consistent with treatment and use of recommended cleansing products.
4. Reassure that most acne medications cause some drying and peeling of the skin.
5. Teach patient about disease process.
6. Advise that treatment may take 4–6 weeks or longer for results.

For more information see Chapter 54 in Smeltzer and Bare: *Brunner and Suddarth's Textbook of Medical Surgical Nursing,* 8th Edition. Philadelphia: Lippincott–Raven, 1996.

ACQUIRED IMMUNODEFICIENCY SYNDROME (AIDS)

AIDS is defined as the most severe form of a continuum of illnesses associated with human immunodeficiency virus (HIV) infection. The virus, a retrovirus, is transmitted by high-risk behaviors such as male homosexual relations, IV drug use (IVDU), and heterosexual relations with an HIV-infected partner or one at risk for infection. Also at risk are persons who received transfusions of blood or blood products contaminated with HIV, children born to mothers with HIV infection, and the breastfed infants of HIV-infected mothers.

CLINICAL MANIFESTATIONS

Symptoms are widespread and may affect any organ system.

Respiratory

1. Shortness of breath, dyspnea, cough, chest pain, and fever.
2. *Pneumocystis carinii* pneumonia (PCP)—most common infection.
3. *Mycobacterium avium* complex (MAC) disease is emerging as a leading cause of respiratory infection.
4. HIV-associated tuberculosis occurs early in the course, precedes diagnosis. If diagnosed early, responds well to antituberculosis therapy.

Gastrointestinal

Anorexia, nausea, vomiting, oral and esophageal candidiasis, and chronic diarrhea; effects of diarrhea can be devastating.

Wasting Syndrome (Cachexia)

Profound involuntary weight loss exceeding 10% of baseline body weight; presents with chronic diarrhea, chronic weakness, and documented intermittent or constant fever with no concurrent illness.

Cancer

1. High incidence of cancer, including Kaposi's sarcoma (KS) and B-cell lymphomas.
2. Carcinomas of the skin, stomach, pancreas, rectum, and bladder.

Neurologic

1. Encephalopathy (AIDS dementia complex [ADC]) occurs in two-thirds of patients with AIDS.
2. *Cryptococcus neoformans,* fungal infection.
3. Progressive multifocal leukoencephalopathy (PML), a central nervous system demyelinating disorder.

Integumentary

KS, herpes simplex and zoster, and various forms of dermatitis.

HIV Infection in Women

1. Persistent recurrent vaginal candidiasis may be the first sign of HIV infection.
2. Ulcerative sexually transmitted diseases (STDs) are more severe.
3. Human papillomavirus (HPV) and cervical cancer have an increased severity.
4. Higher incidence of menstrual abnormalities (amenorrhea or bleeding between periods).

Chronic Illness

1. Develops when opportunistic diseases and symptoms of HIV do not resolve.
2. Unexplained fatigue, headache, profuse night sweats, unexplained weight loss, dry cough, shortness of breath, extreme weakness, diarrhea, and persistent lymphadenopathy.

DIAGNOSTIC EVALUATION

Confirm presence of HIV antibodies: enzyme-linked immunosorbent assay (ELISA) test, Western blot assay, and indirect immunofluorescence assay (IFA).

MANAGEMENT

Goals of treatment include treatment of HIV-associated infections and malignancies, arresting HIV growth and replication through antiviral agents, and augmentation and restoration of the immune system through the use of immunomodulators.

Medications for HIV-Related Infections

1. PCP: treat with trimethoprimsulfamethoxazole (TMP/SMZ), an antibacterial agent. Pentamidine, an antiprotozoal, is an alternative agent.
2. MAC: treatment has not been clearly established and involves multidrug regimens administered over a prolonged period.
3. Cryptococcal meningitis: treat with IV amphotericin B with or without fluconazole, an antifungal agent.
4. Retinitis: treat with ganciclovir.

Malignancies

KS: treat with alpha-interferon or chemotherapeutic agents, i.e., Adriamycin, bleomycin, vincristine (ABV); vinblastine for intraoral lesions.

Antiretroviral Agents

1. Zidovudine (ZDV), formerly azidothymidine (AZT).
2. Dideoxyinosine (ddI).
3. Dideoxycytidine (ddC).

Immunomodulators

Alpha-interferon.

Vaccines

Research continues to work on development of a vaccine for HIV.

Supportive Care and Alternative Therapies

1. Spiritual or psychological: e.g., laughter, hypnosis, faith healing, guided imagery.
2. Nutritional: e.g., vegetarian, macrobiotic diets, vitamin C or betacarotene supplements, Chinese herbs.
3. Drug and biologic: e.g., medicines not approved by the FDA.

4. Physical forces and devices: e.g., acupuncture, massage therapy, yoga, reflexology, crystals.

NURSING PROCESS

Assessment

Identify potential risk factors including sexual and IV drug use history.

NUTRITIONAL STATUS

1. Obtain a dietary history.
2. Identify factors that may interfere with oral intake, i.e., anorexia, nausea, vomiting, oral pain, or difficulty swallowing.
3. Measure nutritional status by weight, tricep skin fold measurement and blood urea nitrogen, serum protein, albumin, and transferrin levels.

SKIN AND MUCOUS MEMBRANE

1. Inspect daily for breakdown, ulceration, and infection.
2. Monitor the oral cavity for redness, ulcerations, and white creamy patches (candidiasis).
3. Assess the perianal area for excoriation and infection.
4. Obtain wound cultures to identify infectious organisms.

RESPIRATORY STATUS

1. Monitor for cough, sputum production, shortness of breath, orthopnea, tachypnea, and chest pain; assess breath sounds.
2. Assess other parameters of pulmonary function, i.e., chest x-rays, arterial blood gases (ABGs), and pulmonary function tests.

NEUROLOGIC STATUS

1. Assess level of consciousness and orientation to person, place, and time, and the occurrence of memory lapses.
2. Observe for sensory deficits, i.e., visual changes, headache, numbness and tingling in the extremities.

3. Observe for motor impairments, i.e., altered gait and paresis.
4. Observe for seizure activity.

FLUID AND ELECTROLYTE STATUS

1. Examine the skin and mucous membranes for turgor and dryness.
2. Assess for dehydration by observing for increased thirst, decreased urine output, or low blood pressure.
3. Monitor electrolyte imbalances (lab studies).
4. Assess for signs and symptoms of electrolyte depletion.

LEVEL OF KNOWLEDGE

1. Evaluate patient's knowledge of disease and transmission.
2. Assess the level of knowledge of family and friends.
3. Explore the patient's reaction to the diagnosis of AIDS.
4. Gain an understanding of how the patient has dealt with illness and major life stressors in the past.
5. Identify the patient's resources for support.

Major Nursing Diagnosis

1. Impaired skin integrity related to cutaneous manifestations of HIV infection, excoriation, and diarrhea.
2. Risk for infection related to immunodeficiency.
3. Activity intolerance related to weakness, fatigue, malnutrition, impaired fluid and electrolyte balance, and hypoxia associated with pulmonary infections.
4. Altered thought processes related to shortened attention span, impaired memory, confusion, and disorientation (HIV encephalopathy).
5. Ineffective airway clearance related to PCP, increased bronchial secretions, and decreased ability to cough related to weakness and fatigue.
6. Altered nutrition, less than body requirements, related to decreased oral intake.

7. Knowledge deficit related to means of preventing HIV transmission and self-care.
8. Social isolation related to stigma of the disease, withdrawal of support systems, isolation procedures, and fear of infecting others.
9. Anticipatory grieving related to changes in lifestyle and roles to unfavorable prognosis.

Collaborative Problems

1. Opportunistic infections.
2. Impaired breathing or respiratory failure.
3. Wasting syndrome and fluid and electrolyte imbalance.
4. Untoward reaction to medications.

Planning and Implementation

Goals include achievement and maintenance of skin integrity, resumption of usual bowel habits, absence of infection, improved activity tolerance, improved thought processes, improved airway clearance, increased comfort, improved nutritional status, increased socialization, expression of grief, increased knowledge regarding disease prevention and self-care, and absence of complications.

Nursing Interventions

PROMOTING SKIN INTEGRITY

1. Assess skin and oral mucosa for changes in appearance, location and size of lesions, and evidence of infection and breakdown.
2. Use devices, i.e., convoluted foam, alternating-pressure mattresses, and low– and high–air-loss beds.
3. Encourage patients to avoid scratching, to use nonabrasive, nondrying soaps, and to use nonperfumed skin moisturizers on dry skin.
4. Avoid excessive use of tape.
5. Advise patients with foot lesions to wear white cotton socks and shoes that do not cause the feet to perspire.

Maintaining Perianal Skin Integrity

1. Assess perianal region for skin integrity and infection.
2. Instruct to keep the area as clean as possible.
3. Promote healing with prescribed topical ointments and lotions.

Promoting Usual Bowel Habits

1. Assess bowel patterns for signs and symptoms of diarrhea.
2. Assess factors that exacerbate the frequency of diarrhea.
3. Counsel the patient about ways to decrease diarrhea, i.e., avoid foods that act as bowel irritants, e.g., raw fruits and vegetables.
4. Administer prescribed medications, i.e., anticholinergic antispasmodics or opiates, antibiotics, and antifungal agents.

Preventing Infection

1. Instruct patient and caregivers to monitor for signs and symptoms of infection.
2. Monitor lab values that indicate the presence of infection, i.e., white blood cell count and differential blood cell count.
3. Advise on strategies to avoid infection.
4. Strongly urge patients and sexual partners to avoid exposure to body fluids and use condoms for any sexual activities.
5. Strongly discourage IV drug use because of risk to the patient from other infections and transmission of HIV infection.
6. Maintain strict aseptic technique for invasive procedures.
7. Observe universal precautions in all patient care.

Improving Activity Tolerance

1. Assess ability to ambulate and perform daily activities.

2. Assist in planning a balance between activity and rest.
3. Decrease anxiety that contributes to weakness and fatigue by using measures, i.e., relaxation and guided imagery.

CLARIFYING THOUGHT PROCESSES

1. Assess for alterations in mental status.
2. Reorient to person, place, and time whenever necessary.
3. Give instructions in a slow, simple, and clear manner.

IMPROVING AIRWAY CLEARANCE

1. Assess daily respiratory status, mental status, and skin color.
2. Note presence of cough, quantity, and characteristics of sputum.
3. Prevent stasis of secretions and promote clearance of airway by providing pulmonary measures, i.e., coughing, deep breathing, postural drainage, percussion, and vibration.
4. Assist the patient in attaining a position (high or semi-Fowler's) that will facilitate breathing and airway clearance.
5. Evaluate fluid volume status; encourage intake of 3–4 liters daily.

RELIEVING PAIN AND DISCOMFORT

1. Assess patient for the quality and quantity of pain associated with impaired perianal skin integrity, lesions of KS, and peripheral neuropathy.
2. Explore the effects of pain on all physical and emotional aspects, along with exacerbating and relieving factors.
3. Use soft cushions or foam pads while sitting.
4. Administer nonsteroidal anti-inflammatory agents (NSAIDS), opiates, and nonpharmacolgic approaches, e.g., relaxation techniques.

IMPROVING NUTRITIONAL STATUS

1. Assess weight, dietary intake, anthropometric measurements, serum albumin, BUN, protein, and transferrin levels.
2. Instruct about ways to supplement nutritional value of meals.

DECREASING THE SENSE OF SOCIAL ISOLATION

1. Provide an atmosphere of acceptance and understanding of AIDS patients, their families, and partners.
2. Assess the patient's usual level of social interaction early to provide a baseline for monitoring changes in behavior.
3. Encourage to express feelings of isolation and aloneness; assure them that these feelings are not unique or abnormal.
4. Assure patients, family, and friends that AIDS is not spread through casual contact.

COPING WITH GRIEF

1. Help patients explore and identify resources for support and mechanisms for coping.

MONITORING AND MANAGING COMPLICATIONS

1. Impaired breathing: monitor ABGs; provide suctioning and oxygen therapy; assist patient on mechanical ventilation to cope with associated stress.
2. Wasting syndrome and fluid and electrolyte disturbances: Monitor weight gains or losses, skin turgor, ferritin levels, hemoglobin and hematocrit, and electrolytes. Assist in selecting foods that will replenish electrolytes. Initiate measures to control diarrhea.
3. Adverse reactions to medications: provide information about purpose, administration, side effects, and strategies to manage or prevent side effects of medications.

✎ Patient Education and Health Maintenance: Care in the Home and Community

Patient Teaching

1. Thoroughly discuss the disease and all fears and misconceptions.
2. Discuss precautions to prevent transmission of HIV, i.e., use of condoms during vaginal or anal intercourse; avoiding oral contact with the penis, vagina, or rectum; avoiding sexual practices that might cause cuts or tears in the lining of the rectum, vagina, or penis; and avoiding sexual contact with multiple partners, those known to be HIV positive, persons who use illicit IV drugs, or sexual partners of persons who use IV drugs.
3. Instruct patients to not donate blood.

Family/Caregiver Teaching

1. Assist families or caregivers in providing supportive care.
2. Teach how to prevent disease transmission, including handwashing and methods of safely handling items soiled with body fluids.
3. Teach medication administration, including IV preparations.
4. Teach guidelines about infection, follow-up care, diet, rest, and activities.
5. Give support and guidance in coping with this disease.

Community Health Nurses and Hospice Nurses

1. Assist in the administration of parenteral antibiotics, chemotherapy, nutrition, complicated wound care, and respiratory care.
2. Provide emotional support to patients and families.
3. Refer patients to community programs, i.e., housekeeping assistance, meals, transportation, shopping, individual and group therapy, support for caregivers, telephone networks for the homebound, and legal and financial assistance.

✚ Clinical Alert: Preventing HIV Transmission

1. Teach health care workers the risk of transmission of AIDS is less likely from contact with feces, nasal secretions, sputum, sweat, breast milk, tears, urine, and vomitus unless they contain visible blood.
2. Apply universal precautions to blood; cerebrospinal fluid; synovial, pleural, peritoneal, pericardial, amniotic, and vaginal fluids; and semen.
3. Consider all body fluids to be potentially hazardous in emergency circumstances when differentiation between fluid types is difficult.
4. Reduce the risk of disease transmission to patients and health care workers by using the Body Substance Isolation System as an alternative to Universal Blood and Body Fluid Precautions, since this system offers a broader strategy of isolation.

For more information, see Chapter 50 of Smeltzer and Bare: *Brunner and Suddarth's Textbook of Medical–Surgical Nursing,* 8th Edition. Philadelphia: Lippincott–Raven, 1996.

ACROMEGALY

See Pituitary Tumors

ACTINIC KERATOSES

See Cancer of the Skin

ACUTE GLOMERULONEPHRITIS

See Glomerulonephritis, Acute

ACUTE LYMPHOCYTIC LEUKEMIA

See Leukemia, Lymphocytic, Acute

ACUTE MYELOGENOUS LEUKEMIA

See Leukemia, Myelogenous, Acute

ACUTE OTITIS MEDIA

See Otitis Media, Acute

ACUTE PANCREATITIS

See Pancreatitis, Acute

ACUTE PHARYNGITIS

See Pharyngitis, Acute

ACUTE PULMONARY EDEMA

See Pulmonary Edema, Acute

ACUTE RENAL FAILURE

See Renal Failure, Acute

ADDISON'S DISEASE

See Chronic Primary Adrenocorticol Insufficiency

ADENOIDITIS

See Tonsillitis and Adenoiditis

ADRENAL HYPERPLASIA

See Cushing's Syndrome

ADULT RESPIRATORY DISTRESS SYNDROME (ARDS)

ARDS (noncardiogenic pulmonary edema) is a clinical syndrome characterized by a progressive decrease in arterial oxygen content occurring after a serious illness or injury. It may have a mortality rate as high as 50–60%. Factors related to the development of ARDS:

1. Aspiration (gastric secretions, drowning, hydrocarbons).
2. Drug ingestion and overdose.
3. Hematologic disorders (disseminated intravascular coagulopathy [DIC], massive transfusions, cardiopulmonary bypass).
4. Prolonged inhalation of high concentrations of oxygen, smoke, or corrosive substances.
5. Localized infection (bacterial, fungal, viral pneumonia).
6. Metabolic disorders (pancreatitis, uremia).
7. Shock (any cause).
8. Trauma (pulmonary contusion, multiple fractures, head injury).
9. Major surgery.
10. Fat or air embolism.
11. Systemic sepsis.

DIAGNOSTIC EVALUATION

Based on clinical manifestations.

CLINICAL MANIFESTATIONS

1. Acute respiratory failure.
2. Bilateral pulmonary infiltrates (reticulogranular pattern) a ground glass appearance on x-ray.
3. Hypoxemia (PaO_2 below 50–60 mmHg) despite (FIO_2) of 50–60%.

MANAGEMENT

1. Early detection, aggressive treatment, prevention of infection.
2. Provide adequate ventilation initially; as disease progresses use positive end-expiratory pressure (PEEP).
3. Provide circulatory support.
4. Provide adequate fluid management; intravenous solutions.
5. Provide nutritional support.

Nursing Interventions

1. Close monitoring because condition can quickly change to life-threatening situation.
2. Facilitate respiratory management, i.e., position to maximize respiration, oxygen, endotracheal intubation, tracheostomy, suctioning, and mechanical ventilation.
3. Provide safety interventions related to ventilator care.
4. Encourage oral fluid intake if patient is not ventilated.
5. Provide emotional support and reduce patient anxiety.

For more information see Chapter 24 in Smeltzer and Bare: *Brunner and Suddarth's Textbook of Medical–Surgical Nursing,* 8th Edition. Philadelphia: Lippincott–Raven, 1996.

AIDS

See Acquired Immunodeficiency Syndrome

ALL

See Leukemia, Lymphocytic, Acute

ALS

See Amyotrophic Lateral Sclerosis

ALZHEIMER'S DISEASE

Alzheimers's disease (AD) is sometimes called primary degenerative dementia or senile dementia of the Alzheimer's type (SDAT). It accounts for at least 50% of all dementias suffered by the elderly. It is a progressive, irreversible, degenerative neurologic disease that begins insidiously. It is characterized by gradual losses of cognitive function and disturbances in behavior and affect. AD is classified as "familial" or "sporadic" (no known family history). Chromosome 21 is implicated in early-onset familial Alzheimer's disease (FAD), which begins in the 50s. Chromosome 14 is linked to FAD, onset in the 40s. Late-onset AD (after age 65) shows a genetic linkage with chromosome 19. Early or late onset are considered to be clinically and pathologically identical. Life expectancy varies from 3 to 20 years. Death occurs as a result of a complicating condition such as pneumonia, malnutrition, or dehydration.

CLINICAL MANIFESTATIONS

Symptoms are highly variable:

1. Early in disease, forgetfulness and subtle memory loss occur.

2. Social skills and behavior patterns remain intact (early).
3. Forgetfulness is manifested in many daily actions with progression of the disease, i.e., lose way in a familiar environment or repeat same stories.
4. Ability to formulate concepts and think abstractly disappears.
5. May exhibit inappropriate impulsive behavior.
6. Personality changes are negative, i.e., may become depressed, suspicious, paranoid, hostile, and even combative.
7. Speaking skills deteriorate to nonsense syllables; agitation and physical activity increase.
8. Voracious appetite may develop because of high activity level.
9. Eventually will need help with all aspects of daily living.
10. Terminal stage may last for months.

DIAGNOSTIC EVALUATION

Diagnosis is one of exclusion and is confirmed by autopsy.

1. Clinical symptoms.
2. Electroencephalography (EEG).
3. Computed tomography (CT scan).
4. Magnetic resonance imaging (MRI).
5. Examination of the blood and cerebrospinal fluid (CSF).

NURSING INTERVENTIONS

Supporting Cognitive Function

1. Provide a calm predictable environment.
2. Minimize confusion and disorientation; give the patient a sense of security with a quiet, pleasant manner, clear simple explanations, and use of memory aids and cues.

Promoting Physical Safety

1. Provide a safe environment to allow patient to move about as freely as possible and relieve family worry about safety.
2. Prevent falls and other accidents by removing obvious hazards.
3. Monitor the patient's intake of medications and food.
4. Allow smoking only with supervision.
5. Reduce wandering behavior with gentle persuasion and distraction.
6. Avoid restraints because they may increase agitation.
7. Secure doors leading from the house.
8. Supervise all activities outside the home to protect the patient.
9. Ensure patient wears an identification bracelet or neck chain.

Reducing Anxiety and Agitation

1. Give constant emotional support to reinforce a positive self-image.
2. Encourage patient to enjoy simple activities.
3. Improve the quality of life with hobbies and activities.
4. Keep the environment simple, familiar, and noise-free.
5. Remain calm and unhurried during a combative, agitated state known as catastrophic reaction (overreaction to excessive stimulation).

Improving Communication

1. Promote the patient's interpretation of messages by remaining unhurried and reducing noises and distractions.
2. Use easy-to-understand sentences to convey messages.

Promoting Independence in Self-Care Activities

1. Simplify daily activities into short achievable steps so that the patient can experience a sense of accomplishment.
2. Maintain personal dignity and autonomy.
3. Encourage to make choices when appropriate and to participate in self-care activities as much as possible.

Providing for Socialization and Intimacy Needs

1. Encourage visits, letters, and phone calls (visits should be brief and nonstressful).
2. Advise that the nonjudgmental friendliness of a pet can provide satisfying activity and an outlet for energy.
3. Encourage the spouse to talk about any sexual concerns and suggest sexual counseling if necessary.

Promoting Adequate Nutrition

1. Keep mealtimes simple and calm without confrontations.
2. Cut food into small pieces to prevent choking.
3. Prevent burns by serving hot food and beverages warm.

Promoting Balanced Activity and Rest

1. Access to the outdoors should be blocked.
2. Help to relax to sleep with music, warm milk, or a backrub.
3. Give sufficient opportunities to participate in exercise activities to enhance nighttime sleep.
4. Discourage long periods of daytime sleeping.

Supporting and Educating Family Caregivers

1. Be sensitive to the highly emotional issues that the family is confronting.
2. Refer to the Alzheimer's Association for family support groups, respite care, and adult day care.

For more information see Chapter 12 in Smeltzer and Bare: *Brunner and Suddarth's Textbook of Medical–Surgical Nursing,* 8th Edition. Philadelphia: Lippincott–Raven, 1996.

AML

See Leukemia, Myelogenous, Acute

AMYOTROPHIC LATERAL SCLEROSIS

Amyotrophic lateral sclerosis (ALS) is a disease of unknown cause in which there is a loss of motor neurons (nerve cells controlling muscles) in the anterior horns of the spinal cord and the motor nuclei of the lower brain stem. As these cells die, the muscle fibers that they supply undergo atrophic changes. The degeneration of the neurons may occur in both the upper and lower motor neuron systems. ALS affects more men than women, with onset occurring usually in the fifth or sixth decade. In the United States it is often referred to as Lou Gehrig's disease. Death occurs from infection, respiratory failure, or aspiration. The average time from onset to death is approximately 3 years.

CLINICAL MANIFESTATIONS

Depends on the location of the affected motor neurons. In the majority of patients, chief symptoms are progressive muscle weakness, atrophy, and fasciculations (twitching).

Symptoms of Patients with Loss of Motor Neurons in the Anterior Horns of the Spinal Cord

1. Progressive weakness and atrophy of the muscles noted in the arms, trunk, or legs.
2. Spasticity is usually present, and stretch reflexes are brisk and overactive.
3. Anal and bladder sphincters are not affected.

Symptoms of Patients with Weakness in the Musculature Supplied by the Cranial Nerves (25% of Patients in Early Stage)

1. Difficulty talking, swallowing, and ultimately breathing.
2. Soft palate and upper esophageal weakness cause liquids to be regurgitated through the nose.
3. Impaired ability to laugh, cough, or blow the nose.

In Patients with Bulbar Muscle Impairment

1. Progressive difficulty in speaking, swallowing, and aspiration.
2. Voice assumes a nasal sound and speech becomes unintelligible.
3. Emotional lability, but intellectual function is not impaired.
4. Respiratory function is compromised eventually.

DIAGNOSTIC EVALUATION

Based on signs and symptoms because no clinical or laboratory tests are specific for this disease.

MANAGEMENT

No specific treatment for ALS is available.

Symptomatic Treatment and Rehabilitative Measures

1. Baclofen or diazepam for spasticity.
2. Quinine for muscle cramps.
3. Nasogastric feedings, cervical esophagostomy, or gastrostomy for patients with aspiration or swallowing difficulties.

Mechanical Ventilation

1. Decision is based on patient and family's understanding of the disease, prognosis, and the implications of initiating such therapy.

NURSING PROCESS

The nursing care of the patient with ALS is generally the same as the basic care plan for patients with degenerative neurologic disorders (see Myasthenia Gravis).

For more information see Chapter 60 in Smeltzer and Bare: *Brunner and Suddarth's Textbook of Medical–Surgical Nursing*, 8th Edition. Philadelphia: Lippincott–Raven, 1996.

ANAPHYLAXIS

Anaphylaxis is an immediate immunologic reaction between a specific antigen and an antibody. This reaction may occur with medications, food, exercise, and cytotoxic antibody transfusions.

Local anaphylactic reactions usually involve urticaria and angioedema at the site of exposure; can be severe but rarely fatal. Systemic reactions occur in major organ systems within about 30 minutes of exposure.

CLINICAL MANIFESTATIONS

Mild

1. Peripheral tingling; a warm sensation; fullness in the mouth and throat.
2. Nasal congestion; periorbital swelling, pruritus; sneezing; tearing of the eyes.
3. Onset of symptoms begins within the first 2 hours of exposure.

Moderate

1. May include any of the mild symptoms plus bronchospasm and edema of the airways or larynx with dyspnea, cough, and wheezing.
2. Flushing, warmth, anxiety, and itching.
3. Onset of symptoms is the same as a mild reaction.

Severe

1. An abrupt onset with the same signs and symptoms described above and progress rapidly to bronchospasm, laryngeal edema, severe dyspnea, and cyanosis.
2. Dysphagia, abdominal cramping, vomiting, diarrhea, and seizures.
3. Cardiac arrest and coma rarely results.

MANAGEMENT

1. Evaluate respiratory and cardiovascular function.
2. Institute CPR if in cardiac arrest.
3. Provide oxygen in high concentrations during CPR or when cyanotic, dyspneic, or wheezing.
4. Give epinephrine, antihistamines, and steroids to prevent recurrences of the reaction and for urticaria and angioedema.
5. Use volume expanders and vasopressor agents to maintain blood pressure and normal hemodynamic status.
6. Educate patients with mild reactions about risk for potential recurrences.
7. Closely observe patients with severe reactions for 12–14 hours.

✎ PATIENT EDUCATION AND HEALTH MAINTENANCE: CARE IN THE HOME AND COMMUNITY

Prevention is the most important aspect of anaphylaxis. Teach individuals sensitive to insect bites and stings; food or drug reactions; idiopathic or exercise-induced anaphylactic reactions:

1. Strategies to avoid exposure to allergens.
2. Carry an emergency kit that contains epinephrine.
3. Provide verbal/written instruction about the emergency kit.
4. Ensure patient's ability to demonstrate correct self-injection.

5. Encourage patient to wear drug allergy identification, e.g., Medic-Alert bracelet.

For more information see Chapter 51 in Smeltzer and Bare: *Brunner and Suddarth's Textbook of Medical–Surgical Nursing,* 8th Edition. Philadelphia: Lippincott–Raven, 1996.

ANEMIA

Anemia is a low red cell count and a below-normal hemoglobin (Hgb) or hematocrit (Hct) level. It reflects a disease state or altered body function. There are many different kinds of anemias. Some causes are inadequate production (erythropoiesis) of red blood cells (RBC); premature or excessive destruction of RBCs (hemolysis); blood loss (most common cause); other etiologic factors, i.e., deficits in iron and nutrients, hereditary factors, and chronic diseases.

CLINICAL MANIFESTATIONS

The more rapidly an anemia develops, the more severe its symptoms.

General Signs and Symptoms

1. Weakness, fatigue, general malaise.
2. Pallor of the skin and mucous membranes.

Symptoms Specific to Hemoglobin Levels

1. Slight tachycardia on exertion (Hgb 9–11 g/dl).
2. Exertional dyspnea (Hgb below 7.5 g/dl).
3. Weakness (Hgb below 6 g/dl).
4. Dyspnea at rest (Hgb below 3 g/dl).
5. Cardiac failure only at the extremely low level of 2–2.5 g/dl.

DIAGNOSTIC EVALUATION

Complete blood studies (i.e., Hgb/Hct), bone marrow aspiration/biopsy; studies for underlying acute or chronic illness.

MANAGEMENT

Reverse the cause and replace blood loss.

NURSING PROCESS

Assessment

OBTAIN A HEALTH HISTORY AND PHYSICAL EXAMINATION

1. Include information about medications that could depress bone marrow activity or interfere with folate metabolism.
2. Question about any loss of blood, i.e., excessive menses or blood in stool.
3. Question family history regarding inherited anemias.
4. Question dietary habits for nutritional deficiencies, i.e., iron, vitamin B_{12}, and folic acid.

ASSESS FOR INCREASED CARDIAC WORKLOAD

1. Tachycardia, palpitations, dyspnea.
2. Dizziness, orthopnea, exertional dyspnea.

ASSESS FOR CONGESTIVE HEART FAILURE

1. Cardiomegaly.
2. Hepatomegaly.
3. Peripheral edema.

ASSESS FOR NEUROLOGICAL DEFICITS

1. Peripheral numbness and paresthesias.
2. Ataxia and poor coordination.
3. Confusion.

ASSESS FOR GASTROINTESTINAL FUNCTION

1. Nausea.
2. Vomiting.

3. Diarrhea.
4. Anorexia.
5. Glossitis.

Major Nursing Diagnosis

1. Activity intolerance related to weakness, fatigue, and general malaise.
2. Altered nutrition, less than body requirements, related to inadequate intake of essential nutrients.

Collaborative Problems

1. Congestive heart failure.
2. Paresthesias.
3. Confusion.

Planning and Implementation

The major goals may include tolerance of normal activity, attainment or maintenance of adequate nutrition, and absence of complications.

Nursing Interventions

TOLERATING NORMAL ACTIVITY

1. Plan care to conserve strength, physical and emotional energy.
2. Encourage frequent rest periods.
3. Elicit family support to promote a restful environment.
4. Encourage ambulation and daily activities as tolerated.
5. Resume activities gradually as blood studies return to normal.
6. Encourage conditioning exercises for increased endurance.
7. Use safety precautions to prevent falls from poor coordination, paresthesias, and weakness.

MONITORING AND MANAGING COMPLICATIONS

1. Decrease activities and stimuli that cause an increase in heart rate and cardiac output.

2. Encourage patient to identify situations that precipitate palpitations and dyspnea.
3. Administer oxygen; elevate head of bed for dyspnea.
4. Monitor vital signs and observe for indications of fluid retention.
5. Monitor for signs of paresthesia, poor coordination, ataxia, and confusion.
6. Implement safety measures to prevent injury.

ATTAINING AND MAINTAINING ADEQUATE NUTRITION

1. Encourage a well-balanced diet high in protein, high caloric foods, fruits, and vegetables.
2. Teach to avoid spicy (irritating) and gas-producing foods.
3. Plan dietary teaching sessions for patient and family.

✪ GERONTOLOGIC CONSIDERATIONS

Anemia is the most common hematologic condition that affects the elderly. Studies show that the aging process does not affect hemopoiesis.

1. The elderly person may be unable to respond adequately to anemia (with increased cardiac output or pulmonary ventilation), causing serious effects on cardiopulmonary function.
2. Identify and treat the cause of anemia rather than consider it a consequence of aging.

For more information see Chapter 32 in Smeltzer and Bare: *Brunner and Suddarth's Textbook of Medical–Surgical Nursing*, 8th Edition. Philadelphia: Lippincott–Raven, 1996.

ANEMIA, APLASTIC

Aplastic anemia (hypoproliferative) is caused by a decrease in precursor cells in the bone marrow and replacement of the marrow with fat. It can be congenital or acquired. It may be idiopathic; result from certain infections; or be caused by drugs, chemicals, or radiation damage. The most common offenders are antimicrobials (chloramphenicol), organic arsenicals, anticonvulsants, phenylbutazone, sulfonamides, and gold compounds. A prompt and complete recovery may be anticipated if patient exposure is terminated early. If exposure to the agent continues after signs of hypoplasia have appeared, bone marrow depression almost certainly progresses to complete and irreversible failure. Diagnosis is made by bone marrow biopsy.

CLINICAL MANIFESTATIONS

1. Gradual onset marked by weakness and pallor; breathlessness on exertion.
2. Abnormal bleeding in one-third of patients.
3. Granulocytic series involvement presents with fever, acute pharyngitis, other form of sepsis, and bleeding.

MANAGEMENT

1. Bone marrow transplantation.
2. Administration of immunosuppressive therapy with antithymocyte globulin (ATG).

Supportive Therapy

1. Discontinue any offending drug.
2. Prevent symptoms with transfusions of red cells and platelets.
3. Protect patients with pronounced leukopenia from contact with people who have infections.

Preventive Management

1. Use potentially toxic medications only when alternative therapies are not available.
2. Monitor blood cell counts in patients receiving potentially bone marrow–toxic drugs, e.g., chloramphenicol.

3. Teach persons taking toxic drugs on a long-term basis the need for periodic blood studies and to know what symptoms to report.

Nursing Interventions

1. Assess for signs of infection, tissue hypoxia, and bleeding.
2. Guard against any wound, abrasion, or ulcer of mucous membrane or skin as a potential site of infection.
3. Provide oral hygiene.
4. Preserve patient's energy by planning care depending on the degree of weakness and fatigue.
5. Avoid minor trauma, including subcutaneous and intramuscular (IM) injections, when thrombocytopenia is present.
6. Teach importance of regular atraumatic bowel movements because hemorrhoids can develop and become infected or bleed.

For more information, see Chapter 32 in Smeltzer and Bare: *Brunner and Suddarth's Textbook of Medical–Surgical Nursing,* 8th Edition. Phildelphia: Lippincott–Raven, 1996.

ANEMIA, IRON DEFICIENCY

Iron deficiency anemia is a condition in which the total body iron content is decreased below a normal level. It is the most common type of anemia. It is found in men and postmenopausal women from bleeding (i.e., ulcers, gastritis, or gastrointestinal tumors), malabsorption or diet very high in fiber (prevents iron absorption). The most frequent cause in premenopausal women is menorrhagia. Chronic alcoholism often causes inadequate iron intake and loss of iron through blood from the gastrointestinal tract.

CLINICAL MANIFESTATIONS

1. Red cells are hypochromic and microcytic.
2. Symptoms of anemia: fatigue, irritability, numbness, and tingling of extremities.
3. If severe, may have a smooth, sore tongue; pica.
4. Hemoglobin proportionately lower than hematocrit and red cell count.
5. Serum iron concentration low.
6. Total iron-binding capacity high; serum ferritin low.
7. White count usually normal; platelet count variable.

MANAGEMENT

1. Search for the cause, which may be a curable gastrointestinal malignancy, uterine fibroids, or cancer.
2. Test stool specimens for occult blood.
3. Administer prescribed oral iron preparations.
4. Avoid tablets with enteric coating; may be poorly absorbed.
5. Continue iron for a year after bleeding has been controlled.

Nursing Interventions

1. Administer IM or IV iron in some cases when oral iron is not absorbed, is poorly tolerated, or is needed in large amounts. (Administer a small test dose prior to IM injection to avoid risk of anaphylaxis (which is greater with IM than IV injections.)
2. Advise to take iron supplements with meals if gastric distress occurs; after symptoms subside, resume between-meal schedule for maximum absorption.
3. Inform iron salts change stool to dark green or black color.
4. Advise frequent oral hygiene because ferrous sulfate is likely to be deposited on the teeth and gums; take liquid iron through a straw and rinse mouth with water.

Patient Education and Health Maintenance: Care in the Home and Community

1. Teach preventive education because iron deficiency anemia is common in menstruating and pregnant women.
2. Educate patients regarding food sources high in iron, i.e., organ and other meats, beans, leafy vegetables, raisins, and molasses.
3. Take iron-rich foods with vitamin C to enhance absorption.
4. Avoid taking antacids with iron; phosphates may form complexes with iron.
5. Provide nutritional counseling for those whose normal diet is inadequate.

For more information see Chapter 32 in Smeltzer and Bare: *Brunner and Suddarth's Textbook of Medical–Surgical Nursing,* 8th Edition. Philadelphia: Lippincott–Raven, 1996.

ANEMIA, SICKLE CELL

Sickle cell anemia is a severe hemolytic anemia resulting from a defective hemoglobin molecule and associated with attacks of pain. It is found predominantly in Mediterranean and African populations and predominates in blacks. The defect is a single amino acid substitution in the β chain of hemoglobin. Sickle hemoglobin acquires a crystal-like formation when exposed to low oxygen tension. The cell containing S hemoglobin becomes deformed, rigid, and sickle shaped when in the venous circulation.

Long rigid cells become lodged in small vessels and blood flow to a region or organ may be slowed, resulting in ischemia or infarction where there may be pain, swelling, or fever.

CLINICAL MANIFESTATIONS

1. Symptoms are secondary to hemolysis and thrombosis.
2. Anemia with hemoglobin values in the 7 to 10 g/dl range.
3. Jaundice most obvious in the sclera.
4. Bone marrow expands in childhood, sometimes causing enlargement of bones of the face and skull.
5. Tachycardia, cardiac murmurs, and often cardiomegaly are associated with the chronic anemia.
6. Dysrhythmias and heart failure in older patients.
7. All tissues and organs are vulnerable and susceptible to hypoxic damage or true ischemic necrosis at any time.

DIAGNOSTIC EVALUATION

Hemoglobin electrophoresis, isoelectric focusing, high performance liquid chromatography techniques. Sickling occurs whether the patient has sickle trait or sickle cell anemia; only electrophoresis shows a distinction.

MANAGEMENT

1. Trial drugs have shown some promising results, e.g., hydroxyurea (increases fetal hemoglobin production), cetiedil citrate (RBC membrane modifier), pentoxifylline (reduces blood viscosity and peripheral vascular resistance), and vanillin (food additive, antisickling properties).
2. Counsel population at risk.
3. Promptly treat infections, which predispose to crises.
4. Instruct patients to avoid high altitudes, anesthesia, and fluid loss because dehydration promotes sickling.
5. Administer folic acid therapy daily for increased marrow requirement.

Sickle Crisis Management

1. Mainstays of therapy are hydration and analgesia.
2. Teach patient to handle minor crises at home, but hospital admission may be necessary after several hours without relief.
3. Differentiate sickle crisis from infection, appendicitis, or cholecystitis.
4. Hydrate with 3–5 L/day of intravenous fluids (adults).
5. Give adequate doses of narcotic analgesics.
6. Use nonsteroidal anti-inflammatory drugs for milder pain.
7. Transfusions are reserved for aplastic crisis, crisis not responsive to therapy, preoperatively to dilute sickled blood, and sometimes the latter half of pregnancy to prevent crises.

NURSING PROCESS

Assessment

1. Assess all body systems with particular emphasis on pain, swelling, and fever (all joint areas and abdomen).
2. Elicit symptoms of cerebral hypoxia by careful neurologic examination.
3. Question patient about symptoms indicative of gallstones.
4. Assess for the presence of any infectious process.
5. Examine the chest and long bones and femoral head, as pneumonia and osteomyelitis are common.
6. Consider chronic anemia (common problem).
7. Question patients in crisis about factors that could have precipitated the crisis and measures used to prevent crises.
8. Discuss history of alcohol intake.

Major Nursing Diagnosis

1. Pain related to agglutination of sickled cells within blood vessels.

2. Knowledge deficit regarding prevention of crisis.
3. Self-esteem disturbance related to altered body image.

Collaborative Problems

1. Infection.
2. Hypoxia and ischemia.
3. Renal failure.
4. Priapism.

Planning and Implementation

The major goals include relief of pain, avoidance of situations that can precipitate crisis, enhanced feelings of self-esteem and power, and absence of potential complications.

Monitor and Manage Potential Complications

1. Help the patient and family adjust to the chronic disease.
2. Understand the importance of hydration and prevention of infection.
3. Practice careful dressing changes and protection from trauma and wound contamination, i.e., leg ulcers.
4. Focus care on patient's strengths to enhance effective coping skills.
5. Teach male patients with episodes of priapism to empty bladder at the onset of the attack, exercise, and take a warm bath; recommend medical attention if attack persists more than 3 hours.

For more information see Chapter 32 in Smeltzer and Bare: *Brunner and Suddarth's Textbook of Medical–Surgical Nursing*, 8th Edition. Philadelphia: Lippincott–Raven, 1996.

ANEMIA, MEGALOBLASTIC (VITAMIN B$_{12}$ DEFICIENCY AND FOLIC ACID DEFICIENCY)

The anemias caused by deficiencies of the vitamins B$_{12}$ and folic acid show identical bone marrow and peripheral blood changes. Both vitamins are essential for DNA synthesis. In each case hyperplasia of the marrow occurs and the precursor erythroid and myeloid cells are large and bizarre. A pancytopenia develops.

VITAMIN B$_{12}$ DEFICIENCY

Vitamin B$_{12}$ deficiency is rare but can occur from inadequate intake in strict vegetarians; faulty absorption from the gastrointestinal tract; absence of intrinsic factor (pernicious anemia); disease involving the ilium or pancreas, which impairs B$_{12}$ absorption; and gastrectomy. Without treatment patients die after several years, usually from congestive heart failure secondary to anemia.

Clinical Manifestations

Symptoms are progressive and may be marked by spontaneous partial remissions and exacerbations.

1. Gradually becomes weak, listless, and pale.
2. Develops a smooth, sore, red tongue and mild diarrhea (pernicious anemia).
3. Spinal cord damage results in confusion, more often parathesias in the extremities and difficulty keeping balance; loses position sense.

Diagnostic Evaluation

Schilling test.

Management

1. Oral supplementation with vitamins or fortified soy milk (strict vegetarians).
2. IM injections of vitamin B_{12} for defective absorption or absence of intrinsic factor.
3. Prevent recurrence with lifetime vitamin B_{12} therapy for patient who has had pernicious anemia or non-correctable malabsorption.

NURSING INTERVENTIONS

1. Support patients during diagnostic tests.
2. Give nursing care for disease aspects: anemia, congestive heart failure, and neuropathy.
3. Prevent pressure ulcers and contracture deformities when incontinent or paralyzed.
4. Assist in urine collections for Schilling test.
5. Teach about the chronicity of the disorder and necessity for monthly injections even when asymptomatic.
6. Teach importance of ongoing medical follow-up (gastric carcinoma risk).

FOLIC ACID DEFICIENCY

Folic acid is a vitamin that is necessary for normal red blood cell production. Deficiency occurs in persons who rarely eat uncooked vegetables or fruits, i.e., primarily elderly people living alone or persons with alcoholism. Alcohol increases folic acid requirements and alcoholics usually have a diet deficient in the vitamin. Folic acid requirements are also increased in hemolytic anemia and pregnancy. Patients on prolonged intravenous feeding or parenteral nutrition may become folate deficient after several months without IM supplement. Some patients with diseases of the small bowel may not absorb folic acid normally.

Clinical Manifestations

All patients have characteristics of megaloblastic anemia along with a sore tongue. Symptoms are similar to these vitamin B_{12} deficiencies; however, neurologic manifestations do not occur.

Management

1. Administration of a nutritious diet and 1 mg of folic acid daily.
2. IM folic acid for malabsorption syndromes.
3. Oral folic acid is given as a separate tablet (except prenatal vitamins).
4. Stop folic acid replacement when hemoglobin returns to normal with the exception of alcoholics who continue consumption.

For more information see Chapter 32 in Smeltzer and Bare: *Brunner and Suddarth's Textbook of Medical–Surgical Nursing*, 8th Edition. Philadelphia: Lippincott–Raven, 1996.

ANEURYSM, AORTIC

An aneurysm is a localized sac or dilatation of an artery formed at a weak point in the vessel wall. Mycotic aneurysms are very small aneurysms due to local infections; saccular aneurysms project from one side of the vessel only; fusiform aneurysms involve dilatation of an entire arterial segment. The most common forms are saccular and fusiform. Aortic aneurysms are usually classified as thoracic, abdominal, or dissecting. The most common cause is atherosclerosis. Other causes include trauma to the wall of the artery, infection (pyogenic or syphilitic), and congenital defects of the artery wall. Rupture can lead to hemorrhage and death.

THORACIC AORTIC ANEURYSM

Thoracic aneurysms are usually caused by atherosclerosis. They occur most frequently in men between the ages of 40 and 70. The thoracic area is the most common site for the development of a dissecting aneurysm. About one-third of patients die from rupture.

CLINICAL MANIFESTATIONS

Symptoms are variable and depend on how rapidly the aneurysm dilates and causes pressure on surrounding structures. Some are asymptomatic.

1. Constant, boring pain, which may occur only when supine.
2. Dyspnea.
3. Cough (paroxysmal and brassy).
4. Hoarseness.
5. Stridor.
6. Weak voice or aphonia.
7. Dysphagia.
8. Dilated superficial veins on the chest, neck, or arms.
9. Edematous areas on the chest wall.
10. Cyanosis.
11. Unequal pupils.

DIAGNOSTIC EVALUATION

Chest x-ray, sonography, and computed tomography (CT) scan.

MANAGEMENT

Surgical Repair

1. The goal of surgery is to remove the aneurysm and restore vascular continuity with a graft.
2. Intensive monitoring in the critical care unit is required.

Medical Management

1. Strict control of blood pressure and reduction in pulsatile flow.
2. Systolic pressure is maintained at 100–120 mmHg with antihypertensive drugs, e.g., nitroprusside.
3. Pulsatile flow is reduced by medications that reduce cardiac contractility, e.g., propranolol.

ABDOMINAL AORTIC ANEURYSM

The most common cause is atherosclerosis. Men are affected four times more often than women. More common among whites and after the age of 60. Most occur below the renal arteries. Forty percent of patients have symptoms. Rupture and death may occur if untreated. Risk factors include genetic predisposition, smoking, and hypertension.

CLINICAL MANIFESTATIONS

1. Patients complain of "heart beating" in abdomen when lying down or a feeling of an abdominal mass or abdominal throbbing.
2. "Blue toe syndrome" is an occlusion of a digital vessel.
3. Severe back pain or abdominal pain is a sign of impending rupture.

DIAGNOSTIC EVALUATION

1. Presence of a pulsatile mass in the middle and upper abdomen.
2. Ultrasonography or CT scan to determine the size of the aneurysm.

MANAGEMENT

1. Surgery is the treatment of choice for abdominal aneurysms larger than 5 cm (2 in.) in diameter or those that are enlarging.
2. Prognosis for a ruptured aneurysm is poor and surgery is performed immediately.

Preoperative Nursing Assessment

1. Guide assessment by the fact that the aneurysm may rupture.
2. Establish functional capacity of all organ systems.
3. Implement medical therapies to stabilize patient.

Postoperative Care

1. Monitor for complications: arterial occlusion, hemorrhage, infection, ischemic colon, renal failure, and impotence.
2. Prescribe an exercise schedule after the acute recovery phase.
3. Discourage prolonged sitting.

✚ CLINICAL ALERT

1. Constant intense back pain, falling blood pressure, and decreasing hematocrit are signs of a rupturing abdominal aortic aneurysm.
2. Hematomas into the scrotum, perineum, flank, or penis indicate retroperitoneal rupture.
3. Signs of heart failure or a loud bruit suggest rupture into the vena cava.
4. Rupture into the peritoneal cavity is rapidly fatal.

DISSECTING ANEURYSM OF THE AORTA

A dissecting aneurysm is caused by rupture in the intimal layer resulting in blood dissecting the vessel layers. It is often associated with poorly controlled hypertension, and is three times more common in men between 50 and 70 years. Early diagnosis is difficult because of a variable clinical picture.

CLINICAL MANIFESTATIONS

1. Onset is sudden with severe and persistent pain described as "tearing" or "ripping" in the anterior chest or back and extends to shoulders, epigastric area, or abdomen.

2. Pallor, sweating, and tachycardia.
3. Elevated blood pressure or markedly different from one arm to the other.
4. Death is usually caused by external rupture of the hematoma.

DIAGNOSTIC EVALUATION

Angiogram, CT scan, ultrasound, and magnetic resonance imaging (MRI).

MANAGEMENT

Medical or surgical treatment depends on the type of aneurysm and follows the general principles for treatment of thoracic aortic aneurysm.

For more information see Chapter 31 in Smeltzer and Bare: *Brunner and Suddarth's Textbook of Medical–Surgical Nursing,* 8th Edition. Philadelphia: Lippincott–Raven, 1996.

ANEURYSM, INTRACRANIAL

An intracranial (cerebral) aneurysm is a dilation of the walls of a cerebral artery that develops as a result of weakness in the arterial wall. Cause is unknown—may be due to atherosclerosis; a congenital defect of the vessel walls; hypertensive vascular disease; head trauma; or advancing age. Most commonly affected are the internal carotid, anterior cerebral, anterior communicating, and middle cerebral arteries. Symptoms are produced when the aneurysm enlarges and presses on nearby cranial nerves or brain substance, or ruptures, causing subarachnoid hemorrhage.

CLINICAL MANIFESTATIONS

1. Rupture of the aneurysm causes sudden, unusually severe headache; often loss of consciousness for a variable period; pain and rigidity of the back of the neck and spine; visual disturbances (visual loss, diplopia, ptosis).

2. Tinnitus, dizziness, and hemiparesis also may occur. If aneurysm leaks blood, patient may show little neurologic deficit, or severe bleeding, resulting in cerebral damage followed rapidly by coma and death.
3. Prognosis depends on the neurologic condition of the patient, age, associated diseases, and the extent and location of the aneurysm.

DIAGNOSTIC EVALUATION

CT scan, lumbar puncture, and cerebral angiography.

MANAGEMENT

1. Allow the brain to recover from the initial insult (bleeding).
2. Prevent or minimize the risk of rebleeding.
3. Prevent or treat other complications: rebleeding, cerebral vasospasm, acute hydrocephalus, seizures, and anxiety.
4. Bed rest with sedation to prevent agitation and stress.
5. Management of the vasospasm with calcium channel blockers (verapamil [Isoptin] and nifedipine [Procardia]).
6. Surgical or medical treatment to prevent rebleeding.
7. Management of increased intracranial pressure (ICP).
   a. Cerebral spinal fluid (CSF) drainage by lumbar puncture or ventricular catheter drainage.
   b. Mannitol to reduce ICP; monitor for signs of dehydration and rebound elevation of ICP.
   c. Antifibrinolytic agents to delay or prevent dissolution of the clot if surgery is delayed or contraindicated.
8. Management of systemic hypertension.
   a. Antihypertensive therapy.
   b. Monitor blood pressure constantly by arterial line.
   c. Anticonvulsive agents administered prophylactically.

d. Use stool softeners to prevent straining and elevation of blood pressure.
e. Analgesics for head and neck pain.
f. Prevent deep vein thrombosis, i.e., graded pressure elastic stockings.

NURSING PROCESS

Assessment

1. Perform a complete neurologic assessment: level of consciousness, pupillary reaction, motor and sensory function, cranial nerve deficits (extraocular eye movements, facial droop, presence of ptosis), speech difficulties, visual disturbance or headache.
2. Document and report neurologic assessment findings and reassess any changes in the patient's condition.
3. Detect subtle changes, especially alterations of level of consciousness (earliest sign of deterioration, i.e., mild drowsiness and slight slurring of speech).

Major Nursing Diagnosis

1. Altered cerebral perfusion due to bleeding from the aneurysm.
2. Sensory/perceptual alteration due to the restrictions of subarachnoid precautions.
3. Anxiety due to illness or restrictions of subarachnoid precautions.

Collaborative Problems

1. Seizures.
2. Vasospasm.

Planning and Implementation

Patient goals include improved cerebral tissue perfusion, relief of sensory/deprivation, relief of anxiety, and the absence of complications.

Interventions

IMPROVING CEREBRAL TISSUE PERFUSION

1. Monitor continually for neurologic deterioration.
2. Check blood pressure, pulse, level of responsiveness, pupillary responses, and motor function hourly.
3. Implement subarachnoid precautions (immediate and absolute bed rest in a quiet, nonstressful setting; restrict visitors).
4. Elevate head of bed moderately or as ordered.
5. Avoid any activity that suddenly increases blood pressure or obstructs venous return, e.g., Valsalva maneuver, eliminate caffeine, administer all personal care, and minimize external stimuli.

RELIEVING SENSORY DEPRIVATION

1. Keep sensory stimulation to a minimum.

RELIEVING ANXIETY

1. Inform patient of plan of care and reassure patient and family.

MONITORING AND MANAGING POTENTIAL COMPLICATIONS (SEIZURE)

1. Maintain seizure precautions.
2. Maintain airway and prevent injury if a seizure occurs.
3. Administer drug treatment as prescribed.

MONITORING AND MANAGING POTENTIAL COMPLICATIONS (VASOSPASM)

Administer calcium blockers or fluid volume expanders as prescribed.

For more information see Chapter 60 in Smeltzer and Bare: *Brunner and Suddarth's Textbook of Medical–Surgical Nursing,* 8th Edition. Philadelphia: Lippincott–Raven, 1996.

ANGINA PECTORIS

Angina pectoris is a clinical syndrome characterized by paroxysms of pain or a feeling of pressure in the anterior chest. The cause is insufficient coronary blood flow. Angina is usually a result of atherosclerotic heart disease and is associated with a significant obstruction of a major coronary artery. Factors affecting anginal pain are physical exertion, exposure to cold, eating a heavy meal, stress or any emotion-provoking situation that increases myocardial workload.

CLINICAL MANIFESTATIONS

1. Pain varies from feeling pressure in the upper chest to agonizing pain.
2. Accompanied by severe apprehension and feeling of impending death.
3. Usually retrosternal, deep in the chest behind the upper or middle third of the sternum.
4. Frequently localized, may radiate to the neck, jaw, shoulders, and inner aspect of the upper extremities.
5. Tightness, choking, or strangling sensation with a viselike, insistent quality.
6. Feeling of weakness or numbness in the arms, wrists, and hands.
7. Important characteristic of anginal pain is that it subsides when the precipitating cause is removed.

DIAGNOSTIC EVALUATION

1. Evaluation of clinical manifestations of pain and patient history.
2. Electrocardiogram (ECG) changes; stress testing.

MANAGEMENT

The goals of medical management are to decrease the oxygen demands of the myocardium and to increase the oxygen supply through pharmacologic therapy and risk factor control. Surgically, the goals of management are met through revascularization of the blood supply to the myocardium. Frequently a combination of medical and surgical therapies is used.

Approaches to Revascularize the Myocardium

1. Coronary artery bypass surgery.
2. Percutaneous transluminal coronary angioplasty (PTCA).
3. Application of intracoronary stents to enhance blood flow.
4. Lasers to vaporize plaques.
5. Percutaneous coronary endarterectomy to extract obstruction.

Pharmacologic Therapy

1. Nitrates remain the mainstay of therapy (nitroglycerin [NTG]).
2. Beta-adrenergic blockers (propranolol hydrochloride [Inderal]).
3. Calcium ion antagonists/channel blockers (nifedipine [Procardia], verapamil [Isoptin, Calan], diltiazem [Cardizem]).

Risk Factor Control

1. Refer to modifiable risk factors in section on coronary artery disease.

NURSING PROCESS

Assessment

1. Observe and record all facets of patient activities that precede and precipitate attacks of anginal pain.
2. Design a logical program of prevention from patient history.

Major Nursing Diagnosis

1. Pain related to myocardial ischemia.
2. Anxiety related to fear of death.
3. Knowledge deficit about the underlying nature of disease and methods for avoiding complications.
4. Potential noncompliance to therapeutic regimen related to nonacceptance of necessary lifestyle changes.

Collaborative Problems

1. Potential complications of angina include myocardial infarction.

Planning and Implementation

Patient goals include prevention of pain, reduction of anxiety, awareness of the underlying nature of the disorder, understanding of the prescribed care, and adherence to the self-care program.

Interventions

PREVENTING PAIN

1. Teach patient to understand the symptom complex and avoid activities known to cause anginal pain.
2. Avoid sudden exertion, exposure to cold, tobacco; eat regularly but lightly, maintain prescribed weight.
3. Teach patient to maintain an unhurried pace throughout the day.
4. Discourage over-the-counter (OTC) drugs, e.g., diet pills, nasal decongestants, or drugs that increase heart rate and blood pressure.

REDUCING ANXIETY

1. Stay with the hospitalized patient to minimize fear of death.
2. Provide essential information about the illness and explain importance of following prescribed directives for the ambulatory patient at home.

✎ PATIENT EDUCATION AND HEALTH MAINTENANCE: CARE IN THE HOME AND COMMUNITY

Understanding of the Illness and Strategies to Avoid Complications

1. Educate the patient about the basic nature of the illness.
2. Furnish the facts needed to reorganize living habits: to reduce the frequency and severity of anginal attacks; delay underlying disease; provide protection from other complications.

Adherence to the Self-Care Program

1. Prepare self-care program in collaboration with the patient, family, or friends.
2. Plan activities to minimize the occurrence of angina episodes.
3. Teach patient that any pain unrelieved by the usual methods should be treated at the closest emergency center.

✪ GERONTOLOGIC CONSIDERATIONS

The elderly person who experiences angina may not exhibit the typical pain profile because of changes in neuroceptors.

Pain is often manifested as weakness or fainting. Advise patient to recognize feelings of weakness as an indication for rest or taking prescribed medications. During cold-temperature exposure the patient may experience anginal symptoms more quickly than younger persons because of less subcutaneous fat to provide insulation. Encourage patient to dress with extra clothing.

For more information see Chapter 28 in Smeltzer and Bare: *Brunner and Suddarth's Textbook of Medical–Surgical Nursing,* 8th Edition. Philadelphia: Lippincott–Raven, 1996.

AORTIC ANEURYSM

See Aneurysm, Aortic

AORTIC INSUFFICIENCY (REGURGITATION)

Aortic insufficiency is caused by inflammatory lesions that deform the flaps of the aortic valve. The lesions prevent complete sealing of the aortic orifice during diastole, allowing a backflow of blood from the aorta into the left ventricle. This disorder may result from rheumatic endocarditis, endocarditis, congenital abnormalities, or diseases such as syphilis and dissecting aneurysm that cause dilation or tearing of the ascending aorta.

CLINICAL MANIFESTATIONS

1. Develops insidiously.
2. Earliest manifestation is increased force of heartbeat, i.e., visible or palpable pulsations over the precordium and in the neck.
3. Exertional dyspnea and easy fatigability.
4. Signs and symptoms of left ventricular failure (orthopnea, paroxysmal nocturnal dyspnea).
5. Pulse pressure widened.
6. Water-hammer pulse (the pulse strikes the palpating finger with quick, sharp strokes and then suddenly collapses).

DIAGNOSTIC EVALUATION

ECG, echocardiogram, and cardiac catheterization.

MANAGEMENT

Treatment of choice is aortic valve replacement. Surgery is recommended when left ventricular hypertrophy is present.

For more information see Chapter 29 in Smeltzer and Bare: *Brunner and Suddarth's Textbook of Medical–Surgical Nursing,* 8th Edition. Philadelphia: Lippincott–Raven, 1996.

AORTIC REGURGITATION

See Aortic Insufficiency

AORTIC STENOSIS

Aortic valve stenosis is the narrowing of the orifice between the left ventricle and the aorta. In adults the stenosis may be congenital, or it may be a result of rheumatic endocarditis or cusp calcification of unknown cause. There is progressive narrowing of the valve orifice over a period of several years to several decades. The heart muscle increases in size (hypertrophy) in response to all degrees of obstruction; heart failure occurs when obstruction is severe.

CLINICAL MANIFESTATIONS

1. Exertional dyspnea.
2. Dizziness and fainting.
3. Angina pectoris.
4. Blood pressure can be low but is usually normal.
5. Low pulse pressure (30 mmHg or less).
6. Physical examination: loud, rough, systolic murmur heard over the aortic area; vibration over the base of the heart resembling the purring of a cat.

DIAGNOSTIC EVALUATION

1. 12-lead ECG and echocardiogram.
2. Left heart catheterization.

MANAGEMENT

Surgical replacement of the aortic valve is favored. Uncorrected condition can lead to irreversible heart failure.

For more information see Chapter 29 in Smeltzer and Bare: *Brunner and Suddarth's Textbook of Medical–Surgical Nursing,* 8th Edition. Philadelphia: Lippincott–Raven, 1996.

AORTIC VALVE STENOSIS

See Aortic Stenosis

APLASTIC ANEMIA

See Anemia, Aplastic

APHASIA

Aphasia is a disturbance of language function resulting from injury or disease of the brain centers. It may involve impairment of the ability to read and write, speak, listen, calculate, comprehend, and understand gestures. Major causes are stroke, head injury, and brain tumor. Broca's area (speech center) is near the left motor area. Many patients paralyzed on the right side (due to damage or injury on the left side of the brain) are unable to speak. Some patients are not affected but these usually are left-handed persons whose speech area is located in the right hemisphere.

NURSING PROCESS

Assessment

1. Assess the communication abilities of the patient in cooperation with the speech-language pathologist and the neurologist.

2. Obtain information regarding the patient's pre-illness speech-language skills and interests.
3. Use formalized, standardized tests and observational methods to evaluate comprehension, mathematical, reading, and residual language skills.
4. Listen to patient, ask to follow simple directions, and observe how patient copes with dysfunction.

Nursing Interventions

DEVELOPING SELF-ESTEEM

1. Give as much psychological security as possible.
2. Practice a kind, unhurried manner combined with encouragement, patience, and a willingness to invest time.
3. Accept the patient's behavior and feelings, relieve embarrassment, and give support by assuring there is nothing wrong with patient's intelligence.
4. Provide a relaxed and permissive environment.
5. Encourage to socialize with family and friends.
6. Return items in the room to their proper place as the aphasic patient has almost an obsession with orderliness.

IMPROVING COMMUNICATION ABILITIES

1. Guide the patient in efforts to improve communication skills.
2. Emphasize listening and speaking skills.
3. Encourage to verbalize needs and to use a communication board (pictures of commonly requested needs and phrases) when unable to express needs.

INCREASING AUDITORY STIMULATION

1. Encourage patient to listen.
2. Give patient time to organize an answer.
3. Provide social contact by talking to the patient while providing care.

HELPING THE FAMILY COPE

1. Talk about the stroke or head injury, acknowledge the changes, focus on the patient's abilities, and inform the patient of support systems.
2. Encourage family members to act naturally and treat the patient in the same manner as before the illness.
3. Inform family that the patient's ability to speak may vary from day to day and fatigue has an adverse effect on speech.
4. Inform that the patient may strike out verbally when emotional controls are lowered; tears and laughter may occur without cause and frequent mood shifts are common.
5. Provide information concerning support groups and group therapy for socialization and motivation.
6. Counsel family to continue a life of their own and seek the aid of health professionals in dealing with their frustrations.

For more information see Chapter 59 in Smeltzer and Bare: *Brunner and Suddarth's Textbook of Medical–Surgical Nursing,* 8th Edition. Philadelphia: Lippincott–Raven, 1996.

APPENDICITIS

The appendix is a small fingerlike appendage, attached to the cecum just below the ileocecal valve. Because it empties inefficiently, and its lumen is small, it is prone to becoming obstructed and is vulnerable to infection (appendicitis). It is the most common cause of acute inflammation in the right lower quadrant of the abdominal cavity and most common cause of emergency abdominal surgery. Males are affected more than females, teenagers more frequently than adults; the highest incidence is in those between the ages of 10 and 30.

CLINICAL MANIFESTATIONS

1. Lower quadrant pain usually accompanied by low-grade fever, nausea, and often vomiting.
2. At McBurney's point (located halfway between the umbilicus and the anterior spine of the ilium) local tenderness with pressure and some rigidity of the lower portion of the right rectus muscle.
3. Rebound tenderness may be present; location of appendix dictates amount of tenderness, muscle spasm, and occurrence of constipation or diarrhea.
4. Rovsing's sign (elicited by palpating left lower quadrant, which causes pain in right lower quadrant).
5. If appendix ruptures, pain becomes more diffuse; abdominal distention develops from paralytic ileus and condition worsens.

DIAGNOSTIC EVALUATION

1. Diagnosis is based on a complete physical examination and laboratory and radiologic tests.
2. Leukocyte count greater than 10,000/mm3; neutrophil count greater than 75%; abdominal x-rays and ultrasound studies reveal right lower quadrant density or localized airflow levels.

MANAGEMENT

1. Surgery is indicated if appendicitis is diagnosed; perform appendectomy as soon as possible to decrease risk of perforation. Methods: low abdominal incision under general or spinal anesthetic; laparoscopy.
2. Administer antibiotics and IV fluids until surgery is performed.
3. Analgesics can be given after diagnosis is made.

COMPLICATIONS OF APPENDECTOMY

1. The major complication is perforation of the appendix, which can lead to peritonitis or an abscess.

2. Perforation generally occurs 24 hours after onset of pain (symptoms include fever, toxic appearance, and continued pain).

Nursing Interventions

1. Nursing goals include relieving pain, preventing fluid volume deficit, reducing anxiety, eliminating infection due to the potential or actual disruption of the gastrointestinal tract, maintaining skin integrity, and attaining optimum nutrition.
2. Preoperatively: prepare for surgery, start IV, give prescribed antipyretic, antibiotic, nasogastric tube (if evidence of paralytic ileus), and ask patient to void.
3. Postoperatively: place in semi-Fowler's position, give narcotic analgesic as ordered, administer oral fluids when tolerated, and food as desired on day of surgery (if tolerated).
4. Provide discharge teaching: inform of follow-up appointment with surgeon, discuss incision care and activity guidelines, teach patient and family wound care and dressing changes/irrigations (if peritonitis complication). Home health nurse to assist with this care and continue monitoring for complications and wound healing.

✪ GERONTOLOGIC CONSIDERATIONS

In the elderly, signs and symptoms of appendicitis may vary greatly. May be very vague and suggestive of bowel obstruction or another process; some may experience no symptoms until appendix ruptures.

Incidence of perforated appendix is higher in the elderly because many of these persons do not seek health care as quickly as younger persons.

For more information see Chapter 37 in Smeltzer and Bare: *Brunner and Suddarth's Textbook of Medical–Surgical Nursing,* 8th Edition. Philadelphia: Lippincott–Raven, 1996.

ARDS

See Adult Respiratory Distress Syndrome

ARF

See Renal Failure, Acute

ARTERIAL EMBOLISM

Arterial emboli arise most commonly from thrombi that develop in the chambers of the heart as a result of atrial fibrillation, myocardial infarction, infective endocarditis, or chronic congestive heart failure. Thrombi become detached and are carried from the left side of the heart into the arterial system where they cause obstruction. The symptoms of arterial emboli depend primarily on the size of the embolus, the organ involved, and the state of the collateral vessels. The immediate effect is cessation of distal blood flow. Secondary vasospasm can contribute to ischemia. Emboli tend to lodge at arterial bifurcations and atherosclerotic narrowing.

CLINICAL MANIFESTATIONS

1. Pain, pallor, pulselessness, paresthesia, and paralysis (5P's).
2. The part of limb below the occlusion is markedly colder and paler than above as a result of ischemia.

MANAGEMENT

Acute Embolic Occlusion

1. Emergency embolectomy is the surgical procedure of choice.

Presence of Collateral Circulation

1. IV anticoagulation with heparin.
2. Thrombolytic agents, e.g., streptokinase, urokinase, tissue-type plasminogen activator (t-PA). Contraindications are internal bleeding, stroke, recent major surgery, uncontrolled hypertension, and pregnancy.

POSTOPERATIVE NURSING MANAGEMENT

1. Encourage movement of the leg to stimulate circulation and prevent stasis.
2. Anticoagulants continued to prevent thrombosis of the affected artery and to diminish development of subsequent thrombi.
3. Assess the surgical incision frequently for hemorrhage.

For more information see Chapter 31 in Smeltzer and Bare: *Brunner and Suddarth's Textbook of Medical–Surgical Nursing,* 8th Edition. Philadelphia: Lippincott–Raven, 1996.

ARTERIAL INFLAMMATION

See Buerger's Disease

ARTERIAL INSUFFICIENCY

See Peripheral Arterial Occlusive Disease

ARTERIAL OCCLUSIVE DISEASE

See Buerger's Disease

ARTERIOSCLEROSIS AND ATHEROSCLEROSIS

Arteriosclerosis is the most common disease of the arteries. It is a diffuse process whereby the muscle fibers and the endothelial lining of the walls of small arteries and arterioles become thickened. Although the pathologic processes of arteriosclerosis and atherosclerosis differ, rarely does one occur without the other. Terms are used interchangeably. Atherosclerosis primarily affects the main arteries throughout the entire arterial tree in varying degrees. The primary lesion, atheroma, is a local area of lipid plaque in a fibrous covering that slowly occludes the lumen of the vessel. These plaques are found predominantly in the abdominal aorta, coronary, popliteal, and internal carotid arteries.

RISK FACTORS

There is no single risk factor as a primary contributor; the greater the number of risk factors, the greater the likelihood of developing the disease.

1. High-fat diet has been strongly implicated.
2. Hypertension.
3. Diabetes.
4. Smoking is one of the strongest risk factors.
5. Obesity, stress, and lack of exercise.

CLINICAL MANIFESTATIONS

Depend on the tissue or organ affected, e.g., heart, brain, peripheral vessels.

MANAGEMENT

Traditional management of atherosclerosis depends on risk factor modification, medication administration, and nursing measures related to the resulting diseases. Several radiological techniques have been shown to be important adjunctive therapies to surgical procedures, such as laser angioplasty and rotational atherectomy.

GERONTOLOGIC CONSIDERATIONS

Atherosclerotic cardiovascular disease is found in 80% of the population over 65 years of age, and is the most common condition of the arterial system in the elderly.

For more information see Chapter 31 in Smeltzer and Bare: *Brunner and Suddarth's Textbook of Medical–Surgical Nursing,* 8th Edition. Philadelphia: Lippincott–Raven, 1996.

ARTHRITIS

See Osteoarthritis

ARTHRITIS, RHEUMATOID

Rheumatoid arthritis (RA) is an inflammatory disorder that primarily involves the synovial membrane of the joints and is commonly characterized by joint pain, stiffness, decreased mobility, and fatigue. RA occurs between ages 30 and 50 with peak incidence between ages 40 and 60. Women are affected two to three times more frequently. RA is believed to be an immune response to unknown antigens. The stimulus may be viral or bacterial. There may be a predisposition to the disease.

CLINICAL MANIFESTATIONS

1. Determined by the stage and severity of the disease.
2. Joint pain, swelling, warmth, erythema, and lack of function are classic clinical features.
3. Palpitation of joints reveals spongy or boggy tissue.
4. Fluid can usually be aspirated from the inflamed joint.

Characteristic Pattern of Joint Involvement

1. Begins with small joints in hands, wrists, and feet.
2. Progressively, the knees, shoulders, hips, elbows, ankles, cervical spine, and temporomandibular joints are involved.
3. Onset is usually acute, bilateral and symmetric.
4. Joints may be hot, swollen, and painful; morning stiffness lasting for more than 30 minutes.
5. Deformities of the hands and feet are common.

Extra-articular Features

1. Fever, weight loss, fatigue, anemia, and lymph node enlargement.
2. Raynaud's phenomenon.
3. Rheumatoid nodules, nontender and movable; found in subcutaneous tissue over bony prominences.

DIAGNOSTIC EVALUATION

1. Several factors contribute to an RA diagnosis: rheumatoid nodules, joint inflammation, laboratory findings.
2. Rheumatoid factor (RF) present in more than 80% of patients.
3. Red blood count and C_4 complement component are decreased.

MANAGEMENT

Goals of management include education, a balance of rest and exercise, and referral to community agencies for support.

1. Early RA: medication management involves therapeutic doses of salicylates or nonsteroidal anti-inflammatory drugs (NSAIDS); antimalarials, gold, penicillamine, or sulfasalazine; methotrexate; analgesics for periods of extreme pain.
2. Moderate, erosive RA: formal program of occupational and physical therapy.

3. Persistent, erosive RA: reconstructive surgery and corticosteroids.
4. Advanced unremitting RA: immunosuppressive agents, such as methotrexate, cyclophosphamide, and azathioprine.
5. RA patients frequently experience anorexia, weight loss, and anemia, requiring careful dietary history to identify usual eating habits and food preferences. (Corticorsteroids may stimulate appetite and cause weight gain.)

NURSING PROCESS

Assessment

1. Assess the patient's self-image related to musculoskeletal changes and determine if the patient is experiencing unusual fatigue, general weakness, pain, morning stiffness, fever, or anorexia.
2. Assess the cardiovascular, pulmonary, and renal systems.
3. Assess the joints by inspecting, palpating, and inquiring about tenderness, swelling, and redness in the affected joints.
4. Assess joint mobility, range of motion, and muscle strength.
5. Focus on identifying patient problems and factors.
6. Assess medication compliance and self-management.
7. Gather information regarding the patient's understanding, motivation, knowledge, coping abilities, past experiences, preconceptions, and unknown fears.

Major Nursing Diagnosis

1. Pain related to inflammation, tissue damage, and joint immobility.
2. Fatigue related to increased disease activity.
3. Impaired physical mobility related to restricted joint movement.

4. Self-care deficits (feeding, bathing, dressing, toileting) related to fatigue and joint stiffness.
5. Sleep pattern disturbance related to pain and fatigue.
6. Disturbance in self-concept related to the physical and psychologic dependency of chronic illness and loss of independence.

Planning and Implementation

Patient goals include relief of pain and discomfort, decreased fatigue, increased mobility, achievement of an optimal, individual level of independence in activities of daily living, improved quality of sleep, increased knowledge regarding self-management, and attainment of a positive self-concept.

Interventions

RELIEVING PAIN AND DISCOMFORT

1. Question carefully to distinguish pain from stiffness.
2. Teach and use pain management techniques for immediate short-term management (i.e., use of heat and cold, joint protection, rest, and analgesics).
3. Educate regarding long-term pain management (i.e., use of anti-inflammatory medications, establishing an exercise regimen for maintaining joint mobility, and relaxation techniques).
4. Provide comfort measures while giving care
5. Set realistic expectations so patient and significant others realize pain can be controlled depending on disease activity.

REDUCING FATIGUE

1. Educate patient on physical and emotional factors related to RA that cause or contribute to fatigue.
2. Teach the patient how to use level of fatigue to monitor the disease and balance physical activities accordingly.

INCREASING MOBILITY AND INDEPENDENCE IN SELF-CARE ACTIVITIES

1. Understand that deformity does not equate with disability and patient's ability to perform self-care.
2. Relieve persistent pain and morning stiffness to increase patient's mobility and self-care.

IMPROVING SLEEP

1. Identify the cause of a sleep problem.
2. Adjust anti-inflammatory and analgesic administration times.

INCREASING KNOWLEDGE REGARDING DISEASE MANAGEMENT

1. Tailor education to patient's previous knowledge base, interest level, degree of comfort, and social or cultural influences.
2. Instruct patient on basic disease management, medications, and necessary adaptations in lifestyle.
3. Encourage patient to practice new self-management skills.

IMPROVING SELF-CONCEPT

1. Try to understand the patient's emotional reactions to the disease.
2. Encourage communication so patient and family verbalize feelings, perceptions, and fears related to the disease.
3. Encourage patient and family to comply with the management program for more positive outcomes.

✎ PATIENT EDUCATION AND HEALTH MAINTENANCE: CARE IN THE HOME AND COMMUNITY

1. The community nurse should visit the home to make sure the patient is able to function as independently as possible.
2. Alert the patient/family to local support services such as local chapters of the Arthritis Foundation.

For more information see Chapter 52 in Smeltzer and Bare: *Brunner and Suddarth's Textbook of Medical–Surgical Nursing,* 8th Edition. Philadelphia: Lippincott–Raven, 1996.

ASTHMA

Asthma is an intermittent, reversible, obstructive airway disease characterized by narrowing of the airways, resulting in dyspnea, cough, and wheezing. Acute exacerbations occur from minutes to hours, interspersed with symptom-free periods.

It can begin at any age; about half develop asthma in childhood and another third before age forty. Asthma is rarely fatal but does affect lifestyle.

Asthma is described as allergic, idiopathic (nonallergic), or mixed. Allergic asthma is caused by a known allergen(s) (e.g., dust pollens, animals, food, molds). Children with asthma often outgrow the condition by adolescence.

Idiopathic or nonallergic asthma is not related to specific allergens. Factors such as a respiratory infection, exercise, emotions, and environmental pollutants may trigger an attack. These attacks become more severe and frequent with time and can progress to chronic bronchitis and emphysema.

Mixed asthma is the most common form of asthma. It has characteristics of both allergic and idiopathic forms.

CLINICAL MANIFESTATIONS

Common Symptoms

1. Cough.
2. Dyspnea.
3. Wheezing.

Asthma Attacks

1. Frequently occur at night.
2. Start suddenly with coughing and a sensation of chest tightness.

3. Then slow, laborious, wheezy breathing.
4. Expiration more strenuous and prolonged than inspiration.
5. Obstructed airflow creates sensation of dyspnea.
6. Cough is tight and dry at first; followed by more forceful cough with distinctive sputum of thin mucus.
7. Total attack may last from 30 minutes to several hours and may subside spontaneously.

Later Signs

1. Cyanosis secondary to severe hypoxia.
2. Symptoms of carbon dioxide retention (e.g., sweating, tachycardia, and a widened pulse pressure).

Related Reactions

1. Eczema.
2. Urticaria.
3. Angioneurotic edema.

DIAGNOSTIC EVALUATION

No single test will confirm a diagnosis of asthma.

MANAGEMENT

Drug Therapy

1. Beta agonists.
2. Methylxanthines.
3. Anticholinergics.
4. Corticosteroids.
5. Mast cell inhibitors.

Prevention

1. Evaluate and identify foreign proteins that precipitate the attacks.
2. Conduct skin test with material from the mattress and pillows if attacks occur at night.
3. Conduct skin tests made with an antigen composed from hair or skin scraping if attacks appear to be associated with an animal.

4. Avoid exposure to offending pollens, i.e., stay in air-conditioned rooms during pollen season or if feasible change climate zone.
5. Prevent exercise-induced asthma (EIA) by inspiring air at 37°C and 100% relative humidity.
6. Cover the nose and mouth with a mask for activities that precipitate attack.

Associated Psychotherapeutic Modalities

Maintain good physical and mental health because attacks may be induced by suggestion alone.

For more information see Chapter 24 in Smeltzer and Bare: *Brunner and Suddarth's Textbook of Medical–Surgical Nursing,* 8th Edition. Philadelphia: Lippincott–Raven, 1996.

ASTHMA: STATUS ASTHMATICUS

Status asthmaticus is severe asthma that is unresponsive to conventional therapy and lasts longer than 24 hours. A vicious self-perpetuating cycle may occur as a result of infection, anxiety, overuse of tranquilizers, nebulizer abuse, dehydration, increased adrenergic block, and nonspecific irritants. An acute episode may be precipitated by hypersensitivity to aspirin. Two predominant pathologic problems occur: a decrease in the diameter of the bronchi and a ventilation-perfusion abnormality.

CLINICAL MANIFESTATIONS

1. Same as those seen in severe asthma.
2. No correlation between severity of attack and number of wheezes.
3. With greater obstruction, wheezing may disappear; frequently a sign of impending respiratory failure.

DIAGNOSTIC EVALUATION

1. Primarily by pulmonary function studies and arterial blood gases (ABGs).
2. Respiratory alkalosis is most common finding.

MANAGEMENT

Emergency Room Setting

1. Treat initially with beta agonists, supplemental oxygen, and intravenous fluids to hydrate.
2. Start with low-flow humidified oxygen (Venturi mask or nasal catheter); the flow rate is determined by ABGs (PaO_2 65–85 mmHg).
3. Sedatives are contraindicated.

Hospitalization Required If

1. No response to repeated treatments.
2. Mechanical ventilation needed if patient is tiring or in respiratory failure.

Interventions

1. Assess for signs of dehydration by checking skin turgor.
2. Combat dehydration with adequate fluid intake, to loosen secretions and facilitate expectoration.
3. Administer prescribed IV fluids to 3000–4000 ml/day unless contraindicated.
4. Monitor respiratory status constantly for the first 12–24 hours, or until status asthmaticus stops.
5. Keep room quiet and free of respiratory irritants (flowers).

✎ PATIENT EDUCATION AND HEALTH MAINTENANCE: CARE IN THE HOME AND COMMUNITY

1. Keep recurrences to a minimum with patient education.
2. Instruct patient as to which signs and symptoms require contact with physician (e.g., awakening during night with an acute attack, incomplete relief from the inhaler, or respiratory infection).
3. Give bronchodilators around the clock.
4. Add or increase medication (i.e., theophylline and corticosteroids) when asthmatic attacks occur.

5. Maintain adequate hydration at home to keep secretions from thickening.
6. Instruct to recognize that infection is to be avoided because it can trigger an attack.
7. Instruct in self-care protocols designed with goals of (1) aborting severe attacks and (2) giving the patient a measure of independence.
8. Instruct patient on the hazards of theophylline overuse (narrow therapeutic level).
9. Use hand-held metered-dose inhaler with β_2 selective adrenergic; if this fails, begin corticosteroid (prednisone).

✪ GERONTOLOGIC CONSIDERATIONS

Asthma may occur as a new problem in the elderly patient. Management of asthma in the elderly may be complex because of preexisting conditions, such as heart disease and the cardiovascular side effects of medications.

➕ CLINICAL ALERT

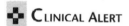

Rising PCO_2 is a danger signal of impending respiratory failure.

For more information see Chapter 24 in Smeltzer and Bare: *Brunner and Suddarth's Textbook of Medical–Surgical Nursing,* 8th Edition. Philadelphia: Lippincott–Raven, 1996.

ATHEROSCLEROSIS, CORONARY

See Coronary Atherosclerosis

BACK PAIN, LOW

Impairment of the back and spine is the third leading cause of disability of people in their employment years. Most low back pain is caused by musculoskeletal problems (e.g., acute lumbosacral strain, unstable lumbosacral ligaments and weak muscles, osteoarthritis of the spine, spinal stenosis, intervertebral disc problems, inequality of leg length). Older patients may have back pain associated with osteoporotic vertebral fractures or bone metastasis. Many other medical and psychosomatic conditions are causes of back pain. Obesity, stress, and occasionally depression may contribute to low back pain. Patients with chronic low back pain may develop a dependence on alcohol or analgesics.

CLINICAL MANIFESTATIONS

1. Patient complains of either acute back pain or chronic back pain (lasting more than 2 months without improvement) and fatigue.
2. Pain radiating along a nerve root (sciatica); accentuated by movement.
3. Pain associated with straight leg raising (spinal root irritation).
4. Paravertebral muscle spasm (greatly increased muscle tone of back postural muscles) with a loss of normal lumbar lordotic curve and possible spinal deformity.
5. Radiculopathy (nerve root problem) or chronic back pain.

DIAGNOSTIC EVALUATION

1. X-ray of spine.
2. Computed tomography (CT scan).

3. Ultrasound.
4. Magnetic resonance imaging (MRI).

MANAGEMENT

The goal is to increase mobility, muscle strength, and flexibility.

Supportive

1. Bed rest, stress reduction, relaxation; self-limiting and resolves within 6 weeks.
2. Position in bed to increase lumbar flexion; elevate head 30° and flex knees slightly; avoid prone position.
3. Physical therapy; intermittent pelvic traction; ice; hot moist packs; infrared radiant heat; ultrasound; diathermy; whirlpool; exercise program; low back supports and braces.

Medications

1. Analgesics.
2. Muscle relaxants.
3. Tranquilizers.
4. Anti-inflammatory agents and nonsteroidal anti-inflammatory agents (NSAIDS).

Transcutaneous Electrical Nerve Stimulation (TENS)

TENS is a noninvasive pain-reduction device thought to give pain relief by overriding pain input and stimulating endorphins.

Exercise Program

Low back supports and braces.

NURSING PROCESS

Assessment

1. Encourage patient to describe the discomfort.
2. Obtain history about previous pain control and how back problem is affecting lifestyle.

3. Observe patient's posture, position changes, and gait.
4. Assess spinal curves, pelvic crest, and shoulder symmetry.
5. Palpate the perispinal muscles, and note spasm and tenderness.
6. Note discomfort and limitations in movement when bending forward and laterally.
7. Evaluate nerve involvement by assessing for abnormal sensations, muscle weakness or paralysis, and back and leg pain with straight leg raises.
8. Assess for obesity and nutritional balance.

Major Nursing Diagnosis

1. Pain related to musculoskeletal problems.
2. Impaired physical mobility related to pain, muscle spasms, and decreased flexibility.
3. Knowledge deficit related to back-conserving body mechanic techniques.
4. Altered nutrition: more than body requirements related to obesity.

Planning and Implementation

The major goals may include relief of pain, improved physical mobility, improved role performance, use of back-conserving body mechanics, and weight reduction.

Interventions

RELIEVING PAIN

1. Encourage to comply with prescribed bed rest and positioning.
2. Modify perceived pain through behavioral therapies, e.g., diaphragmatic breathing, relaxation, and guided imagery.
3. Use gentle, soft-tissue massage to decrease muscle spasm, increase circulation, relieve congestion, and reduce pain.
4. Assess patient's response to each medication prescribed.

5. TENS if not contraindicated by cardiac pacemaker.

IMPROVING PHYSICAL MOBILITY

1. Encourage patient to alternate lying, sitting, and walking activities and advise to avoid sitting, standing, and walking for long periods; resume activities and exercise as pain subsides.
2. Plan for recumbent rest periods several times throughout day.
3. Encourage patient adherence to prescribed exercise program.

PROMOTING PROPER BODY MECHANICS

1. Prevent recurrence of acute low back pain; teach how to stand, lie, and lift properly; shift weight frequently when standing.
2. Practice protective and defensive postures, positions, and body mechanics for natural strengthening of the back and to diminish chance of recurrence of back pain.

MODIFYING NUTRITION FOR WEIGHT REDUCTION

1. Provide a sound nutritional plan that includes a change in eating habits to maintain desirable weight.
2. Monitor weight loss, note achievement, provide encouragement and positive reinforcement, and facilitate adherence.

✎ PATIENT EDUCATION AND HEALTH MAINTENANCE: CARE IN THE HOME AND COMMUNITY

1. Standing: avoid prolonged standing and walking; avoid forward flexion work position.
2. Sitting: avoid prolonged sitting; sit in straight-back chair with back well supported; avoid knee and hip extension; maintain back support; guard against extension strains, i.e., reaching, pushing, sitting with legs straight out; alternate periods of sitting with walking.

3. Lying: rest at intervals; place a firm bedboard under mattress; avoid sleeping in prone position; use a pillow under head, between the legs when lying on side, and when supine, place a pillow under the knees to decrease lordosis.

4. Lifting: keep back straight, hold load close to body, lift with large leg muscles; squat with back straight; avoid twisting the trunk, lifting above waist level, reaching up for long periods.

5. Exercise: daily, walking outdoors with progression in distance and pace; do prescribed back exercises twice daily, increasing exercises gradually and avoid jumping.

For more information see Chapter 63 in Smeltzer and Bare: *Brunner and Suddarth's Textbook of Medical–Surgical Nursing,* 8th Edition. Philadelphia: Lippincott–Raven, 1996.

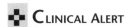 **C**LINICAL **A**LERT

TENS should not be used with a cardiac pacemaker because of the risk of causing dysrhythmias.

BACTERIAL ENDOCARDITIS

See Endocariditis, Infective

BASAL CELL CARCINOMA

See Cancer of the Skin

BASOPHILIC TUMORS

See Pituitary Tumors

BELL'S PALSY

B

Bell's palsy (facial paralysis) is due to peripheral involvement of the seventh cranial nerve on one side, which results in weakness or paralysis of the facial muscles. The cause is unknown, but possible causes may include vascular ischemia, viral disease (herpes simplex, herpes zoster), autoimmune disease, or a combination. Bell's palsy represents a type of pressure paralysis causing a distortion of the face, increased lacrimation (tearing), and painful sensations in the face, behind the ear, and eye. The patient may experience speech difficulties and be unable to eat on the affected side.

MANAGEMENT

The goals of management are to maintain muscle tone of the face and to prevent or minimize denervation.

1. Reassure patient that no stroke has occurred and spontaneous recovery occurs within 3–5 weeks in most patients.
2. Steroid therapy may be given to reduce inflammation and edema, which will reduce vascular compression and permit restoration of blood circulation to the nerve. Early steroid administration appears to diminish severity, relieve pain, and minimize denervation.
3. Facial pain is controlled with analgesics or heat applied to the involved side of face.
4. Electrical stimulation may be applied to the face to prevent muscle atrophy.
5. Surgical exploration may be done if tumor is suspected; surgical decompression of the facial nerve; or surgical rehabilitation of a paralyzed face.

PATIENT EDUCATION AND HEALTH MAINTENANCE: CARE IN THE HOME AND COMMUNITY

Eye Care

1. Because the blink reflex is diminished, the involved eye may not close completely and will need to be protected.
2. Inform of potential complications: corneal irritation and ulceration, overflow of tear (epiphora) from keratitis from dry cornea, and absence of blink reflex.
3. Cover eye with a protective shield at night.
4. Apply eye ointment to keep eyelids closed during sleep.
5. Teach patient to close the paralyzed eyelid manually before going to sleep.
6. Wear wrap-around sunglasses or goggles to decrease normal evaporation from the eye.

Maintain Muscle Tone

1. Massage face with gentle upward motion several times daily.
2. Use facial exercises such as wrinkling the forehead, blowing out the cheeks and whistling, and keep the face warm.

For more information see Chapter 60 in Smeltzer and Bare: *Brunner and Suddarth's Textbook of Medical–Surgical Nursing,* 8th Edition. Philadelphia: Lippincott–Raven, 1996.

BENIGN PROSTATIC HYPERPLASIA/PROSTATECTOMY

Benign prostatic hyperplasia (BPH) is enlargement, or hypertrophy, of the prostate. The prostate gland enlarges, extending upward into the bladder and obstructing the outflow of urine; hydronephrosis and

B

hydroureter may result. The cause is uncertain, but evidence suggests hormonal involvement. BPH is a common occurrence in males over 50.

CLINICAL MANIFESTATIONS

1. On examination the prostate is large, rubbery, and nontender.
2. Fatigue, anorexia, nausea and vomiting, and epigastric discomfort.
3. Ultimately, azotemia and renal failure can occur with chronic urinary retention and large residual volumes.

Prostatism (Obstructive and Irritative Symptom Complex)

1. Hesitancy in starting urination, increased frequency of urination, nocturia, urgency, abdominal straining.
2. Decrease in size and force of urinary stream, interruption of urinary stream, dribbling.
3. Sensation of incomplete emptying of the bladder, acute urinary retention (more than 60 ml), and recurrent urinary tract infections.

DIAGNOSTIC EVALUATION

1. Physical examination including a digital rectal examination.
2. Urinalysis and urodynamic studies to determine obstructive flow.

MANAGEMENT

The plan of treatment depends on the cause, severity of obstruction, and condition of the patient.

1. Immediate catheterization is necessary if patient is unable to void. A suprapubic cystostomy is sometimes necessary.
2. Hormonal manipulation with antiandrogen (finasteride [Proscar]) to decrease the size of the prostate and improve urinary flow.

3. Surgery (prostatectomy) to remove the hypertrophied portion of the prostate gland.
   a. Transurethral resection of the prostate (TUR or TURP); urethral endoscopic procedure is most common approach.
   b. Suprapubic prostatectomy; abdominal incision.
   c. Perineal prostatectomy; perineal incision and incontinence, impotence, or rectal injury may be complications.
   d. Retropubic prostatectomy; low abdominal incision.

NURSING PROCESS

Refer to the nursing process for the patient undergoing prostatectomy under Cancer of the Prostate.

For more information see Chapter 47 in Smeltzer and Bare: *Brunner and Suddarth's Textbook of Medical–Surgical Nursing,* 8th Edition. Philadelphia: Lippincott–Raven, 1996.

BLADDER CANCER

See Cancer of the Bladder

BLADDER INFECTION

See Cystitis

BLEEDING DISORDERS

See Hemophilia

BONE CANCER

See Bone Tumors

BONE TUMORS

B

Neoplasms of the musculoskeletal system are of a variety of types. They include osteogenic, chondrogenic, fibrogenic, muscle, and marrow cell tumors as well as nerve, vascular, and fatty cell tumors. They may be primary tumors or metastatic tumors from primary cancers elsewhere in the body (e.g., breast, lung, prostate, kidney). Metastatic bone tumors are more common than primary bone tumors.

TYPES OF BONE TUMORS

Benign Bone Tumors

1. Slow growing and well circumscribed, present few symptoms, and not a cause of death.
2. Benign primary neoplasms of the musculoskeletal system include osteochondroma, enchondroma, osteoid osteoma, bone cyst, rhabdomyoma, and fibroma.
3. Benign tumors of the soft tissue are more common than malignant tumors.
4. Bone cysts are expanding lesions within the bone (e.g., aneurysmal and unicameral).
5. Osteochondroma is the most common benign bone tumor.
6. Enchondroma is a common tumor of the hyaline cartilage.
7. Osteoid osteoma is a painful tumor that occurs in children and young adults.
8. Osteoclastoma (giant cell tumors) are benign for long periods, but may invade local tissue and cause destruction; may undergo malignant transformation and metastasize.

Malignant Bone Tumors

1. Primary malignant musculoskeletal tumors are relatively rare and arise from connective and supportive

tissue cells (sarcomas) or bone marrow elements (myelomas). Soft tissue sarcomas include liposarcoma, fibrosarcoma, and rhabdomyosarcoma. Metastasis to the lungs is common.

2. Osteogenic sarcoma (osteosarcoma) is the most common and often fatal (early hematogenous metastasis to the lungs). It appears most frequently in males between 10 and 25 years. It is manifested by pain, swelling, limitation of motion, and weight loss. The bony mass may be palpable, tender, and fixed. Common sites are distal femur, proximal tibia, and proximal humerus.

3. Chondrosarcomas, second most common primary malignant bone tumor, are large, bulky, slow-growing tumors that affect adults (men more frequently). Tumor sites may include pelvis, ribs, femur, and humerus. They may recur after treatment.

Metastatic Bone Cancer (Secondary Bone Tumor)

More common than any primary malignant bone tumor. Tumors that metastasize to bone most frequently include carcinomas of the kidney, prostate, lung, breast, ovary, and thyroid. Metastatic tumors frequently attack the skull, spine, pelvis, femur, and humerus.

CLINICAL MANIFESTATIONS

Presents with a wide range of associated problems:

1. Asymptomatic or pain (mild/occasional to constant/severe).
2. Varying degrees of disability; and at times obvious bone growth.
3. Weight loss, malaise, and fever may be present.

DIAGNOSTIC EVALUATION

1. May be diagnosed incidentally after pathologic fracture.
2. Computerized tomography, bone scans, magnetic resonance imaging, arteriography, and x-ray.

3. Biochemical assays of the blood and urine (alkaline phosphatase frequently elevated with osteogenic sarcoma; serum acid phosphatase elevated with metastatic carcinoma of the prostate; hypercalcemia present with breast, lung, and kidney cancer bone metastasis).
4. Surgical biopsy for histologic identification; staging is based on tumor size, grade, location, and metastasis.

MANAGEMENT

The goal of treatment is to destroy or remove the tumor. This may be accomplished by surgical excision (ranging from local incision to amputation and disarticulation), radiation, or chemotherapy.

1. Soft-tissue sarcomas treated with radiation, limb-sparing excision, and adjuvant chemotherapy.
2. Metastatic bone cancer treatment is palliative, and therapeutic goal is to relieve pain and discomfort as much as possible.
3. Internal fixation of pathologic fractures minimizes associated disability and pain.

NURSING PROCESS

Assessment

1. Encourage patient to discuss problem and course of symptoms. Note patient and family's understanding of disease, coping with the problem, and management of pain.
2. Palpate mass gently on physical examination. Note size and associated soft-tissue swelling, pain, and tenderness.
3. Assess neurovascular status and range of motion of extremity.
4. Evaluate mobility and ability to perform activities of daily living.

Major Nursing Diagnosis

1. Knowledge deficit about the disease process and the therapeutic regimen.
2. Pain related to pathologic process and surgery.
3. Risk for injury: pathologic fracture related to tumor.
4. Ineffective coping related to fear of the unknown, perception of disease process, and inadequate support system.
5. Disturbance in self-esteem related to loss of body part or alteration in role performance.

Collaborative Problems

1. Delayed wound healing.
2. Nutritional deficiency.
3. Infection.

Planning and Implementation

The major goals include knowledge of disease process and treatment regimen, control of pain, absence of pathologic fractures, effective patterns of coping, improved self-esteem, and absence of complications.

Interventions: Preoperative

1. Explain diagnostic test, treatments, and expected results.
2. Reinforce and clarify information provided by the physician.
3. Encourage independence and function as long as possible.

Interventions: Postoperative

1. Monitor vital signs; assess blood loss and development of complications, i.e., deep vein thrombosis, pulmonary emboli, infection, contracture, and disuse atrophy.
2. Elevate operative part to control swelling; assess neurovascular status of extremity; immobilize the area by splints, casts, or elastic bandages until the bone heals.

CONTROLLING PAIN

1. Use psychologic and pharmacologic management techniques.
2. Work with patient to design the most effective pain management.
3. Prepare patient and give support during painful procedures.

PREVENTING PATHOLOGIC FRACTURE

1. Support affected bones and handle gently during nursing care.
2. Use external supports (e.g., splints) for additional protection.
3. Follow prescribed weight-bearing restrictions.
4. Teach how to use ambulatory devices safely and how to strengthen unaffected extremities.

COPING EFFECTIVELY

1. Encourage patient and family to verbalize feelings honestly.
2. Support and accept them as they deal with the impact of the malignant bone tumor.
3. Expect feelings of shock, despair, and grief.
4. Refer to health professionals for specific psychological help.

IMPROVING SELF-ESTEEM

1. Support family in working through adjustments that must be made; recognize changes in body image due to surgery and possible amputation.
2. Provide realistic reassurance about the future and resumption of role-related activities; encourage self-care and socialization.
3. Involve patient and family throughout treatment to promote a sense of being in control of one's life.

MONITORING AND MANAGING POTENTIAL PROBLEMS

1. Minimize pressure on wound site to promote circulation.

2. Promote healing with an aseptic, nontraumatic wound dressing.
3. Monitor and report laboratory findings to facilitate treatment.
4. Reposition patient frequently to prevent skin breakdown.

ACHIEVING ADEQUATE NUTRITIONAL STATUS

1. Give antiemetics and provide relaxation techniques to reduce gastrointestinal reaction.
2. Control stomatitis with anesthetic or antifungal mouthwash.
3. Provide adequate hydration; nutritional supplements or total parenteral nutrition.

MANAGING OSTEOMYELITIS AND WOUND INFECTIONS

1. Use prophylactic antibiotics and strict aseptic dressing techniques.
2. Prevent other infections (e.g., upper respiratory) so hematogenous spread does not result in osteomyelitis.
3. Monitor white blood cell count and instruct patient to avoid persons with colds and infections.

✎ PATIENT EDUCATION AND HEALTH MAINTENANCE: CARE IN THE HOME AND COMMUNITY

1. Prepare and coordinate continuing health care and direct patient education toward medications, dressings, treatment regimens, and physical and occupational therapy programs.
2. Teach signs and symptoms of possible complications to patient and family.
3. Emphasize the need for long-term health supervision to ensure cure or to detect tumor recurrence or metastasis.

For more information see Chapter 63 in Smeltzer and Bare: *Brunner and Suddarth's Textbook of Medical–Surgical Nursing,* 8th Edition. Philadelphia: Lippincott–Raven, 1996.

BOWEL OBSTRUCTION, LARGE

B

Large bowel obstruction results in an accumulation of intestinal contents, fluid, and gas proximal to the obstruction. Obstruction in the colon can lead to severe distention and perforation unless gas and fluid can flow back through the ileal valve. If the blood supply is cut off, intestinal strangulation and necrosis occur; this condition is life threatening.

CLINICAL MANIFESTATIONS

Symptoms develop and progress relatively slowly.

1. Constipation may be the only symptom for days (obstruction in sigmoid or rectum).
2. Abdomen becomes markedly distended, loops of large bowel become visibly outlined through the abdominal wall, and the patient suffers from crampy lower abdominal pain.
3. Fecal vomiting develops; symptoms of shock may occur.

DIAGNOSTIC EVALUATION

Symptoms and radiologic studies (barium studies contraindicated).

MANAGEMENT

1. Colonoscopy to untwist and decompress the bowel, if obstruction is high in the colon.
2. Cecostomy may be performed for those patients who are poor surgical risks and urgently need relief from the obstruction.
3. Rectal tube to decompress an area that is lower in the bowel.
4. Usual treatment is surgical resection to remove the obstructing lesion; a temporary or permanent colostomy may be necessary.

Nursing Interventions

1. Monitor symptoms indicating worsening intestinal obstruction.
2. Provide emotional support and comfort.
3. Administer IV fluids and electrolyte replacement.
4. Prepare patient for surgery if no response to medical treatment.
5. Teach patient as the condition indicates.
6. Give routine and abdominal wound care postoperatively.

For more information see Chapter 37 in Smeltzer and Bare: *Brunner and Suddarth's Textbook of Medical–Surgical Nursing*, 8th Edition. Philadelphia: Lippincott–Raven, 1996.

BOWEL OBSTRUCTION, SMALL

An accumulation of intestinal contents, fluid, and gas develops above the intestinal obstruction. Distention and retention reduce the absorption of fluids and stimulate gastric secretion. Fluids and electrolytes are lost. A decrease in venous and arteriolar capillary pressure is caused, resulting in edema, congestion, necrosis, and eventual rupture or perforation of the intestinal wall. Reflux vomiting may also occur. Dehydration and acidosis develop because of water and sodium loss. With acute fluid losses, hypovolemic shock may occur.

CLINICAL MANIFESTATIONS

1. The initial symptom is crampy pain, wavelike and colicky; may pass blood and mucus but no fecal matter or flatus; vomiting occurs.
2. Peristaltic waves become extremely vigorous and assume a reverse direction, propelling intestinal contents toward the mouth, if the obstruction is complete.

3. If the obstruction is in the ileum, fecal vomiting takes place.
4. Dehydration results in intense thirst, drowsiness, generalized malaise, and aching.
5. Tongue and mucous membranes become parched: abdomen becomes distended (the lower the obstruction in the gastrointestinal [GI] tract, the more marked is the distention).
6. If uncorrected, shock occurs due to dehydration and loss of plasma volume.

DIAGNOSTIC EVALUATION

Symptoms, radiologic, and laboratory studies.

MANAGEMENT

1. Decompression of the bowel through a nasogastric or small-bowel tube.
2. When bowel is completely obstructed, possibility of strangulation warrants surgical intervention. Surgical treatment depends on the cause of obstruction.
3. IV therapy to replace water, sodium, chloride, and potassium.

For more information see Chapter 37 in Smeltzer and Bare: *Brunner and Suddarth's Textbook of Medical–Surgical Nursing,* 8th Edition. Philadelphia: Lippincott–Raven, 1996.

BPH

See Benign Prostatic Hyperplasia

BRAIN ABSCESS

A brain abscess is a collection of infectious material within the tissue of the brain. It may occur by direct invasion of the brain from intracranial trauma or surgery; by spread of infection from nearby sites, i.e., sinuses, ears, and teeth; or by spread of infection from other organs (lung abscess, infective endocarditis); and can be a complication associated with some forms of meningitis. It can be a complication in patients whose immune systems have been suppressed through therapy or disease. To prevent brain abscesses, treat otitis media, mastoiditis, sinusitis, dental infections, and systemic infections promptly.

CLINICAL MANIFESTATIONS

1. Generally result from edema, brain shift, infection, or the location of the abscess.
2. Headache, usually worse in morning, is the most continuing symptom.
3. Vomiting, focal neurologic signs (weakness of an extremity, decreasing vision, seizures) may occur depending on the site of the abscess.
4. Change in mental status, e.g., lethargic, confused, irritable, or disoriented behavior.
5. Fever may or may not be present.

DIAGNOSTIC EVALUATION

CT scan locating the site of the abscess.

MANAGEMENT

The goal of management is to eliminate the abscess.
1. Antimicrobial therapy, surgical incision, or aspiration.
2. Corticosteroids to reduce the inflammatory cerebral edema.
3. Anticonvulsant medications for prophylaxis against seizures.
4. Monitor abscess resolution with CT scans.
5. Neurologic deficits after treatment may include hemiparesis, seizures, visual defects, and cranial nerve palsies.
6. Relapse is common with a high mortality rate.

For more information see Chapter 60 in Smeltzer and Bare: *Brunner and Suddarth's Textbook of Medical–Surgical Nursing,* 8th Edition. Philadelphia: Lippincott–Raven, 1996.

BRAIN TUMORS

A brain tumor is a localized intracranial lesion that occupies space within the skull. In adults, most brain tumors originate in glial cells. The highest incidence of brain tumors in adults occurs between the fifth and seventh decades with a slightly higher incidence in men. Brain tumors rarely metastasize outside the central nervous system, but cause death by impairing vital functions. Brain tumors are classified as follows: (1) those arising from the coverings of the brain, i.e., dural meningioma; (2) those developing in or on the cranial nerves, i.e., acoustic neuroma; (3) those originating in the brain tissue, i.e., various gliomas; (4) metastatic lesions originating elsewhere in the body. Tumors of the pineal gland and pituitary and of cerebral blood vessels are also included in the types of brain tumors. Tumors may be benign or malignant. A benign tumor may occur in a vital area and have effects as serious as a malignant tumor.

Specific Tumors

1. Gliomas, the most frequent brain neoplasm, cannot be totally removed because they spread by infiltrating into the surrounding neural tissue.
2. Pituitary adenomas may cause symptoms due to mass (pressure) effects on adjacent structures or to hormonal changes.
3. Angiomas are found in or on the surface of the brain; may never cause symptoms, or may give rise to symptoms of brain tumor. The walls of the blood vessels in angiomas are thin, increasing a risk for cerebral vascular accident (stroke).

4. Acoustic neuroma is a tumor of the eighth cranial nerve (hearing and balance). It may grow slowly and attain considerable size before it is correctly diagnosed.

CLINICAL MANIFESTATIONS

Increasing Intracranial Pressure (ICP) Symptoms

1. Headache, although not always present, is most common in the early morning and is made worse by coughing, straining, or sudden movement. Headaches are usually described as deep or expanding or as dull but unrelenting. Frontal tumors produce a bilateral frontal headache; pituitary gland tumors produce bitemporal pain; in cerebellar tumors the headache may be located in the suboccipital region at the back of the head.
2. Vomiting, seldom related to food intake, is usually due to irritation of the vagal centers in the medulla.
3. Papilledema is associated with visual disturbances.
4. Mental changes (e.g., dullness and giddiness) are often general but can be localized.

Localized Symptoms

The progression of the signs and symptoms is important, because it indicates tumor growth and expansion.

1. Tumor of the motor cortex: convulsive movements localized on one side of the body.
2. Occipital lobe tumors: visual manifestations, i.e., contralateral homonymous hemianopsia (visual loss in one-half of the visual field on the opposite side of tumor) and visual hallucinations.
3. Tumors of the cerebellum: dizziness, ataxic or staggering gait with tendency to fall toward side of lesion, marked muscle incoordination, and nystagmus.
4. Tumors of the frontal lobe: personality disorders, changes in emotional state and behavior, and a disinterested mental attitude.

DIAGNOSTIC EVALUATION

1. History of the illness and manner the symptoms evolved.
2. Neurologic examination indicates areas involved.
3. CT imaging, MRI, computer-assisted stereotactic (three-dimensional) biopsy, cerebral angiography, electroencephalogram, and cytologic studies of the cerebral spinal fluid.

MANAGEMENT

The objective of management is to remove all of the tumor or as much as possible without increasing the neurologic deficit (paralysis, blindness) or to achieve relief of symptoms by partial tumor removal (decompression), radiation therapy, chemotherapy, or a combination of these. Evaluation and treatment should be done as soon as possible before irreversible neurologic damage occurs. Most patients undergo neurosurgical procedure, followed by radiation and possibly chemotherapy.

Other Therapies

1. Corticosteroids to prevent postoperative swelling.
2. Intravenous autologous bone marrow transplantation for marrow toxicity associated with high dosages of drugs and radiation.
3. Radioisotopes (^{125}I) implanted directly into the brain tumor.

Nursing Interventions

1. Evaluate gag reflex and ability to swallow preoperatively.
2. Teach patient to direct food and fluids toward the unaffected side, placing the patient upright to eat, offering a semisoft diet, and having suction readily available if diminished gag response.
3. Reassess function postoperatively, as changes can occur.

4. Perform neurologic checks; monitor vital signs; maintain a neurologic flow record; space nursing interventions to prevent rapid increase in ICP.
5. Reorient patient when necessary to person, time, and place.
6. Use orienting devices (personal possessions, photographs, lists, clock), supervise and assist with self-care, and monitor and intervene for prevention of injury.
7. Carefully monitor patients with seizures.
8. Check motor function at intervals; assess sensory disturbances.
9. Evaluate speech; assess eye movement, pupil size, and reaction.

For more information see Chapter 60 in Smeltzer and Bare: *Brunner and Suddarth's Textbook of Medical–Surgical Nursing,* 8th Edition. Philadelphia: Lippincott–Raven, 1996.

BREAST CANCER

See Cancer of the Breast

BROCA'S APHASIA

See Aphasia

BRONCHIECTASIS

Bronchiectasis is a chronic dilation of the bronchi and bronchioles, which causes a variety of conditions, including pulmonary infections and obstruction of the bronchus; aspiration of foreign bodies, vomitus, or material from the respiratory tract; and extrinsic pressure from tumors, dilated blood vessels, and enlarged lymph nodes. A person may be predisposed to bronchiectasis.

After surgery, bronchiectasis may also develop when the patient's cough is ineffective.

CLINICAL MANIFESTATIONS

1. Chronic cough and production of copious purulent sputum, which has a quality of "layering out" into three layers on standing: a frothy top layer, a middle clear layer, and a dense particulate bottom layer.
2. Hemoptysis, clubbing of the fingers, and repeated episodes of pulmonary infection.

DIAGNOSTIC EVALUATION

Definite diagnostic clue is prolonged history of productive cough, with sputum consistently negative for tubercle bacilli.

MANAGEMENT

The objectives of treatment are to prevent and control infection and to promote bronchial drainage.

1. Antimicrobial therapy guided by sputum sensitivity studies.
2. Year-round regimen of antibiotics, alternating types of drugs at intervals.
3. Vaccinate against influenza and pneumococcal pneumonia
4. Remove bronchial secretions using expectorants, percussion, postural drainage, or bronchoscopy.
5. Bronchodilators; sympathomimetics (β-adrenergic); and aerosolized nebulizer treatments (face tent to provide extra humidification for aerosols) to promote bronchial drainage.
6. Increase oral fluid intake.
7. Advise smoking cessation.
8. Surgical intervention used infrequently.

For Nursing Management and Patient Education, see Chronic Obstructive Pulmonary Disease.

For more information see Chapter 24 in Smeltzer and Bare: *Brunner and Suddarth's Textbook of Medical–Surgical Nursing,* 8th Edition. Philadelphia: Lippincott–Raven, 1996.

BRONCHITIS

See Chronic Obsructive Pulmonary Disease

BRONCHITIS, CHRONIC

Chronic bronchitis is defined as the presence of a productive cough that lasts 3 months a year for 2 consecutive years. It is primarily associated with cigarette smoking or exposure to pollution. Patients have increased susceptibility to recurring infections of the lower respiratory tract.

CLINICAL MANIFESTATIONS

1. Chronic, productive cough in winter months, earliest sign; cough is exacerbated by cold weather, dampness, and pulmonary irritants.
2. History of cigarette smoking, frequent respiratory infections.

MANAGEMENT

The main objectives of treatment are to maintain the patency of the peripheral bronchial tree, facilitate removal of bronchial exudates, and prevent disability.

1. Note changes in the sputum pattern (nature, color, amount, thickness) and in the cough pattern.
2. Treat recurrent bacterial infections with antibiotic therapy.
3. Facilitate removal of bronchial exudates (bronchodilators).
4. Provide for postural drainage and chest percussion.

B

5. Give fluids orally or parenterally to liquify secretions.
6. Use steroid therapy when conservative measures fail.
7. Patient must stop smoking (causes bronchocon-striction).
8. Counsel patient to avoid respiratory irritants (e.g., tobacco smoke).
9. Immunize against common viral agents (influenza, S. pneumoniae).
10. Provide proper treatment for acute upper respiratory infections (antimicrobial therapy and sensitivity studies).

For Nursing Management and Patient Education, see Nursing Process: The Patient with COPD.

For more information see Chapter 24 in Smeltzer and Bare: *Brunner and Suddarth's Textbook of Medical–Surgical Nursing,* 8th Edition. Philadelphia: Lippincott–Raven, 1996.

BUERGER'S DISEASE (THROMBOANGIITIS OBLITERANS)

Buerger's disease is a recurring inflammation of the intermediate and small arteries and veins of the lower and, rarely, upper extremities. It results in thrombus formation and occlusion of the vessels. The cause is unknown. It occurs most often in men between the ages of 20 and 35, and has been reported in all races in many areas of the world. There is considerable evidence that heavy smoking is either a causative or aggravating factor. Arteriography confirms arterial occlusive disease.

CLINICAL MANIFESTATIONS

1. Pain is the outstanding symptom; complaints of cramps in the feet (arches) or legs after exercise (intermittent claudication); relieved by rest.

2. Burning pain aggravated by emotional disturbances, smoking, or chilling; rest pain in the fingers or toes; a feeling of coldness or sensitivity to cold may be early symptoms.
3. Types of paresthesia may develop; pulses diminished or absent.
4. Color changes may affect only one extremity or certain digits.
5. Ulceration with gangrene eventually occurs.

MANAGEMENT

The main objectives are to improve circulation to the extremities, prevent the progression of the disease, and protect the extremities from trauma and infection.

1. Stop smoking completely.
2. Vasodilators are rarely prescribed (cause dilation of healthy vessels only).
3. Regional sympathetic block or ganglionectomy.

PROGNOSIS

1. If gangrene of a toe develops, usually a below-knee amputation, or occasionally an above-knee, is necessary.
2. Indications for amputation are worsening gangrene (especially if moist); severe rest pain; or sepsis secondary to gangrene.

For more information see Chapter 31 in Smeltzer and Bare: *Brunner and Suddarth's Textbook of Medical–Surgical Nursing,* 8th Edition. Philadelphia: Lippincott–Raven, 1996.

BURN INJURY

Burns are caused by a transfer of energy from a heat source to the body. Burns can be categorized as thermal, radiation, electrical, or chemical. Young children and the elderly are at particularly high risk for burn injury. Four major goals relating to burns are prevention; institution of life-saving measures for the severely burned person; prevention of disability and disfigurement; and rehabilitation. Persons under 5 and over 40 years are at risk of mortality following burn trauma.

BURN DEPTH

Burns are classified according to the depth of tissue destruction:

1. Superficial (first degree), e.g., sunburn; skin involvement includes the epidermis only.
2. Partial thickness (second degree), e.g., scald; skin involvement includes the epidermis and part of the dermis.
3. Full thickness (third degree), e.g., flame, electric current; skin involvement includes the epidermis, entire dermis, and sometimes subcutaneous tissue.

EXTENT OF SURFACE AREA BURNED

Determination of how much surface area is affected is achieved by one of the following methods:

1. Rule of Nines: an estimation of the total body surface area (BSA) burned by dividing the body into multiples of nine.
2. Lund and Browder Method: a more precise method of estimating extent of burned BSA that recognizes the percentage of BSA surface of various anatomic parts (head and legs) changes with growth.
3. Palm method: a method to estimate percentage of scattered burns, using the size of the patient's palm (approximately 1% of BSA) for assessing extent of burn injury.

NURSING PROCESS: BURN CARE DURING THE EMERGENT/RESUSCITATIVE PHASE

Assessment

1. Initial assessment data obtained by prehospital providers.

2. Focus on the major priorities of any trauma patient, with the wound as a secondary consideration.
3. Monitor for patent airway; evaluate apical, carotid, and femoral pulses.
4. Start cardiac monitoring.
5. Check vital signs frequently using an ultrasound device if necessary.
6. Check peripheral pulses on burned extremities hourly.
7. Insert large-bore IV catheters and indwelling urinary catheter.
8. Monitor fluid intake and output and measure hourly; assess urine specific gravity, pH, protein, and hemoglobin.
9. Note presence of increased hoarseness, stridor, abnormal respiratory rate and depth, or mental changes from hypoxia.
10. Assess body temperature, body weight, history of preburn weight, allergies, tetanus immunization, past medical/surgical problems, current illnesses, and use of medication.
11. Assess depth of the wound and identify areas of full- and partial-thickness injury.
12. Assess neurologic status: consciousness; psychologic status, pain and anxiety levels, and behavior.
13. Assess patient's and family's understanding of injury/treatment.

Major Nursing Diagnosis

1. Impaired gas exchange related to carbon monoxide poisoning, smoke inhalation, and upper airway obstruction.
2. Ineffective airway clearance related to edema and effects of smoke inhalation.
3. Fluid volume deficit related to increased capillary permeability and evaporative fluid loss from the burn wound.

4. Hypothermia related to loss of skin microcirculation and open wounds.
5. Pain related to tissue and nerve injury and emotional impact of injury.
6. Anxiety related to fear and the emotional impact of injury.

Collaborative Problems

1. Acute respiratory failure.
2. Distributive shock.
3. Acute renal failure.
4. Compartment syndrome.
5. Paralytic ileus.
6. Curling's ulcer.

Planning and Implementation

The major goals for the emergent/resuscitative phase include maintenance of a patent airway, ventilation, and tissue oxygenation; establishment of optimal fluid and electrolyte balance and perfusion of vital organs; maintenance of normal body temperature; minimal pain and anxiety; and absence of potential complications.

Interventions

PROMOTING GAS EXCHANGE AND AIRWAY CLEARANCE

1. Note respiratory rate, quality, and depth; auscultate lungs for adventitious sounds.
2. Institute aggressive pulmonary care measures; turning, coughing, deep breathing, periodic forceful inspiration using spirometry, and tracheal suctioning.
3. Maintain proper positioning to decrease the work of breathing and promote optimal chest expansion; administer humidified oxygen or initiate mechanical ventilation.
4. Maintain asepsis to prevent contamination of the respiratory tract and infection that increases metabolic requirements.

Restoring Fluid and Electrolyte Balance

1. Assess vital signs and urinary output, central venous pressure, pulmonary artery pressure, and cardiac output.
2. Provide intravenous (IV) fluids as prescribed and titrate with urinary output; document intake and output and daily weight.
3. Monitor serum electrolyte levels; recognize developing fluid and electrolyte imbalances.

Maintaining Normal Body Temperature

1. Adjust room temperature according to patient's needs (prone to hypothermia or chilling because of loss of skin).
2. Maintain comfort with cotton blankets, ceiling mounted heat lamps, and aluminum insulated blankets.
3. Use efficient approach for removing dressings and wound care to shorten time exposed to ambient temperature.

Minimizing Pain and Anxiety

1. Perform a respiratory assessment before giving analgesics; use IV route for medication administration (other routes give unpredictable absorption).
2. Give IV sedatives as needed.
3. Assess family dynamics, coping strategies, and anxiety levels to plan individualized interventions.
4. Provide emotional support and simple explanations about procedures.
5. Give antianxiety medications if patient remains highly anxious and agitated after psychologic interventions.

Monitoring and Managing Potential Complications

1. Acute respiratory failure: assess for signs of inhalation injury; report to physician and prepare to assist with intubation or escharotomy.

2. Distributive shock: monitor for early signs of hypovolemic shock or fluid overload; manage by increasing IV fluids and monitoring fluid status.

3. Acute renal failure: monitor urine output and quality; blood, urea, nitrogen (BUN), and creatinine levels.

4. Compartment syndrome: assess neurovascular status of extremities; report any extremity pain, loss of peripheral pulses or sensation.

5. Paralytic ileus: insert nasogastric (NG) tube; assess abdomen regularly for distention and bowel sounds; begin oral feedings as soon as possible when ileus is resolved.

6. Curling's ulcer: assess gastric pH; maintain at a level less acidic by using antacid therapy (histamine blockers, e.g., Zantac); check NG aspirate and stools for occult blood.

NURSING PROCESS: BURN CARE DURING THE ACUTE/INTERMEDIATE PHASE

The acute or intermediate phase begins 42–72 hours after the burn injury. Burn wound care and pain control are priorities at this stage.

Assessment

1. Focus on hemodynamic alterations, wound healing, pain and psychosocial responses, and early detection of complications.

2. Measure vital signs frequently.

3. Assess peripheral pulses for first few days postburn.

4. Observe ECG for dysrhythmias resulting from potassium imbalance, preexisting cardiac disease, or the effects of electrical injury or burn shock.

5. Assess residual gastric volumes and pH on patients with NG tubes (clues to early sepsis or need for antacid therapy).

6. Note blood in gastric fluid or stool and report.

7. Assess wound, i.e., size, color, odor, eschar, exudate, abscess formation under the eschar, epithelial buds, bleeding, granulation tissue appearance, progress of graphs and donor sites, and quality of surrounding skin.
8. Focus on pain and psychosocial responses, daily body weight, caloric intake, general hydration, and serum electrolyte, hemoglobin, and hematocrit levels.
9. Assess for excessive bleeding adjacent to areas of surgical exploration and debridement.

Major Nursing Diagnosis

1. Fluid volume excess related to resumption of capillary integrity and fluid shift from interstitial to intravascular compartment.
2. Risk for infection related to loss of skin barrier and impaired immune response.
3. Altered nutrition: less than body requirements related to hypermetabolism and wound healing needs.
4. Impaired skin integrity related to open burn wounds.
5. Pain related to exposed nerves, wound healing, and treatment.
6. Impaired physical mobility related to burn wound edema, pain, and joint contractures.
7. Ineffective individual coping related to fear and anxiety, grieving, and forced dependence on health care providers.
8. Altered family processes related to burn injury.
9. Knowledge deficit about the course of burn treatment.

Planning and Implementation

The major goals may include restoration of normal fluid balance; absence of infection; attainment of anabolic state and normal weight; improved skin integrity; reduction of pain and discomfort; optimal physical mobility; adequate patient and family coping; adequate patient and family knowledge of burn treatment; and absence of complications.

Interventions

RESTORING NORMAL FLUID BALANCE

1. Monitor IV and oral fluid intake; use IV infusion pumps.
2. Measure intake and output and daily weight.
3. Report changes in hemodynamics.
4. Administer low-dose dopamine to increase renal perfusion and diuretics to promote increased urine output; monitor patient's response.
5. Promote lung expansion and gas exchange by positioning comfortably and raising head of bed; report increased difficulty with respiration promptly.

PREVENTING INFECTION

1. Protect patient from sources of cross-contamination.
2. Practice aseptic technique for wound care and invasive procedures.

MAINTAINING ADEQUATE NUTRITION

1. Initiate oral fluids slowly when bowel sounds resume.
2. Collaborate with dietitian to plan diet acceptable to patient; encourage family to bring nutritious favorite foods.
3. Document caloric intake; insert NG tube if caloric goals cannot be met by oral feeding (for continuous or bolus feedings).
4. Weigh patients daily; encourage and support patient with anorexia to increase food intake; total parenteral nutrition (TPN) may be required.

IMPROVING SKIN INTEGRITY THROUGH WOUND CARE

1. Assess wound status; use creative approaches to wound dressing; support during emotionally distressing and painful wound care.

2. Coordinate complex aspects of wound care and dressing changes.
3. Assess and record any changes and progress in wound healing; inform all members of the health care team of changes in the wound or treatment.
4. Instruct patient and family by instruction, support, and encouragement to take an active part in dressing changes/wound care.
5. Anticipate home care needs early; assess strengths of patient and family and use in preparing for discharge and home care.

Relieving Pain and Discomfort

1. Teach the patient relaxation techniques; give some control over wound care and analgesia; provide frequent reassurance.
2. Provide guided imagery in altering patient perceptions and responses to pain; hypnosis, biofeedback, and behavioral modification are also useful.
3. Administer minor antianxiety medications and analgesics before pain becomes too severe; assess frequently for pain and discomfort.
4. Work quickly to complete treatments and dressing changes; encourage to use analgesic medications before painful procedures.
5. Promote comfort during healing phase by using oral antipruritic agents, a cool environment, lubrication of the skin, exercise and splinting to prevent skin contracture, and diversional activities.

Promoting Physical Mobility

1. Prevent complications (atelectasis, pneumonia, edema, pressure ulcers, and contractures) resulting from immobility by deep breathing, turning, and proper repositioning.
2. Modify interventions to meet the individual patient needs; encourage early sitting and ambulation; when legs are involved, apply elastic pressure bandages before the patient is placed in an upright position.

3. Make aggressive efforts to prevent contractures and hypertrophic scarring of the wound area after wound closure for a year or more.

4. Initiate passive and active range-of-motion (ROM) exercises from admission until after grafting within prescribed limitations.

5. Apply splints or functional devices to extremities for contracture control; monitor for signs of vascular insufficiency and nerve compression.

STRENGTHENING COPING STRATEGIES

1. Assist patient in developing effective coping strategies by setting specific expectations for behavior, promoting trust, helping patient practice coping strategies, and giving positive feedback.

2. Enlist a noninvolved person for patient to vent feelings without fear of retaliation.

3. Include patient in decisions regarding care; set realistic expectations for self-care.

SUPPORTING PATIENT AND FAMILY PROCESSES

1. Support and address patient and family's verbal and nonverbal concerns.

2. Instruct family in ways to support the patient.

3. Make psychologic or social work referrals as needed.

MONITORING AND MANAGING POTENTIAL COMPLICATIONS

1. Congestive heart failure: assess for decreased cardiac output, oliguria, jugular vein distention, edema, or onset of S_3 or S_4 heart sounds.

2. Pulmonary edema: assess for increasing central venous pressure (CVP), pulmonary artery (PA) and wedge pressures, and crackles.

3. Sepsis: assess for increased temperature, increased pulse, widened pulse pressure, and flushed, dry skin in unburned areas (early signs); perform wound and blood cultures; give scheduled antibiotics on time.

4. Acute respiratory failure and adult respiratory distress syndrome (ARDS): monitor respiratory status for dyspnea, change in respiratory pattern and onset of adventitious sounds; assess for decrease in tidal volume and lung compliance in patients on mechanical ventilation. The hallmark of onset of ARDS is hypoxemia on 100% oxygen, decreased lung compliance, and significant shunting.

5. Visceral damage (from electrical burns): monitor ECG and report dysrhythmias; pay attention to pain related to deep muscle ischemia and report. Early detection may minimize severity of this complication; fasciotomies may be necessary to relieve swelling and ischemia in the muscles and fascia.

✎ Patient Education and Health Maintenance: Care in the Home and Community

1. Recognize that family roles are disrupted when patients are sent to burn centers; many centers are far from home, compounding role disruption.

2. Give patient and family thorough information about the burn care and expected course of treatment.

3. Assess patient's and family's abilities to process the educational content; do not provide information before they can cope with it.

NURSING PROCESS: BURN CARE FOR THE REHABILITATION/LONG-TERM PHASE

It is important that rehabilitation begin immediately after the burn has occurred. Wound healing, psychosocial support, and restoring maximum functional activity remain priorities.

Assessment

1. Obtain information about the patient's educational level, occupation, leisure activities, cultural background, religion, and family interactions.

2. Assess self-concept, mental status, emotional response to injury and hospitalization, level of intellectual functioning, previous hospitalizations, response to pain and pain relief measures, and sleep pattern.
3. Assess rehabilitation goals including ROM of affected joints, functional abilities in activities of daily living (ADLs).
4. Document participation in wound care and abilities in ambulation and feeding to demonstrate self-care.
5. Assess specific complications and treatments, e.g., postoperative assessment of patient undergoing primary excision.

Major Nursing Diagnosis

1. Activity intolerance related to pain on exercise, limited joint mobility, muscle wasting, and limited endurance.
2. Body image disturbance related to altered physical appearance and self-concept.
3. Knowledge deficit of postdischarge home care and follow-up needs.

Collaborative Problems

1. Contractures.
2. Inadequate psychologic adaptation to burn injury.

Planning and Implementation

The goals include increased participation in ADLs; increased understanding of the injury, treatment, and planned follow-up care; adaption and adjustment to alterations in body image, self-concept, and lifestyle, and absence of potential complications.

Interventions

PROMOTING ACTIVITY TOLERANCE

1. Schedule care to have periods of uninterrupted sleep.
2. Communicate plan of care to family and other caregivers.

3. Give hypnotics for sleep.
4. Listen and reassure patient when nightmares, or other fears about the outcome of the injury, cause insomnia.
5. Reduce metabolic stress by relieving pain, preventing chilling or fever, and promoting physical integrity of all body systems to help conserve energy.
6. Incorporate physical therapy exercises to prevent muscular atrophy and maintain mobility required for daily activities.
7. Improve psychologic outlook and increase tolerance for activity by scheduling activities in periods of increasing duration.

IMPROVING BODY IMAGE AND SELF-CONCEPT

1. Refer patients to a support group to meet others with similar experiences and develop coping strategies to deal with losses.
2. Assess patient's psychosocial reactions; provide support and develop a plan to help the patient handle these feelings.
3. Promote a healthy body image and self-concept by helping patients practice responses to people who stare or ask about their injury.
4. Recognize patient through small gestures such as providing a birthday cake, combing patient's hair before visitors, sharing information on cosmetic resources to enhance appearance.
5. Teach patient to direct attention away from a disfigured body to the self within.
6. Coordinate consultants such as psychologists, social workers, vocational counselors, and teachers during rehabilitation.

MONITORING AND MANAGING POTENTIAL COMPLICATION

1. Contractures: provide early and aggressive physical and occupational therapy; intervene with surgery to achieve full range of motion if needed.

2. Impaired psychologic adaptation to the burn injury: obtain psychologic or psychiatric referral as soon as evidence of major coping problems appear.

✎ Patient Education and Health Maintenance: Care in the Home and Community

1. Increase participation of patient in care by making aware of the consequences of injury, goals of planned treatment, and patient's role in ongoing care.
2. Include families in planning and carrying out care according to their interest, ability and patient's needs.
3. Educate patients and families during the course of the hospital stay to care for the burn wound by early active participation.
4. Encourage and support patients and families to handle follow-up wound care; coordinate all aspects of care.
5. Refer to a community health nurse to provide assistance with wound care and exercises for patients with inadequate support systems.
6. Inform and review with patient-specific exercises and use of elastic pressure garments and splints; provide written instruction.
7. Evaluate patient status periodically by burn team for modification of home care instructions and planning for reconstructive surgery.

✪ Gerontologic Considerations

The elderly are at higher risk for burn injury because of reduced mobility, changes in vision, and decreased sensation in feet and hands. The morbidity and mortality associated with burns are often much greater than with younger patients.

Thinning and loss of elasticity of the skin in the elderly predispose them to a deep injury from a thermal insult that might cause a less severe burn in a younger person. Chronic illness decreases the aged person's ability to withstand the multisystem stressors of burn injury and requires very close observation with even relatively small burns, during the emergent and acute phases.

Acute oliguric renal failure is more common in the elderly than in those under 40 years. Suppressed immunologic response, high incidence of malnutrition, and inability to withstand metabolic stressors (cold environment) further compromise the patient's ability to heal. Eschar separation in full-thickness burns is delayed.

Nursing assessment should include particular attention to pulmonary function, response to fluid resuscitation, and signs of mental confusion or disorientation; careful history of preburn medications and preexisting illnesses is essential.

Contact social and community nursing services to provide for optimal care upon hospital discharge.

For more information see Chapter 55 in Smeltzer and Bare: *Brunner and Suddarth's Textbook of Medical–Surgical Nursing,* 8th Edition. Philadelphia: Lippincott–Raven, 1996.

CAD

See Coronary Artery Disease

CANCER OF THE BLADDER

Cancer of the urinary bladder is seen more frequently in persons age 50 onward and affects men more than women (3:1). There are two forms of bladder cancer: superficial (which tends to recur) and invasive. Tumors usually arise at the base of the bladder and involve the ureteral orifices and bladder neck. Risk factors include cigarette smoking and carcinogens in the work environment, i.e., dyes, rubber, leather, ink, or paint. There may be a relationship between coffee drinking and bladder cancer. Chronic schistosomiasis (parasitic infection that irritates the bladder) is also a risk factor. Cancers arising from the prostate, colon, and rectum in males and from the lower gynecologic tract in females may metastasize to the bladder.

CLINICAL MANIFESTATIONS

1. Gross painless hematuria, most common symptom.
2. Infection of the urinary tract; common complication producing frequency, urgency, and dysuria.
3. Any alteration in voiding or change in the urine is indicative.
4. Pelvic or back pain may indicate metastasis.

DIAGNOSTIC EVALUATION

Biopsies of the tumor and adjacent mucosa are definitive, but the following procedures are also used:

1. Excretory urography.
2. CT scans.
3. Ultrasonography.
4. Cystoscopy.
5. Bimanual examination under anesthesia.

MANAGEMENT

Treatment of bladder cancer depends on the grade of tumor, the stage of tumor growth, and the multicentricity of the tumor. Age and physical, mental, and emotional status are considered in determining treatment modalities.

1. Transurethral resection (TUR) or fulguration for simple papillomas.
2. Benign papillomas should be followed with cytology and cystoscopy periodically for the rest of patient's life.
3. Chemotherapy with a combination of methotrexate, vinblastine, doxorubicin (Adriamycin), and cisplatin (M-VAC).
4. Topical chemotherapy applied directly to the bladder wall.
5. Irradiate tumor preoperatively to reduce microextension and viability.
6. Radiation therapy in combination with surgery to control inoperable tumors.
7. Simple cystectomy or radical cystectomy for invasive or multifocal bladder cancer.
8. Cytotoxic agent infusions through the arterial supply of the involved organ.
9. Hydrostatic therapy: for advanced bladder cancer or patients with intractable hematuria (following radiation therapy).
10. Formalin, phenol, or silver nitrate instillations to achieve relief of hematuria and strangury (slow and painful discharge of urine) in some patients.

For more information see Chapter 43 in Smeltzer and Bare: *Brunner and Suddarth's Textbook of Medical–Surgical Nursing,* 8th Edition. Philadelphia: Lippincott–Raven, 1996.

CANCER OF THE BLOOD

See Leukemia, Acute

CANCER OF THE BRAIN

See Brain Tumors

CANCER OF THE BREAST

One of every eight women in the United States has a lifetime risk of developing breast cancer. The incidence is increasing while mortality remains the same. The most common type of breast cancer is infiltrating ductal carcinoma (75% of cases). These tumors are hard on palpation, usually metastasize to the axillary nodes, and have a poorer prognosis than other types of breast cancer. Infiltrating lobular carcinoma accounts for 5–10% of cases. These tumors present with ill-defined thickening and multicentric tumors. Axillary node involvement is similar to infiltrating ductal carcinoma, but sites of distant metastases differ. Ductal carcinomas usually spread to bone, lung, liver, or brain, while lobular carcinomas metastasize to meningeal surfaces or other unusual sites. Many other types of breast cancer exist with varied presentation and prognosis. At this time there is no cure for breast cancer. There is no one specific cause; rather a series of genetic, hormonal, and environmental events may contribute to its development. If lymph nodes are unaffected, prognosis is better. The key to improved cure rates is early diagnosis before metastasis.

RISK FACTORS

1. Previous breast cancer; risk of developing cancer in the other breast increases 1% each year.

2. History of first-degree relatives increases risk 2–3 times.
3. Nulliparity or first birth after age 30.
4. Prolonged exposure to hormonal stimulation, i.e., early menarche prior to age 12 and late menopause after age 55.
5. Exposure to ionizing radiation after puberty and before age 30.
6. Obesity, oral contraceptives, hormone replacement therapy, alcohol intake, and possibly high-fat diet.
7. History of benign breast disease.

CLINICAL MANIFESTATIONS

1. Symptoms are insidious; generally the lesions are nontender, fixed, and hard with irregular borders; majority occur in the upper outer quadrant, more often on the left breast.
2. Pain is usually absent except in later stages; some women have no symptoms and no palpable lump but have an abnormal mammogram.
3. Without detection and treatment: dimpling or peau d'orange (orange-peel skin); asymmetry and an elevation of the affected breast; nipple retraction; breast more or less fixed on the chest wall; ulceration and metastasis.

DIAGNOSTIC EVALUATION

Fine-needle aspiration; excisional biopsy; core biopsy, needle localization.

STAGING OF BREAST CANCER

Tumors are staged I–IV depending on size, lymph node involvement, and metastasis. (Other staging is expressed in TNM symbols: T = primary tumor, N = lymph node involvement, M = metastasis.)

1. Stage I: small tumor less than 2 cm, negative lymph nodes, no detectable metastases.
2. Stage II: tumor greater than 2 cm but less than 5 cm,

negative or positive unfixed lymph nodes, no detectable metastases.

3. Stage III: large tumor greater than 5 cm, or a tumor of any size with invasion of the skin or chest wall or positive fixed lymph nodes in the clavicular area without evidence of metastases.

4. Stage IV: tumor of any size with lymph nodes positive or negative with distant metastases.

MANAGEMENT

1. Modified radical mastectomy: the entire breast tissue is removed along with axillary lymph nodes.

2. Breast-conserving surgery: lumpectomy, segmental mastectomy, or quadrantectomy, and axillary node dissection followed by radiation therapy to residual microscopic disease.

3. Mastectomy provides maximum opportunity to remove the tumor and the affected nodes.

4. A course of external beam radiation therapy to the tumor mass to decrease chance of recurrence and eradicate residual cancer.

5. Chemotherapy is given to eradicate micrometastatic spread of the disease, i.e., Cytoxan (C), methotrexate (M), fluorouracil (F), and Adriamycin (A).

6. A CMF or CAF regimen is a common treatment protocol.

7. Autologous bone marrow transplant (ABMT) is increasingly being used; current use of growth factors to stimulate the bone marrow have led to an overall decline in mortality.

8. Hormonal therapy based on the index of estrogen and progesterone receptors. Tamoxifen is the primary hormonal agent used to suppress hormonal-dependent tumors. Other hormonal agents are Megace, DES, Halotestin, and Cytadren.

9. Elective reconstructive surgery provides considerable psychologic benefit, but is contraindicated if cancer is locally advanced, metastatic, or inflammatory.

NURSING PROCESS

Assessment: Preoperative

1. Assess the reaction of the patient to the diagnosis and ability to cope with it.
2. Take a complete health and gynecologic history.
3. Ask pertinent questions that include the following: coping skills, support systems, knowledge deficit, and presence of discomfort.
4. Perform a complete physical assessment with particular attention to breasts and related mass signs and symptoms.

Assessment: Postoperative

1. Monitor pulse and blood pressure for signs of shock and hemorrhage.
2. Avoid blood pressure readings, injections, IVs, and venipunctures on the operative side to prevent infection and compromised circulation.
3. Inspect dressings for bleeding on regular basis; monitor drainage; turn and encourage deep breathing; assess graft areas for unusual redness, pain, swelling, or drainage.

Major Nursing Diagnosis: Preoperative

1. Knowledge deficit about breast cancer and treatment options.
2. Fear and ineffective coping related to the diagnosis of cancer, its treatment, and the prognosis.

Major Nursing Diagnosis: Postoperative

1. Pain and discomfort.
2. Impaired skin integrity due to surgical incision.
3. Body image disturbance related to mastectomy and the side effects of radiation and chemotherapy.
4. Potential sexual dysfunction related to the loss of a body part, change in self-image, and fear of partner's reaction to this loss.

C

Collaborative Problems

Lymphedema.

Planning and Implementation

The major goals may include increased knowledge about disease and its treatment, reduction of preoperative and postoperative fear, emotional stress, and anxiety; pain relief and maintenance of skin integrity; improved self-concept; improved self-care; improved sexual function; and absence of complications.

Interventions

RELIEVING PAIN AND DISCOMFORT

1. Provide patient-controlled analgesia (PCA).
2. Elevate the involved extremity moderately.

MAINTAINING SKIN INTEGRITY

1. Maintain patency of surgical drain to prevent fluid accumulation under the chest wall incision.
2. Inform of decreased sensation in the operative area because of nerve disruption; teach signs of infection or irritation.
3. Teach to gently massage healed surgical site with vitamin E or other lotions to promote circulation and increased skin elasticity.

REDUCING STRESS AND IMPROVING COPING SKILLS

1. Preoperatively, give patient time to absorb significance of diagnosis and give information to help evaluate available treatment options.
2. Promote the best preoperative physical, psychologic, and nutritional conditions possible; consider the patient as an active member of the health care team and allow to discuss concerns with those who will be administering care.
3. Avoid forcing patient to look at incision site if not ready.

4. Elicit assistance from supportive family or friends to promote acceptance of body alteration.
5. Recognize that spouse or partner is often in need of guidance, support, and education to cope with the crisis.

PROMOTING SELF-CARE

1. Provide information about development of postoperative surgical edema and strategies to prevent it; cuts, bruises, and infections on the operative side are dangerous precursors to problems.
2. Encourage ambulation when free of postanesthesia nausea and is tolerating fluids; initiate passive range-of-motion exercises to promote circulation and muscle strength, and prevent stiffness.
3. Encourage self-care and exercises such as "climbing the wall" with fingers to prevent contractures; pain other than mild discomfort should not occur with therapeutic exercise; radical mastectomy causes greater difficulty.
4. Encourage normal household and work-related arm activities, arm movements when walking, cleanliness of operative site, avoidance of injury to operative side, and loose nonconstrictive clothing.

IMPROVING SEXUAL FUNCTION

1. Discuss how patient sees self and possible decreased libido related to fatigue, nausea, or anxiety.
2. Clarify misconceptions, i.e., cancer can be transmitted sexually.
3. Encourage open discussion about fears.
4. Suggest variations in time of day for sexual activity (when least tired) or positions that are most comfortable, and alternate options, i.e., hugging, kissing, manual stimulation.

MANAGING LYMPHEDEMA

1. Facilitate development of collateral or auxiliary lymph drainage by promoting movement and exercise through postoperative education.

2. Elevate arm on pillow so that the elbow is higher than shoulder.
3. Wear custom-made elastic sleeves from wrist to shoulder during active hours in cases of persistent swelling.

CORRECTING KNOWLEDGE DEFICIT

1. Teach follow-up with phone calls for concerns about incision, pain management, and patient and family adjustment; get patient's permission to initiate community nurse service contacts if needed.
2. Teach how to empty reservoir and measure drainage if discharged with a drain in place.

For more information see Chapter 46 in Smeltzer and Bare: *Brunner and Suddarth's Textbook of Medical–Surgical Nursing*, 8th Edition. Philadelphia: Lippincott–Raven, 1996.

CANCER OF THE CERVIX

Cancer of the cervix, a primary uterine cancer, is less common than it once was because of early detection by Pap test. It is still the third most common reproductive cancer in women, excluding breast cancer. It occurs most commonly between ages 30 and 45, but can occur as early as 18 years of age. Sexual activity has a relationship to the incidence: before age 25, it is more prevalent in those who have had multiple sexual partners and several early pregnancies. Studies conclude that this type of cancer is a STD. Invasive cervical cancer has been identified as an HIV-defining condition.

Risk factors, aside from early first intercourse, early childbearing, and multiple partners, include exposure to HPV, HIV infection, smoking, and exposure to diethylstilbestrol (DES) in utero. Chronic cervical infections seem to play a significant part in cervical cancer.

CLINICAL MANIFESTATIONS

Most often asymptomatic. When discharge or irregular bleeding is present:

1. Discharge increases in amount and becomes watery. It is dark and foul smelling because of necrosis and infection of the tumor mass.
2. Bleeding occurs at irregular intervals between periods or after menopause; slight enough to just spot undergarments, and usually noted after mild trauma (intercourse, douching, or defecation).
3. As disease continues, bleeding may persist and increase.
4. As cancer advances, tissues outside the cervix are invaded, including lymph glands anterior to the sacrum. Nerve involvement producing excruciating pain in the back and legs.
5. The final stage: extreme emaciation and anemia, often with fever due to secondary infection and abscesses in the ulcerating mass, and fistula formation.

DIAGNOSTIC EVALUATION

1. Abnormal Pap test with dysplasia or persistent atypical smears, followed by biopsy identifying cervical intraepithelial neoplasia (CIN) of a high-grade squamous intraepithelial lesion (HGSIL).
2. Clinical staging of the disease (International Classification staging system or TNM [tumor, nodes, metastases] classification).

MANAGEMENT

1. Conservative nonsurgical removal for precursor lesions; cryotherapy (freezing with nitrous oxide) or laser therapy also effective.
2. Conization for carcinoma in situ.
3. Simple hysterectomy if preinvasive cervical cancer occurs after childbearing.
4. Radiation or radical hysterectomy or both for invasive cancer.

NURSING PROCESS FOR THE PATIENT UNDERGOING HYSTERECTOMY

Assessment

Assess the health history, physical and pelvic exam, and laboratory studies; additional data include psychosocial responses.

Major Nursing Diagnosis

1. Anxiety related to the diagnosis of cancer, fear of pain, perceived loss of femininity, and disfigurement.
2. Body image disturbance related to altered sexuality, fertility, and relationships with partner and family.
3. Pain related to surgery and other adjuvant therapy.
4. Knowledge deficit of the perioperative aspects of hysterectomy and self-care.

Collaborative Problems

1. Hemorrhage.
2. Deep vein thrombosis.
3. Bladder dysfunction.

Planning and Implementation

The major goals may include relief of anxiety, self-acceptance after loss of the uterus, absence of pain or discomfort, increased knowledge of self-care requirements, and prevention of complications.

Interventions

RELIEVING ANXIETY

Determine how this experience affects the patient; allow to verbalize feelings and identify strengths.

IMPROVING BODY IMAGE

1. Assess how the patient feels about having a hysterectomy related to the nature of diagnosis, significant others, religious beliefs, and prognosis.

2. Acknowledge concerns: ability to have children, loss of femininity, impact on sexual relations.
3. Educate about sexual relations: sexual satisfaction, orgasm arises from clitoral stimulation, sexual feeling or comfort related to shortened vagina.
4. Understand and teach that depression and heightened emotional sensitivity are expected due to upset hormonal balances.
5. Exhibit interest, concern, and willingness to listen to fears.

RELIEVING PAIN

1. Analgesics to relieve pain and promote early ambulation.
2. Observe nasogastric tube patency (if tube present).
3. Resume food and fluids gradually when persistalis auscultated.

MONITORING AND MANAGING COMPLICATIONS

1. Hemorrhage: count perineal pads used and assess extent of saturation; monitor vital signs; check abdominal dressings for drainage; give guidelines for restricting activity to promote healing and prevent bleeding.
2. Deep vein thrombosis: apply elastic antiembolism stockings; encourage and assist in changing positions frequently; assist with early ambulation; monitor leg pain and positive Homans' sign; instruct to avoid prolonged pressure at the knees and immobility.
3. Bladder dysfunction: monitor urinary output and assess for abdominal distention after catheter is removed; initiate measures to encourage voiding.

✎ PATIENT EDUCATION AND HEALTH MAINTENANCE: CARE IN THE HOME AND COMMUNITY

1. Tailor according to needs, i.e., no menstrual cycles, need for hormones.

2. Instruct to resume activities gradually; no sitting for long periods.
3. Teach that showers are preferable to tub baths to reduce risk of infection and injury getting in and out of tub.
4. Avoid lifting, straining, sexual intercourse, or driving until advised by physician.
5. Report vaginal discharge, foul odor, excessive bleeding, leg redness or pain, or elevated temperature to health care professional promptly.
6. Reinforce information regarding resumption of sexual intercourse.

For more information see Chapter 45 in Smeltzer and Bare: *Brunner and Suddarth's Textbook of Medical–Surgical Nursing,* 8th Edition. Philadelphia: Lippincott–Raven, 1996.

CANCER OF THE ENDOMETRIUM

Diagnosis of cancer of the uterine endometrium (fundus or corpus) has increased partly because people are living longer and there is more accurate reporting. This cancer is the fourth most common in women and the most common pelvic neoplasm. Treatment consists of total hysterectomy and bilateral salpingo-oophorectomy. Intercavitary radiation or external pelvic radiation may be part of the treatment. One-third of women with postmenopausal bleeding have cancer of the uterus. Obese women have a slightly higher risk due to increased levels of estrone from excess weight. This exposes the uterus to unopposed estrogen. Unopposed estrogen given in replacement therapy is also a risk factor. Other risk factors include nulliparity and late menopause. Most uterine cancers are adenocarcinomas and originate in the lining of the uterus. Treatment is based on the stage of the disease and almost always begins with a total hysterectomy and bilateral salpingo-oophorectomy. External radiation and brachytherapy may follow, depending on stage.

For more information see Chapter 45 in Smeltzer and Bare: *Brunner and Suddarth's Textbook of Medical–Surgical Nursing,* 8th Edition. Philadelphia: Lippincott–Raven, 1996.

CANCER OF THE ESOPHAGUS

In the United State carcinoma of the esophagus occurs more than twice as often in men as in women; more frequently in blacks than in whites; usually occurs in fifth decade of life and has a much higher incidence in other parts of the world (China and northern Iran).

Risk factors include chronic irritation, use of alcohol and tobacco. In other parts of the world there has been association with use of opium pipes; ingestion of exceptionally hot beverages; and nutritional deficiencies, mainly lack of fruits and vegetables.

CLINICAL MANIFESTATIONS

The delay between the onset of early symptoms and the time when the patient seeks medical advice is often 12–18 months; usually presents with advanced ulcerated lesion of the esophagus.

1. Dysphagia, initially with solid foods and eventually liquids.
2. Feeling of a lump in the throat and painful swallowing.
3. Substernal pain or fullness; regurgitation of undigested food with foul breath and hiccoughs later.
4. Hemorrhage may take place, and progressive loss of weight and strength due to starvation.

DIAGNOSTIC EVALUATION

1. Diagnosis is confirmed in 95% of the cases by esophagogastroduodenoscopy (EGD) with biopsy and brushings.
2. Other studies: bronchoscopy, mediastinoscopy.

MANAGEMENT

Treatment goals of esophageal cancer may be directed toward cure if found in an early stage; it is often found in late stages, making palliation the goal of therapy. Because the ideal method of treating esophageal cancer has not yet been found, each patient is approached in a way that appears best for that individual.

1. Surgery, radiation, chemotherapy, or a combination of these modalities.
2. Palliative treatment done to maintain esophageal patency: dilatation of the esophagus, laser therapy, radiation, and chemotherapy.
3. Esophagectomy is standard surgical management; carries a relatively high mortality rate.

Nursing Interventions

1. Improving nutritional and physical condition in preparation for surgery, radiation therapy, or chemotherapy.
2. Weight gain program based on high-caloric and high-protein diet in liquid or soft form.
3. Educate about the nature of the postoperative equipment that will be used, e.g., chest drainage, nasogastric suction, parenteral fluid therapy, and gastric intubation.
4. Place patient in semi-Fowler's, and later Fowler's, position after waking from anesthesia to prevent reflux of gastric secretions.
5. Observe carefully for regurgitation, dyspnea, and aspiration pneumonia.
6. Observe for aspiration postoperatively; monitor temperature.
7. If grafting was done, check for graft viability hourly, for first 12 hours.
8. Assess graft for color and presence of pulse (with Doppler).
9. If an endoprosthesis has been inserted or anasto-mosis performed, mark nasogastric tube for posi-

tion immediately postoperative and notify physician if displacement occurs.

10. Encourage small sips of water, later pureed small feedings once feeding begins; involve family.
11. Administer antacids for gastric distress; liquid supplements may be more easily tolerated.
12. Discontinue parenteral fluids when food intake is sufficient.
13. Keep patient upright for at least 2 hours after each meal to assist in movement of food.
14. If patient drools, place a wick-type piece of gauze at corner of the mouth to direct secretions to dressing or emesis basin.
15. Assess for aspiration of saliva into the tracheo-bronchial tree (danger of pneumonia).

✎ PATIENT EDUCATION AND HEALTH MAINTENANCE: CARE IN THE HOME AND COMMUNITY

Instruct family in how to promote nutrition; what to observe; how to handle signs of complications; how to keep patient comfortable; and how to obtain needed physical and emotional support.

For more information see Chapter 34 in Smeltzer and Bare: *Brunner and Suddarth's Textbook of Medical–Surgical Nursing,* 8th Edition. Philadelphia: Lippincott–Raven, 1996.

CANCER OF THE KIDNEYS (RENAL TUMORS)

Cancer of the kidney accounts for 2% of all cancers in adults in the United States; it affects almost twice as many men as women. Risk factors include tobacco use, occupational exposure to industrial chemicals, obesity, and dialysis. The most common type of renal tumor is renal cell or renal adenocarcinoma. These tumors may metastasize early to the lungs, bones, liver, brain, and contralateral kidney. One-fourth to one-half of patients will have metastatic disease at the time of diagnosis.

CLINICAL MANIFESTATIONS

1. Many renal tumors produce no symptoms and are discovered on a routine physical examination as a palpable abdominal mass.
2. Classic triad, occurring late in the course of the disease, blood in the urine (hematuria), pain, and a mass in the flank.
3. The usual sign that first calls attention to the tumor is painless hematuria, either intermittent and microscopic or continuous and gross.
4. Dull pain in the back from pressure from compression of the ureter, extension of the tumor, or hemorrhage into the kidney.
5. Colicky pains occur if a clot or mass of tumor cells passes down the ureter.
6. Symptoms from metastasis may be the first manifestation of renal tumor including unexplained weight loss, increasing weakness, and anemia.

DIAGNOSTIC EVALUATION

Intravenous urography, cystoscopic examination, nephrotomograms, renal angiograms, ultrasonography, or computed tomography (CT scan).

MANAGEMENT

The goal of management is to eradicate the tumor before metastasis occurs.

1. Radical nephrectomy is the preferred treatment, including removal of the kidney, adrenal gland, and surrounding fat and lymph nodes.
2. Radiation therapy, hormonal therapy, or chemotherapy may be used with surgery; immunotherapy may be helpful.

3. Renal artery embolization may be used in metastasis to occlude the blood supply to the tumor and kill the tumor cells.
4. Biologic therapy with interleukin-2 (IL-2).
5. Interferon is also under investigation as a mode of therapy for advanced renal cancer.

NURSING PROCESS

Interventions

1. Assist patient physiologically and psychologically in preparation for extensive diagnostic and therapeutic procedures; monitor carefully for signs of dehydration and exhaustion.
2. Following surgery give frequent analgesia for pain and muscle soreness.
3. Provide assistance with turning; encourage to turn, cough, and take deep breaths to prevent atelectasis and other pulmonary complications.
4. Support patient and family in coping with diagnosis and uncertainties about outcome.
5. Give follow-up care to detect signs of metastases; reassure the patient and family about patient's well-being.
6. Tell patient a yearly physical examination and chest x-ray throughout life is required for patients who have had surgery for renal carcinoma.
7. Evaluate all subsequent symptoms with possible metastases in mind as late metastases are not uncommon.

For more information see Chapter 43 in Smeltzer and Bare: *Brunner and Suddarth's Textbook of Medical–Surgical Nursing,* 8th Edition. Philadelphia: Lippincott–Raven, 1996.

CANCER OF THE LARGE INTESTINE (COLON AND RECTUM)

Cancer of the colon and rectum is now the second most common type of internal cancer in the United States. Colon cancer affects more than twice as many people as rectal cancer. The incidence increases with age (most patients are over 55), and is higher in persons with a family history of colon cancer or polyps; chronic inflammatory bowel disease; and a diet high in fat, protein, and beef and low in fiber. Almost three out of four patients could be saved by early diagnosis and prompt treatment. Most people are asymptomatic for long periods and seek medical help only when they notice a change in bowel habits or rectal bleeding. The low 5-year survival rate of 40–50% is due primarily to late diagnosis.

CLINICAL MANIFESTATIONS

1. Changes in bowel habits (the most common presenting symptom), passage of blood in the stools (second most common symptom).
2. Unexplained anemia, anorexia, weight loss, and fatigue.
3. Right-sided lesions: dull abdominal pain and melena.
4. Left-sided lesions: abdominal pain and cramping, narrowing stools, constipation and distention, bright red blood in the stool.
5. Rectal lesions: tenesmus (rectal pain, feeling of incomplete evacuation after a bowel movement), alternating constipation and diarrhea, and blood.

DIAGNOSTIC EVALUATION

1. Rectal exam, fecal occult blood testing, barium enema, proctosigmoidoscopy, and colonoscopy.
2. Carcinoembryonic antigen (CEA) studies (best as indicator for prognosis and recurrence).

Medical Management

1. Treatment depends on stage of disease and related complications.
2. Staging is determined by endoscopy, ultrasonography, and laparoscopy.
3. Adjuvant: chemotherapy, radiation therapy, and/or immunotherapy.

Surgical Management

Surgery is the primary treatment for most colon and rectal cancers; type of surgery depends on location and size of tumor; may be curative or palliative.

1. Cancers limited to one site are removable through a colonoscope.
2. Laparoscopic colotomy with polypectomy may be used.
3. Nd:YAG laser is effective in some lesions.
4. Bowel resection.
5. Due to improved surgical techniques, colostomies are performed on less than one-third of patients with colorectal cancer.

NURSING PROCESS

Assessment

1. Obtain a health history.
2. Note presence and character of abdominal or rectal pain; past and present elimination patterns; current drug therapy; past medical history; description of color, odor, consistency of stool and presence of blood or mucus; weight loss; dietary habits including alcohol use; unusual fatigue.
3. Auscultate abdomen for bowel sounds; palpate for areas of tenderness, distention, solid masses; and inspect stool for blood.

Major Nursing Diagnosis

1. Constipation related to obstructing lesion.

2. Pain related to tissue compression secondary to obstruction.
3. Risk for fluid volume deficit related to vomiting and dehydration.
4. Anxiety related to impending surgery and the diagnosis of cancer.
5. Knowledge deficit concerning the diagnosis, the surgical procedure, and self-care after discharge.
6. Body image disturbance related to colostomy.

Collaborative Problems

1. Intraperitoneal infection.
2. Complete large-bowel obstruction.
3. GI bleeding/hemorrhage.
4. Bowel perforation.
5. Peritonitis/abscess/sepsis.

Planning and Implementation

The major goals may include adequate elimination of body waste products, reduction/alleviation of pain, increased activity tolerance, attainment of an optimal level of nutrition, maintenance of fluid and electrolyte balance, reduction in anxiety, acquisition of information about the diagnosis, surgical procedure, self-care after discharge, maintenance of optimal tissue healing, adequate protection of periostomal skin, exploration and verbalization of feelings and concerns about colostomy and impact on self, and absence of potential complications.

Nursing Interventions: Preoperative

Maintaining elimination

Monitor frequency and consistency of bowel movements; administer laxatives and enemas as prescribed.

Relieving pain

1. Administer analgesics as prescribed.
2. Make the environment conducive to relaxation.
3. Offer comfort measures, e.g., back rub, position changes.

MAINTAINING FLUID AND ELECTROLYTE BALANCE

1. Record intake and output and restrict fluids and oral food to prevent vomiting.
2. Administer antiemetics as prescribed.
3. Monitor serum electrolytes to detect hypokalemia and hyponatremia.
4. Assess vital signs to detect signs of hypovolemia: tachycardia, hypotension, and decreased pulse volume.
5. Assess hydration status and report decreased skin turgor, dry mucous membranes, concentrated urine, and increased urine specific gravity.

REDUCING ANXIETY

1. Assess the patient's level of anxiety and coping mechanisms used to deal with stress.
2. Provide privacy if desired; instruct in relaxation exercises and biofeedback; listen to patient who wishes to express feelings.
3. Arrange meetings with a member of the clergy if desired.
4. Provide meetings for patient and family with physicians and nurses to discuss the treatment/prognosis; a meeting with an enterostomal therapist may be useful.
5. Promote patient comfort by a relaxed and empathetic attitude.
6. Explain all tests and procedures in language the patient understands.
7. Assess patient's needs and desires for information.

PREVENTING INFECTION

Administer antibiotics as ordered to reduce intestinal bacteria in preparation for bowel surgery.

Nursing Interventions: Postoperative

PROVIDING WOUND CARE

Examine frequently during first 24 hours, checking for infection, dehiscence, hemorrhage, and excessive edema.

MAINTAINING POSITIVE BODY IMAGE

1. Encourage to verbalize feelings and concerns.
2. Provide a supportive environment and attitude to promote patient's adaptation to lifestyle changes related to stoma care.

MONITORING AND MANAGING COMPLICATIONS

Pre- and postoperatively observe for symptoms of complications; report and institute necessary care.

✎ PATIENT EDUCATION AND HEALTH MAINTENANCE: CARE IN THE HOME AND COMMUNITY

1. Provide patients being discharged with specific information, individualized to their needs, about ostomy care and complications to observe for: obstruction, infection, stoma stenosis, retraction or prolapse, and periostomal skin irritation.
2. Provide dietary instructions to help patients identify and eliminate irritating foods that can cause diarrhea or constipation.
3. Provide patients with a list of medications prescribed for them, with information on action, purpose, and possible side effects.
4. Review treatments and dressing changes, and encourage the family to participate.
5. Provide patient with specific directions about when to call the physician and what complications require prompt attention, i.e., bleeding, abdominal distention and rigidity, diarrhea, and the "dumping syndrome."
6. Review side effects of radiation therapy (anorexia, vomiting, diarrhea, and exhaustion) if necessary.

✪ GERONTOLOGIC CONSIDERATIONS

These cancers are considered the most common malignancies in old age except for prostatic cancer in men.

Symptoms are often insidious; fatigue is almost always present, due primarily to iron deficiency anemia. Other commonly reported symptoms are abdominal pain, obstruction, tenesmus, and rectal bleeding.

Colon cancer in the elderly has been closely associated with dietary carcinogens, lack of fiber, and excess fat.

Decreased vision and hearing, as well as difficulty with skills that require fine motor coordination, may require the patient to have help in handling ostomy equipment and periostomal care. Most elderly require 6 months before they feel comfortable with their ostomy care.

Arteriosclerosis causes decreased blood flow to the wound and stoma site. As a result, healing time may be prolonged. Some patients experience delayed elimination after irrigation because of decreased peristalsis and mucus production.

For more information see Chapter 37 in Smeltzer and Bare: *Brunner and Suddarth's Textbook of Medical–Surgical Nursing,* 8th Edition. Philadelphia: Lippincott–Raven, 1996.

CANCER OF THE LARYNX

Cancer of the larynx represents 1% of all cancers and occurs more frequently in men. Contributing factors are tobacco (smoke, smokeless) and alcohol and their combined effects, vocal straining, chronic laryngitis, industrial exposure to carcinogens, nutritional deficiencies (riboflavin), and family predisposition.

CLINICAL MANIFESTATIONS

1. Hoarseness noted early in glottic area.
2. Pain and burning in the throat when drinking hot liquids and citrus juices.
3. Lump may be felt in the neck.
4. Later symptoms include dysphagia, dyspnea, hoarseness, and foul breath.

5. Enlarged cervical nodes, weight loss, general debility, and pain radiating to the ear may suggest metastasis.

DIAGNOSTIC EVALUATION

Direct laryngoscopic examination under general anesthesia.

MANAGEMENT

Treatment varies with the extent of malignancy; options include radiation therapy and surgery.

1. Complete dental exam to rule out oral disease.
2. Dental problems resolved prior to scheduling surgery.
3. Radiation therapy achieves excellent results when only one cord is affected and mobile.
4. Partial laryngectomy is recommended in early stages, especially in intrinsic cancer of the larynx.
5. Supraglottic (horizontal) laryngectomy is used for some extrinsic tumors. The chief advantage to this operation is preservation of the voice.
6. Hemivertical laryngectomy performed when the tumor extends beyond the vocal cord, but is less than 1 cm in the subglottic area.
7. Total laryngectomy for extrinsic cancer (extension beyond the vocal cords)

Patient will have loss of voice, but will have normal swallowing.

NURSING PROCESS FOR THE PATIENT UNDERGOING LARYNGECTOMY

Assessment

1. Assess for hoarseness, sore throat, dyspnea, dysphagia, or pain and burning in the throat.
2. Palpate the neck for swelling.
3. Assess patient's ability to hear, see, read, and write.

4. Determine the psychological preparedness of the patient and evaluate patient's and family's coping methods and give effective support.

MAJOR NURSING DIAGNOSIS

1. Knowledge deficit about the surgical procedure and postoperative course.
2. Anxiety related to the diagnosis of cancer and impending surgery.
3. Ineffective airway clearance related to surgical alterations in the airway.
4. Impaired verbal communication related to removal of larynx and edema.
5. Altered nutrition: less than body requirements, related to swallowing difficulties.
6. Disturbance in body image, self-concept, and self-esteem related to major neck surgery.
7. Self-care deficit related to postoperative care.
8. Potential for noncompliance with rehabilitative program and home maintenance management.

Collaborative Problems

1. Infection.
2. Hemorrhage.
3. Nerve damage.
4. Tracheostomal stenosis.
5. Respiratory distress (hypoxia, airway obstruction, tracheal edema).

Planning and Implementation

The major goals may include attainment of an adequate level of knowledge, reduction in anxiety, maintenance of patent airway, improvement in communication, attainment of optimal levels of nutrition and hydration, improvement in body image and self-esteem, management of self-care, adherence to rehabilitative program, home maintenance management, and prevention of complications.

Nursing Interventions: Preoperative

PROVIDING PATIENT EDUCATION

1. Give patient and family educational materials (written and audiovisual) for review and reinforcement.
2. Explain to patient natural voice will be lost.
3. Assure patient that much can be done through a rehabilitation program.
4. Review equipment/treatments that will be part of the postoperative care.
5. Teach coughing/deep breathing exercises; provide for return demonstration.

REDUCING ANXIETY AND DEPRESSION

1. Assess psychological preparation and give opportunity to verbalize feelings and share perceptions; give complete, concise answers to questions.
2. Arrange a visit from a postlaryngectomy patient to help patient cope with situation and know successful rehabilitation is possible.

Nursing Interventions: Postoperative

MONITORING AND MANAGING POTENTIAL COMPLICATIONS

1. Observe for signs and symptoms of respiratory distress and hypoxia, i.e., restlessness, irritation, agitation, confusion, tachypnea, use of accessory muscles, and decreased oxygen saturation.
2. Rule out obstruction immediately by suctioning and having patient cough and take deep breaths.
3. Contact physician immediately if nursing measures do not improve respiratory status.
4. Contact physician immediately if any active bleeding.
5. Monitor vital signs for changes, i.e, increase in pulse, decrease in blood pressure, or rapid, deep respirations.
6. Observe for early signs and symptoms of infection.

MAINTAINING A PATENT AIRWAY

1. Position in semi-Fowler's or Fowler's position after recovery from anesthesia.
2. Avoid medications that depress respirations.
3. Encourage to turn and deep breathe; suction if necessary; early ambulation.
4. Care for the laryngectomy tube the same way as a tracheostomy tube.
5. Keep stoma clean by daily cleansing as prescribed.
6. Observe wound drainage, measure, and record.

PROMOTING COMMUNICATION AND SPEECH REHABILITATION

1. Implement a system of communication, e.g., "magic slate," hand signals.
2. Use nonwriting arm for IV infusions.
3. Consider visual or illiteracy deficits that create communication problems.
4. Inform patient of alternative communication methods; most common are esophageal speech, the electrolarynx, and tracheal esophageal puncture.

PROMOTING ADEQUATE NUTRITION

1. Inform NPO for 10–14 days; alternative sources will be provided, i.e., IV fluids, enteral feedings, and total parenteral nutrition (TPN).
2. Explain that oral feedings will start with thick fluids such as Ensure and gelatin for easy swallowing; instruct to avoid sweet foods, which increase salivation and suppress appetite.
3. Instruct to rinse mouth with warm water or mouthwash and brush teeth frequently.

PROMOTING A POSITIVE BODY IMAGE AND INCREASING SELF-ESTEEM

1. Use a positive approach; allow to participate in care and review tubes, dressings, and drains with patient and family.
2. Be a good listener and a support to the family.

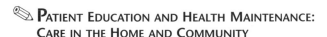

3. Refer to a support group, such as the American Laryngectomy Association and I Can Cope.

✎ **PATIENT EDUCATION AND HEALTH MAINTENANCE: CARE IN THE HOME AND COMMUNITY**

1. Provide discharge instruction as soon as able.
2. Give specific information about what to expect from tracheostomy and stomal care.
3. Assure patient that frequent mucus-producing cough and brassy sounds will diminish in time.
4. Keep orifice clean and clear of mucus; wash skin around stoma at least twice daily; if crusting occurs, lubricate stoma with a non-oil-based ointment.
5. Provide adequate humidification of the environment.
6. Inform to expect a diminished sense of taste and smell after surgery.
7. Teach patient to take precautions when showering to prevent getting water into the stoma.
8. Discourage swimming because the patient with a laryngectomy can drown.
9. Recommend avoidance of hairsprays, loose hair, and powders getting into stoma.
10. Stress activity in moderation; when tired, patient has more difficulty speaking with new voice.
11. Encourage patient to visit physician regularly for physical examinations and advice.
12. Recommend carrying proper ID to alert first-aider to special requirements of CPR.

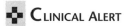 **CLINICAL ALERT**

Postoperatively, the nurse must be alert for the possible serious complications of rupture of the carotid artery. Should this occur, apply direct pressure over the artery, summon assistance, and provide psychological support until the vessel can be ligated.

For more information see Chapter 23 in Smeltzer and Bare: *Brunner and Suddarth's Textbook of Medical–Surgical Nursing,* 8th Edition. Philadelphia: Lippincott–Raven, 1996.

CANCER OF THE LIVER

Hepatic tumors may be malignant or benign. Oral contraceptive use has increased the incidence of benign tumors. Few cancers originate in the liver. Primary tumors ordinarily occur in patients with chronic liver disease (cirrhosis). Hepatocellular carcinoma (HCC) is the most common type of primary liver tumor. It is usually nonresectable because of rapid extension and metastasis elsewhere. Other types include cholangiocellular carcinoma (CCC) and combined HCC and CCC. If found early, resection may be possible; however, early detection is rare.

Cirrhosis, hepatitis B, and exposure to certain chemical toxins have been implicated in the etiology of HCC. Cigarette smoking, especially when combined with alcohol use, has also been identified as a risk factor. Other substances that have been implicated include aflatoxins or carcinogens in herbal medicines and nitrosamines. Half of all late cancer cases are metastases from other primary sites.

CLINICAL MANIFESTATIONS

1. Early manifestations include signs and symptoms of any cancer that interferes with nutrition: recent loss of weight, loss of strength, anorexia, and anemia.
2. Abdominal pain may be present, accompanied by rapid liver enlargement and irregular surface upon palpation.
3. Jaundice is present only if larger bile ducts are occluded.
4. Ascites occurs if portal veins are obstructed or tumor tissue is seeded in the peritoneal cavity.

DIAGNOSTIC EVALUATION

Diagnosis is made on the basis of clinical signs and symptoms, history and physical examination, and results of laboratory and x-ray findings.

NONSURGICAL MANAGEMENT

Radiation Therapy

1. Intravenous injection of antibodies that specifically attack tumor-associated antigens.
2. Percutaneous placement of a high-intensity source for interstitial radiation therapy.

Chemotherapy

1. Systemic chemotherapy and regional infusion used to administer antineoplastic agents.
2. An implantable pump is used to deliver a high-concentration chemotherapy to the liver through the hepatic artery.

Percutaneous Biliary Drainage

1. Used to bypass biliary ducts obstructed by the liver, pancreatic, or bile ducts in patients with inoperable tumors.
2. Complications include sepsis, leakage of bile, hemorrhage, and reobstruction of the biliary system.
3. Observe patients for fever and chills, bile drainage around the catheter, changes in vital signs, and evidence of biliary obstruction, including increased pain or pressure, pruritus, and recurrence of jaundice.

Other Nonsurgical Treatment Modalities

1. Hyperthermia: heat is directed to tumors to cause necrosis of the tumors while sparing normal tissue.
2. Cryosurgery and laser therapy are newer treatment modalities.
3. Embolization of the arterial blood flow to the tumor; effective in small tumors.

4. Immunotherapy: lymphocytes with antitumor reactivity are administered to the patient.

SURGICAL MANAGEMENT

Hepatic lobectomy can be performed when the primary hepatic tumor is localized or when the primary site can be completely excised and the metastasis is limited. Capitalizing on the regenerative capacity of the liver cells, 90% of the liver has been successfully removed. The presence of cirrhosis limits the ability of the liver to regenerate.

Preoperative Evaluation and Preparation

1. Evaluate and address patient's nutritional, fluid, emotional, and physical needs prior to surgery.
2. Prepare the intestinal tract with cathartics, colonic irrigation, and intestinal antibiotics.

Surgical Intervention

Anatomic (surgical) division of the lobes with resection.

Liver Transplantation to Treat Liver Tumors

1. Removal of the liver and its replacement by a healthy donor organ has been successful.
2. Recurrence of primary liver malignancy after transplantation is 80–85%; recommended that patient be treated with systemic chemotherapy or radiation therapy along with liver transplantation.

Nursing Interventions: Postoperative

1. Assess for potential problems related to cardiopulmonary involvement, vascular complications, and respiratory and liver dysfunction.
2. Give careful attention to metabolic abnormalities.
3. Give constant close monitoring and care for the first 2 or 3 days.
4. Encourage early ambulation.

✎ PATIENT EDUCATION AND HEALTH MAINTENANCE: CARE IN THE HOME AND COMMUNITY

C

Instruct family to assess and report complications and side effects of the chemotherapy.

Instruct about the importance of follow-up visits to permit frequent checks on the response of the patient and the tumor to chemotherapy, condition of the site of the pump insertion, and occurrence of toxic effects.

Encourage patient to resume activities as soon as possible but warn to avoid activities that may damage the pump.

The home care nurse serves a vital role in assisting the patient and family to cope with the symptoms that may occur and with the prognosis.

1. Collaborate with the health care team, patient, and family to identify and implement pain management strategies and approaches to management of other problems: weakness, pruritus, inadequate dietary intake, jaundice, and symptoms associated with metastasis to other sites.
2. Assist patient and family in decision making about hospice care and initiation of referrals.
3. Provide reassurance and instructions to patient and family to reduce fear that the percutaneous biliary drainage catheter will fall out.
4. Provide verbal and written instruction as well as demonstration of biliary catheter care to patient and family; instruct in techniques to keep catheter site clean and dry and to assess the catheter and its insertion site.
5. Instruct regarding signs of complications and encourage to notify nurse or physician if problems or questions occur.

For more information see Chapter 38 in Smeltzer and Bare: *Brunner and Suddarth's Textbook of Medical–Surgical Nursing*, 8th Edition. Philadelphia: Lippincott–Raven, 1996.

CANCER OF THE LUNG (BRONCHOGENIC CARCINOMA)

Bronchogenic carcinoma is a malignant tumor arising from the bronchial epithelium. Survival rate is low because of spread to regional lymphatics by the time of diagnosis. Four major cell types of lung cancer include epidermoid (squamous cell) carcinoma, small-cell (oat cell) carcinoma, adenocarcinoma, and large-cell (undifferentiated) carcinoma. Many tumors contain more than one cell type; different approaches to treatment may be indicated by the cell type. The stage of the tumor refers to the anatomic extent of the tumor, spread to the regional lymph nodes, and metastatic spread. Prognosis appears most favorable for epidermoid and adenocarcinoma; undifferentiated small-cell (oat cell) tumors have poor prognosis. Risk factors include tobacco smoke, secondhand smoke, air pollution, occupational exposure, radon, and vitamin A deficiency. Other factors include genetic predisposition and other underlying respiratory diseases, i.e., COPD and tuberculosis.

CLINICAL MANIFESTATIONS

1. Begins insidiously over several decades and often is asymptomatic until late in its course.
2. Signs and symptoms depend on location, tumor size, degree of obstruction, and existence of metastases.
3. Most frequent symptom is a cough, hacking, nonproductive; later progresses to producing thick, purulent sputum. A cough that changes in character should arouse suspicion of lung cancer.
4. Wheezing occurs when the bronchus becomes partially obstructed; expectoration of blood-tinged sputum is common in the morning.
5. A recurring fever may exist in some patients.
6. Pain is a late symptom; often related to bone metastasis.

7. Chest pain, tightness, hoarseness, dysphagia, head and neck edema, and symptoms of pleural or pericardial infusion exist if the tumor spreads to adjacent structures and lymph nodes.
8. Common sites of metastases are lymph nodes, bone, brain, contralateral lung, and adrenal glands.
9. Weakness, anorexia, weight loss, and anemia appear late.

DIAGNOSTIC EVALUATION

1. Chest films, sputum exam, bronchoscopy, fluorescent bronchofibroscopy, and injected hematoporphyrin.
2. Various CT scans and magnetic resonance imaging (MRI).

MANAGEMENT

The objective of management is to provide the maximum likelihood of cure. Treatment depends on cell type, stage of the disease, and physiologic status. Treatment may involve surgery, radiation therapy, chemotherapy, and immunotherapy used separately or in combination.

Monitor and Manage Potential Complications

1. Surgery: respiratory failure.
2. Radiation: diminished cardiopulmonary function.
3. Chemotherapy: pulmonary toxicity, leukemia; pneumonitis (when chemotherapy and radiation are combined).

Nursing Interventions

1. Maintain airway patency; remove secretions.
2. Encourage deep breathing, aerosol therapy, oxygen therapy; mechanical ventilation may be necessary.
3. Assess psychological aspects and assist patient to cope.

GERONTOLOGIC CONSIDERATIONS

Cancer of the lung is not unusual in the elderly. Presence of coronary artery disease or pulmonary insufficiency may be contraindications to surgical intervention. If the patient's cardiovascular status and pulmonary function are satisfactory, surgery is generally well tolerated.

For more information see Chapter 24 in Smeltzer and Bare: *Brunner and Suddarth's Textbook of Medical–Surgical Nursing,* 8th Edition. Philadelphia: Lippincott–Raven, 1996.

CANCER OF THE ORAL CAVITY

Cancer of the oral cavity may occur in any part of the mouth or throat and is highly curable if discovered early. It is associated with use of alcohol and tobacco. Age is also a risk factor in persons over 60. It is increasing in persons under age 30 because of the use of smokeless tobacco. Other predisposing factors may be chronic irritation by a warm pipe stem or prolonged exposure to sun and wind.

CLINICAL MANIFESTATIONS

1. Most common complaint: painless sore/mass that will not heal.
2. Typical lesion is a painful indurated ulcer with raised edges.
3. As the cancer progresses patient may complain of tenderness; difficulty in chewing, swallowing, and speaking; coughing of blood-tinged sputum or enlarged cervical lymph nodes.

DIAGNOSTIC EVALUATION

Oral exam, assessment of lymph nodes, and biopsies on suspicious lesions (not healed within 2 weeks).

MANAGEMENT

Management varies with the nature of the lesion, preference of the physician, and patient choice. Resectional surgery, radiation therapy, chemotherapy, or a combination may be effective.

1. Lip cancer: small lesions are excised liberally; larger lesions may be treated by radiation therapy.
2. Tongue cancer: treated aggressively, recurrence rate is high.
3. Radical neck dissection for metastases of oral cancer to lymphatic channel in the neck region.

NURSING PROCESS

Assessment

1. Assess patient's history to determine teaching and learning needs and symptoms requiring medical evaluation. Include questions related to oral cavity, e.g., oral and dental hygiene; alcohol and tobacco use, also smokeless chewing tobacco; lesions or irritated areas in the mouth, tongue, or throat; recent history of sore throat or bloody sputum; discomfort caused by certain foods.
2. Perform physical exam; inspect and palpate internal and external structures of the mouth and throat; examine for moisture, color, texture, symmetry, and presence of lesions; examine neck for enlarged lymph nodes.

Major Nursing Diagnosis

1. Altered oral mucous membrane related to pathologic condition, infection, or chemical/mechanical trauma (e.g., medications, ill-fitting dentures).
2. Altered nutrition, less than body requirements, related to inability to ingest adequate nutrients secondary to oral/dental conditions.
3. Body image disturbance related to a physical change in appearance resulting from a disease condition or its treatment.

4. Pain related to oral lesion or treatment.
5. Impaired verbal communication related to treatment.
6. Risk for infection related to disease or treatment.
7. Knowledge deficit about disease process and treatment plan.

Planning and Implementation

The major goals may include improvement in the condition of the oral mucous membrane, improvement in nutritional intake, attainment of a positive self-image, attainment of comfort, alternative communication methods, and no infection.

Nursing Interventions

PROMOTING MOUTH CARE

1. Identify patients at risk for oral complications and assist with methods to decrease complications.
2. Instruct the patient in importance and techniques of preventive mouth care, e.g., soft toothbrush, floss, or irrigating solution.

COMBATTING XEROSTOMIA (DRYNESS OF MOUTH)

1. Advise to avoid dry, bulky, and irritating foods and fluids, as well as alcohol and tobacco.
2. Encourage to increase fluids; use a humidifier during sleep.
3. Use synthetic saliva if helpful.

RELIEVING STOMATITIS OR MUCOSITIS

Start prophylactic mouth care as soon as chemotherapy or radiation therapy begins, e.g., benzydamine hydrochloride rinse.

ASSURING ADEQUATE FOOD AND FLUID INTAKE

1. Perform dietary assessment and recommend changes in consistency of foods and frequency of eating based on disease condition and patient preferences.

2. Help attain and maintain desirable body weight and level of energy; promote the healing of tissue.

SUPPORTING A POSITIVE SELF-IMAGE

1. Encourage to verbalize perceived change in body appearance; realistically discuss actual changes or losses.
2. Offer support while verbalizing fears and negative feelings (withdrawal, depression, anger).
3. Reinforce strengths, achievements, and positive attributes.
4. Be alert to signs of grieving and record emotional changes.

MINIMIZING DISCOMFORT AND PAIN

1. Provide patient with an analgesic, i.e., viscous lidocaine (Xylocaine Viscous 2%).
2. Avoid foods that are spicy, hot, or hard.

PROMOTING EFFECTIVE COMMUNICATION

1. Assess patient's ability to communicate in writing preoperatively.
2. Provide a magic slate or pen and paper to communicate postoperatively.
3. Provide a communication board if unable to write; involve a speech therapist postoperatively.

PROMOTING INFECTION CONTROL

1. Evaluate laboratory results frequently; check temperature every 6–8 hours for elevation that may indicate infection.
2. Prohibit visitors who may transmit micro-organisms.
3. Avoid trauma to sensitive skin tissues; use strict aseptic technique when changing dressings.
4. Report signs of wound infection; use antibiotics prophylactically.

✎ PATIENT EDUCATION AND HEALTH MAINTENANCE:
CARE IN THE HOME AND COMMUNITY

Assess patient's need to breathe, obtain nourishment, avoid infection, and be alert for adverse signs and symptoms.

1. Prepare an individualized plan of care.
2. Determine what equipment is needed, i.e., suction or tracheostomy tube, and where items can be obtained.
3. Give consideration to humidification and aeration of patient's room and measures to control odors.
4. Instruct patient and family in use of enteral or parenteral feedings (if unable to take foods orally).
5. Provide information regarding signs of obstruction, hemorrhage, infection, depression, and withdrawal to caregivers.
6. Instruct in the importance of follow-up visits to determine progression or regression, and to receive directions about modifications in medications or general care.

For more information see Chapter 34 in Smeltzer and Bare: *Brunner and Suddarth's Textbook of Medical–Surgical Nursing*, 8th Edition. Philadelphia: Lippincott–Raven, 1996.

CANCER OF THE OVARY

Ovarian cancer is difficult to diagnosis and unique in that it gives rise to many primary cancers and may be the site of metastases from other cancers. Peak incidence is in the fifth decade. It is the fourth most prevalent cause of cancer deaths in women. No definitive causative factors have been determined, but oral contraceptives provide a protective effect. No screening mechanism exists; tumor markers are being explored. Serous adenocarcinoma is the most frequent type of tumor. Risk factors: high-fat diet; smoking; alcohol; use of talcum powder on perineal area; history of breast, colon, or endometrial cancer and family history of breast or ovarian cancer. Nulliparity, infertility, and anovulation are additional risks. Seventy-five percent of ovarian cancers have metastasized outside the ovary by the time of diagnosis.

CLINICAL MANIFESTATIONS

1. Irregular menses, increasing premenstrual tension, menorrhagia with breast tenderness, early menopause, abdominal discomfort, dyspepsia, pelvic pressure, and urinary frequency.
2. Flatulence, fullness after a light meal, and increasing abdominal girth are significant symptoms.

DIAGNOSTIC EVALUATION

Any enlarged ovary must be investigated; pelvic examination will not detect early ovarian cancer.

MANAGEMENT

1. Surgical removal is the treatment of choice.
2. Preoperative work-up can include barium enema, proctosigmoidoscopy, upper GI series, chest radiograph, and IVP.
3. Staging of the tumor is done to direct treatment accordingly.
4. Total abdominal hysterectomy with bilateral salpingo-oophorectomy and omentectomy for early disease.
5. Radiation therapy and intraperitoneal isotopes.
6. Hormonal regulation with tamoxifen.
7. Chemotherapy is the most common form of treatment for advanced disease, i.e., cisplatin, Taxol.
8. Internal (intercavitary) irradiation.
9. Immunotherapy.
10. Intracavity brachytherapy.

Nursing Management

1. Nursing measures include treatment related to surgery, radiation, chemotherapy, and palliation.
2. Emotional support provided by giving comfort measures, showing attentiveness and caring. Allow patients to express feelings about condition and death.

For more information see Chapter 45 in Smeltzer and Bare: *Brunner and Suddarth's Textbook of Medical–Surgical Nursing,* 8th Edition. Philadelphia: Lippincott–Raven, 1996.

CANCER OF THE PANCREAS

Carcinoma of the pancreas is the fourth leading cause of cancer deaths in the United States and occurs most frequently in the sixth and seventh decades of life. Risk factors include exposure to industrial chemicals or toxins in the environment, a high-fat diet, and cigarette smoking. Risk is also increased in persons with hereditary pancreatitis, diabetes mellitus, and chronic pancreatitis. Cancer may arise in any portion of the pancreas, producing symptoms that vary, depending on the location of the lesion and whether or not functioning insulin-secreting pancreatic islet cells are involved. Tumors that originate in the head of the pancreas are the most common; functioning islet cell tumors are responsible for the syndrome of hyperinsulinism. The pancreas can also be the site of metastasis from other tumors. Pancreatic carcinoma has the lowest 5-year survival rate of 60 cancer sites surveyed.

CLINICAL MANIFESTATIONS

1. Weight loss, abdominal pain, and jaundice are the classic signs and may develop only when the disease is far advanced.
2. Rapid, profound, and progressive weight loss.

3. Vague upper or midabdominal pain or discomfort unrelated to any gastrointestinal function; radiates as a boring pain in the midback; is more severe at night; formation of ascites is common.
4. Onset of symptoms of insulin deficiency: glucosuria, hyperglycemia, and abnormal glucose tolerance; diabetes may be an early sign of carcinoma.

DIAGNOSTIC EVALUATION

Endoscopic retrograde cholangiopancreatography (ERCP).

MANAGEMENT

1. Surgical procedure is extensive to remove resectable localized tumors.
2. Treatment is usually limited to palliative measures. Total excision of the lesion often is not feasible because of the extensive growth when the lesion is diagnosed and the probable widespread metastases, especially to the liver, lungs, and bones.
3. Radiation and chemotherapy may be used; intraoperative radiation therapy (IORT) is used for relief of pain.

Nursing Interventions

1. Provide pain management and attention to nutrition.
2. Provide skin care and measures to relieve pain and discomfort associated with jaundice, anorexia, and profound weight loss.
3. Consider patient-controlled analgesia (PCA) for severe escalating pain.

For more information see Chapter 40 in Smeltzer and Bare: *Brunner and Suddarth's Textbook of Medical–Surgical Nursing,* 8th Edition. Philadelphia: Lippincott–Raven, 1996.

CANCER OF THE PROSTATE

Cancer of the prostate is the most common cancer in men; the second most common cause of cancer deaths in American men older than 55; and the most prevalent cancer overall in African-American men. About 1 in 11 men in the United States will develop prostate cancer.

CLINICAL MANIFESTATIONS

Early Stage

1. Usually asymptomatic.
2. Nodule felt within the substance of the gland or extensive hardening in the posterior lobe.

Advanced Stage

1. Lesion is "stony hard" and fixed.
2. Obstructive symptoms occur late in the disease; difficulty and frequency of urination, urinary retention, decreased size and force of the urinary stream.
3. Metastasizes to bone, lymph nodes, brain, and lungs.
4. Symptoms of metastases include backache, hip pain, perineal and rectal discomfort, anemia, weight loss, weakness, nausea, and oliguria; hematuria may result from urethral or bladder invasion.

Early Detection

Every man over age 40 should have a digital rectal examination as part of his regular health checkup—key to a higher cure rate.

DIAGNOSTIC EVALUATION

Confirmed by histologic examination of tissue, open prostatectomy, fine-needle aspiration.

MANAGEMENT

Treatment is based on the stage of the disease and on the patient's age and symptoms. Prostate-specific antigen (PSA) concentration is used to monitor patient response to cancer therapy and detect local progression and early recurrence.

Radical Prostatectomy

1. Removal of the prostate and seminal vesicles.
2. For patients who have potentially curable disease and life expectancy of 10 years of more.
3. May be followed by bilateral orchiectomy.
4. Sexual impotency follows radical prostatectomy and various degrees of urinary incontinence.

Radiation Therapy

1. If cancer is in the early stage, treatment may be curative radiation therapy.
2. There is better preservation of sexual potency and young patients may prefer this treatment modality.

Hormonal Therapy

1. Method of control rather than cure.
2. Accomplished by either orchiectomy or administration of estrogens.
3. Diethylstilbestrol (DES) is the most widely used estrogen.
4. Luteinizing hormone releasing hormone (LHRH) agonists and antiandrogen drugs such as flutamide also used.

Other Therapies

1. Cryosurgery for those who cannot physically tolerate surgery or for recurrence.
2. Chemotherapy, i.e., doxorubicin, cisplatin, and cyclophosphamide.
3. Repeated transurethral resections (TUR) to keep urethra patent; suprapubic or transurethral catheter drainage when TUR is impractical.

Sexual Dysfunction

1. Showing sensitivity to issues of sexuality as a result of disease or therapy assists in the rehabilitation process.
2. Help patient and family to cope with diagnosis, alterations in usual activities, uncertainty of the future.

NURSING PROCESS FOR THE PATIENT UNDERGOING PROSTATECTOMY

Assessment

Take complete history with emphasis on urinary function.

Major Nursing Diagnosis: Preoperative

1. Anxiety related to the inability to void.
2. Pain related to bladder distention.
3. Knowledge deficit about factors related to the problem and the treatment protocol.

Major Nursing Diagnosis: Postoperative

1. Pain related to the surgical incision, catheter placement, and bladder spasms.
2. Knowledge deficit about postoperative and convalescent management.

Collaborative Problems

1. Hemorrhage and shock.
2. Infection.
3. Thrombosis.
4. Catheter obstruction.

Planning and Implementation

The major preoperative goals may include reduced anxiety and teaching the patient about his prostate problem and the perioperative experience. The major postoperative goals may include correction of fluid volume disturbances, relief of pain and discomfort, prevention of infection, ability to perform self-care activities, and absence of complications.

Nursing Interventions: Preoperative
Reducing anxiety

1. Provide a trusting and professional relationship.
2. Encourage verbalization of feelings and concerns.

REDUCING PAIN

1. Place on bed rest; administer analgesics; initiate measures to relieve anxiety.
2. Insert indwelling catheter if urinary retention is present.

✎ PATIENT EDUCATION AND HEALTH MAINTENANCE: CARE IN THE HOME AND COMMUNITY

1. Explain diagnostic tests, surgery procedure, drainage system.
2. Answer questions and provide patient support.
3. Explain rationale for preoperative antiembolism stockings.

Nursing Interventions: Postoperative
RELIEVING PAIN

1. Distinguish cause and location of pain; give analgesics for incisional pain and smooth muscle relaxants for bladder spasm.
2. Irrigate drainage system to correct obstruction.

MONITORING AND MANAGING COMPLICATIONS

1. Hemorrhage: observe catheter drainage, note bright red bleeding with increased viscosity and clots; may require return to surgery.
2. Infection: assess for urinary tract infection and epididymitis; administer antibiotics as prescribed.
3. Thrombosis: assess for deep vein thrombosis and pulmonary embolism; apply antiembolism stockings.

4. Obstructed catheter: provide for patent drainage system; perform gentle irrigation as prescribed to remove blood clots.

✎ PATIENT EDUCATION AND HEALTH MAINTENANCE: CARE IN THE HOME AND COMMUNITY

1. Encourage patient to walk and not sit for prolonged periods.
2. Teach perineal exercises to help regain urinary control.
3. Teach patient not to engage in any Valsalva effort (will increase venous pressure and may produce hematuria).
4. Avoid long motor trips and strenuous exercise, which increases tendency to bleed.
5. Encourage fluids to avoid dehydration and clot formation.

For more information see Chapter 47 in Smeltzer and Bare: *Brunner and Suddarth's Textbook of Medical–Surgical Nursing,* 8th Edition. Philadelphia: Lippincott–Raven, 1996.

CANCER OF THE SKIN

Skin cancer is the most common form of cancer in the United States. It is the most successfully treated type of cancer. Exposure to the sun is the leading cause; incidence is related to the total amount of exposure to the sun. Those at greatest risk are fair, blue-eyed, red-haired persons of Celtic ancestry or persons with ruddy or light complextions. Others at risk are outdoor workers, elderly persons with sun-damaged skin, workers exposed to chemical agents (e.g., arsenic, coal, tar); conditions causing scarring or chronic irritation may also lead to cancer. Genetic factors are also involved. Types of skin cancer: (1) basal cell carcinoma (BCC) arises from the basal cell layer of the epidermis or hair follicles; most common and rarely metastasizes; recurrence is common; (2) squamous cell carcinomas (SCC), a malignant proliferation arising from the epidermis; an invasive carcinoma.

C

CLINICAL MANIFESTATIONS

1. BCC: generally appears on sun-exposed areas of the body; presents as a small, waxy nodule with rolled translucent pearly borders; telangiectatic vessels may present. Other lesions may appear as shiny, flat, gray, or yellowish plaques.
2. SCC: usually appears on sun-damaged skin; may arise from normal skin or preexisting lesions. Appears as a rough, thickened, scaly tumor; asymptomatic or may involve bleeding.

DIAGNOSTIC EVALUATION

Biopsy and histologic evaluation.

MANAGEMENT

The goal of treatment is to eradicate or completely destroy all the tumor. Method of treatment depends on the tumor location, cell type, cosmetic desires, history of previous treatment, whether or not the tumor is invasive, and presence of metastatic nodes.

Excision, micrographic surgery, electrosurgery, cryosurgery, and radiation therapy are possible treatment methods.

NURSING INTERVENTIONS

The role of the nurse is that of teaching the patient postoperative self-care activities and patient education.

1. Teach patient to protect the wound from physical trauma, external irritants, and contamination.
2. Advise regarding dressing protocols; watch for excessive bleeding.
3. Instruct to drink liquids through a straw if lesion is in the oral area; limit excessive talking and facial movement.

4. Educate regarding unnecessary exposure to the sun, use of sunscreens, and protective clothing if patient must be in sun.
5. Educate to have a follow-up evaluation throughout lifetime; watch for development of new lesions.

For more information see Chapter 54 in Smeltzer and Bare: *Brunner and Suddarth's Textbook of Medical–Surgical Nursing,* 8th Edition. Philadelphia: Lippincott–Raven, 1996.

CANCER OF THE STOMACH

Cancer of the stomach usually occurs in people over the age of 40 and occasionally in younger people. Most stomach cancers occur in the lesser curvature or antrum of the stomach and are adenocarcinomas. The incidence of gastric cancer is much greater in Japan. Diet appears to be a significant factor, i.e., high in smoked foods and lacking in fruits and vegetables. Other factors related to the incidence include chronic inflammation of the stomach, pernicious anemia, achlorhydria, gastric ulcers, *Helicobacter pylori* bacteria, and heredity. Prognosis is poor, as most patients have metastases at the time of diagnosis.

CLINICAL MANIFESTATIONS

Early symptoms are often indefinite, because most tumors begin on the lesser curvature where they cause little disturbance to gastric functions.

1. Early stages: symptoms may be absent; may resemble those of patients with benign ulcers, i.e., pain relieved with antacids.
2. Symptoms of progressive disease: indigestion, anorexia, dyspepsia, weight loss, abdominal pain (usually a late symptom), constipation, anemia, and nausea and vomiting.

DIAGNOSTIC EVALUATION

1. X-ray of upper GI with barium.

2. Endoscopy for biopsy and cytologic washings.
3. Computed tomography (CT) scan, bone scan, and liver scan because metastasis frequently occurs before warning signs.
4. Complete x-ray examination of the gastrointestinal tract if dyspepsia of more than 4 weeks duration in any person over age 40.

MANAGEMENT

There is no successful treatment of gastric carcinoma except removal of the tumor. If tumor can be removed while still localized to the stomach, the patient can be cured.

1. Effective palliation (to prevent symptoms such as obstruction) by resection of the tumor; radical subtotal gastrectomy; total gastrectomy.
2. Chemotherapy to further control disease or palliation if surgical treatment does not offer cure.
3. Radiation may be used for palliation.

NURSING PROCESS

Assessment

1. Elicit history of diet (high intake of smoked or cured foods and low intake of fruits and vegetables).
2. Identify weight loss and amount.
3. Obtain cigarette smoking history; how many a day, how long has patient been smoking, any stomach discomfort during or after smoking?
4. History of alcohol intake; how much?
5. Obtain family history of cancer.
6. Obtain patient's marital status (someone to provide emotional and financial support?).

Physical Examination

1. Possible palpation of mass.
2. Observe for presence of ascites.
3. Examine other organs for tenderness or masses.

Major Nursing Diagnosis

1. Anxiety related to the disease and anticipated treatment.
2. Altered nutrition, less than body requirements, related to anorexia.
3. Pain related to the presence of abnormal epithelial cells.
4. Anticipatory grieving related to the diagnosis of cancer.
5. Knowledge deficit regarding self-care activities.

Planning and Implementation

The major goals may include reduction of anxiety, attainment of optimum nutrition, relief of pain, and adjustment to the diagnosis and to anticipated lifestyle changes.

Interventions

REDUCING ANXIETY

1. Provide a relaxed, nonthreatening atmosphere so patient can express fears, concerns, and possibly anger.
2. Encourage family in efforts to support the patient, offering assurance and supporting positive coping measures.
3. Advise about any procedures and treatments; suggest patient discuss feelings with support person, e.g., clergy, if desired.

PROMOTING OPTIMAL NUTRITION

1. Encourage small, frequent feedings of nonirritating foods to decrease gastric irritation.
2. Facilitate tissue repair by assuring food supplements high in calories and vitamins A, C, and iron.
3. Administer parenteral vitamin B_{12} indefinitely if a total gastrectomy is performed.
4. Monitor the rate and frequency of intravenous therapy.
5. Record intake, output, and daily weights.

6. Assess signs of dehydration (thirst, dry mucous membranes, poor skin turgor, tachycardia).
7. Review results of daily laboratory studies to note any metabolic abnormalities (sodium, potassium, glucose, blood urea nitrogen).
8. Administer antiemetics as prescribed.

RELIEVING PAIN

1. Administer analgesics as prescribed (continuous infusion of a narcotic).
2. Assess frequency, intensity, and duration of pain to determine effectiveness of analgesic.
3. Work with patient to help manage pain (e.g., position changes, decreased environmental stimuli, restricted visiting).
4. Suggest nonpharmacologic methods for pain relief (i.e., imagery, distraction, relaxation tapes, back rubs and massage).
5. Encourage periods of rest and relaxation.

PROVIDING PSYCHOSOCIAL SUPPORT

1. Help patient express fears and concerns about the diagnosis.
2. Allow patient freedom to grieve; answer patient's questions honestly.
3. Encourage to participate in treatment decisions.
4. Support patient's disbelief and time needed to accept diagnosis.
5. Offer emotional support and involve family members and significant others whenever possible; reassure that emotional responses are normal and expected.
6. Be aware of mood swings and defense mechanisms (denial, rationalization, displacement, regression).
7. Provide professional services as necessary (i.e., clergy, psychiatric clinical nurse specialists, psychologists, social workers, and psychiatrists).

PATIENT EDUCATION AND HEALTH MAINTENANCE: CARE IN THE HOME AND COMMUNITY

1. Advise patient it may take 6 months before regular meals can be eaten after a partial gastric resection.
2. Explain the possibility of dumping syndrome exists with any enteral feeding, and teach ways to manage it.
3. Explain to the patient necessity of daily periods of rest and frequent visits to physician after discharge.
4. Give patient information concerning chemotherapy and radiation therapy: length of treatments, expected reactions (nausea, vomiting, anorexia, fatigue).
5. Start nutritional counseling in the hospital and reinforce at home.
6. Supervise any enteral or parenteral feeding by visiting nurse who teaches patient and family members how to use equipment and formulas as well as how to detect complications.
7. Teach patient to record daily intake, output, and weight.
8. Educate patient how to cope with pain, nausea, vomiting, and bloating.
9. Teach patient to recognize and report those complications that require medical attention, such as bleeding (overt or covert hematemesis, melena), obstruction, perforation, or any symptoms that become consistently worse.
10. Teach patient how to care for the incision and how to examine the wound for signs of infection.
11. Explain chemotherapy/radiation regimen and the care needed during and after treatments.

For more information see Chapter 36 in Smeltzer and Bare: *Brunner and Suddarth's Textbook of Medical–Surgical Nursing,* 8th Edition. Philadelphia: Lippincott–Raven, 1996.

CANCER OF THE TESTIS

C

Testicular cancer ranks first in cancer deaths among men in the 20–35-year age group. Such cancers are classified as germinal or nongerminal. Most neoplasms are germinal, arising from the germinal cells of the testes (seminomas, teratocarcinomas, and embryonal carcinomas). Nongerminal tumors arise from the epithelium. The cause of testicular tumors is unknown but cryptorchidism, infections, and genetic and endocrine factors appear to play a part in their development. Testicular tumors are usually malignant and tend to metastasize early, spreading from the testicles to the lymph nodes in the retroperitoneum and to the lungs.

CLINICAL MANIFESTATIONS

1. Symptoms appear very gradually with a mass or lump on the testicle. Testicular self-examination is an effective early detection method.
2. Painless enlargement of the testis, may complain of heaviness in the scrotum, inguinal area, or lower abdomen.
3. Backache, pain in the abdomen, loss of weight, and general weakness may result from metastasis.

DIAGNOSTIC EVALUATION

1. The enlargement of the testis without pain is a significant finding.
2. Elevated alpha-fetoprotein and human chorionic gonadotropin (tumor markers).
3. Tumor marker levels are used for diagnosis, staging, and monitoring the response to treatment.

MANAGEMENT

The goals of management are to eradicate the disease and achieve a cure. Treatment selection is based on cell type and anatomic extent of the disease.

1. Orchiectomy and retroperitoneal lymph node dissection (RPLND).
2. Sperm banking may be considered.
3. Postoperative irradiation of the lymph nodes from the iliac region to the diaphragm is used in treating seminomas.
4. Multiple chemotherapy: good results may be obtained by combining different types of treatments, including surgery, radiation therapy, and chemotherapy.

✎ PATIENT EDUCATION AND HEALTH MAINTENANCE: CARE IN THE HOME AND COMMUNITY

1. Address issues related to body image and sexuality.
2. Give encouragement to maintain a positive attitude during course of therapy.
3. Teach patient radiation therapy will not necessarily cause infertility, nor does unilateral excision of a tumor necessarily decrease virility.
4. Highly encourage follow-up evaluation as a patient with a history of one tumor of the testis has a greater chance of developing subsequent tumors.

For more information see Chapter 47 in Smeltzer and Bare: *Brunner and Suddarth's Textbook of Medical–Surgical Nursing,* 8th Edition. Philadelphia: Lippincott–Raven, 1996.

CANCER OF THE THYROID

Cancer of the thyroid is less prevalent than other forms of cancer. The most common type, papillary adenocarcinoma, accounts for over half of thyroid malignancies. This starts in childhood or early adult life, remains localized, and eventually metastasizes. If papillary adenocarcinoma occurs in the elderly, it is more aggressive. Risks include external radiation of the head, neck, or chest in infancy and childhood; familial history of thyroid cancer. Follicular adenocarcinoma appears usually over age 40.

It is encapsulated and feels elastic or rubbery on palpation. This tumor eventually spreads by hematogenous routes to bone, liver, and lung. Prognosis is not as favorable as for papillary adenocarcinoma.

Lesions that are single, hard, and fixed on palpation suggest malignancy. Other less common types of cancer are medullary and anaplastic. These tumors have an extremely poor prognosis.

DIAGNOSTIC EVALUATION

1. Needle biopsy of the thyroid gland.
2. Ultrasound, MRI, CT scans, thyroid scans, radioactive iodine uptake studies, and thyroid suppression tests.

MANAGEMENT

1. Treatment of choice is surgical removal (total or near total thyroidectomy).
2. Modified or extensive radical neck dissection if lymph node involvement.
3. ^{131}I to eradicate residual thyroid tissue.
4. Thyroid hormone is administered in suppressive doses following surgery to lower the levels of TSH to a euthyroid state.
5. Thyroxine required permanently if remaining thyroid tissue is inadequate to produce sufficient hormone.
6. Radiation therapy is administered by several routes.
7. Chemotherapy is used only occasionally.

✎ PATIENT EDUCATION AND HEALTH MAINTENANCE: CARE IN THE HOME AND COMMUNITY

1. Provide instructions about the need to take exogenous thyroid hormone.
2. Encourage follow-up for recurrence of cancer. Total body scans annually for 3 postoperative years, less frequently thereafter. Prior to planned total body scans, stop thyroid hormones for 1 month.

3. Monitor T_4, TSH, serum calcium, and phosphorus levels to determine if thyroid supplementation is adequate and maintain calcium balance.
4. Surgery combined with radioiodine produces a higher survival rate than surgery alone.
5. Instruct in assessment and management of side effects of radiation therapy.

For more information see Chapter 40 in Smeltzer and Bare: *Brunner and Suddarth's Textbook of Medical–Surgical Nursing,* 8th Edition. Philadelphia: Lippincott–Raven, 1996.

CANCER OF THE VAGINA

Cancer of the vagina usually results from metastasized choriocarcinoma or from cancer of the cervix or adjacent organs, such as the uterus, vulva, bladder, or rectum. Primary cancer of the vagina is uncommon. Risk factors include cervical cancer, in utero exposure to diethylstilbestrol (DES), previous vaginal or vulvar cancer, previous radiation therapy, history of human papillomavirus (HPV) or of pessary use.

CLINICAL MANIFESTATIONS

Spontaneous bleeding, vaginal discharge, pain, urinary and/or rectal symptoms.

MANAGEMENT

Laser treatment, surgery, and radiation therapy, depending on the extent of the disease.

NURSING PROCESS

Interventions

1. Encourage close cooperation with health care personnel.
2. Provide emotional support.

3. Specific vaginal dilating procedures may be initiated for those who have had vaginal reconstructive surgery.
4. Inform patient that water-soluble lubricants are helpful in reducing dyspareunia.
5. Assist patient to explore all aspects and effects of radiation therapy, chemotherapy, or surgery on an individual basis.
6. Provide education on early detection of vaginal and vulvar cancer.

For more information see Chapter 45 in Smeltzer and Bare: *Brunner and Suddarth's Textbook of Medical–Surgical Nursing,* 8th Edition. Philadelphia: Lippincott–Raven, 1996.

CANCER OF THE VULVA

Primary cancer of the vulva is seen mostly in post-menopausal women; its incidence in younger women is rising. More whites than nonwhites are afflicted. Squamous cell carcinoma accounts for most primary vulvar tumors. Little is known about what causes this disease. The median age for cancer limited to the vulva is 44 years; median age for invasive vulvar cancer is 61 years. Risk factors are hypertension, obesity, and diabetes.

CLINICAL MANIFESTATIONS

1. Longstanding pruritus is the most common symptom.
2. Bleeding, foul-smelling discharge, and pain are signs of advanced disease.
3. Early lesions appear as chronic dermatitis; later a lump that continues to grow and becomes a hard, ulcerated cauliflower-like growth.

DIAGNOSTIC EVALUATION

Biopsy.

MANAGEMENT

1. Preinvasive (vulvar carcinoma in situ): local excision, laser vaporization, chemotherapeutic creams (fluorouracil), or cryosurgery.
2. Invasive: wide excision or vulvectomy (primary treatment), radiation (unresectable tumors), pelvic exenteration.

NURSING PROCESS FOR THE PATIENT UNDERGOING A VULVECTOMY

Assessment

1. Develop a rapport between patient and nurse; ascertain health habits and receptivity for learning.
2. Give preoperative preparation and psychological encouragement.

Major Nursing Diagnosis

1. Anxiety related to the diagnosis and surgery.
2. Alteration in skin integrity related to wound drainage.
3. Pain related to surgical incision and subsequent wound care.
4. Sexual dysfunction related to change in body part.

Collaborative Problems

1. Wound infection and sepsis.
2. Deep vein thrombosis.
3. Hemorrhage.

Planning and Implementation

The major goals may include acceptance of and preparation for surgical intervention, recovery of optimal sexual function, ability to perform adequate and appropriate self-care, and prevention of complications.

Nursing Interventions: Preoperative

RELIEVING ANXIETY

1. Allow patient time to talk and ask questions.
2. Advise patient that the possibility of having sexual relations is good and pregnancy is possible after a simple vulvectomy.

Nursing Interventions: Postoperative

RELIEVING PAIN AND DISCOMFORT

1. Administer analgesics.
2. Position patient to relieve tension on incision and give soothing back rubs.

IMPROVING SKIN INTEGRITY

1. Provide air mattress or egg crate pad.
2. Install overbed trapeze.
3. Protect intact skin from drainage and moisture.
4. Assess and document surgical site characteristics and drainage.

SUPPORTING POSITIVE SEXUALITY AND SEXUAL FUNCTION

1. Establish a trusting nurse–patient relationship.
2. Encourage patient to share and discuss concerns with sexual partner.

MONITORING AND MANAGING COMPLICATIONS

1. Monitor closely for local and systemic signs and symptoms of infection: purulent drainage, redness, increased pain, fever, increased white blood cell count.
2. Assist in obtaining tissue specimens for culture.
3. Administer antibiotics as prescribed.
4. Avoid cross-contamination; carefully handle catheters, drains, and dressings.
5. Provide a low-residue diet to prevent straining on defecation and wound contamination.
6. Discourage sitz bath because of risk of infection.

7. Assess for signs and symptoms of deep vein thrombosis and pulmonary embolism; apply elastic antiembolism stockings.
8. Monitor closely for signs of hemorrhage and hypovolemic shock.

PATIENT EDUCATION AND HEALTH MAINTENANCE: CARE IN THE HOME AND COMMUNITY

1. Encourage to share concerns as patient recovers.
2. Encourage participation in dressing changes and cleansing self.
3. Give complete instructions to family member or other who will provide posthospital care.
4. Encourage communication with home care nurse to ensure continuity of care.

For more information see Chapter 45 in Smeltzer and Bare: *Brunner and Suddarth's Textbook of Medical–Surgical Nursing*, 8th Edition. Philadelphia: Lippincott–Raven, 1996.

CARDIAC ARREST

Cardiac arrest occurs when the heart suddenly stops beating, resulting in the cessation of effective circulation. All heart action may stop, or asynchronized muscular twitchings (ventricular fibrillation) may occur. There is an immediate loss of consciousness and absence of pulses and audible heart sounds. Dilation of the pupils begins within 45 seconds. Seizures may or may not occur.

CLINICAL MANIFESTATIONS

There is an interval of approximately 4 minutes between cessation of circulation and development of irreversible brain damage. Interval varies with age of the patient. During this period, the diagnosis of cardiac arrest must be made and circulation restored. The most reliable sign of arrest is the absence of a carotid pulsation.

MANAGEMENT

1. Initiate immediate cardiopulmonary resuscitation.
2. Follow-up monitoring once the patient is successfully resuscitated.

For more information see Chapter 28 in Smeltzer and Bare:
*Brunner and Suddarth's Textbook of Medical–Surgical
Nursing,* 8th Edition. Philadelphia: Lippincott–Raven, 1996.

CARDIAC FAILURE

Cardiac failure (congestive heart failure) is the inability
of the heart to pump sufficient blood to meet the needs
of the tissues for oxygen and nutrients. The term *congestive heart failure* is most commonly used when refer-
ring to left-sided and right-sided failure.

The underlying mechanism of cardiac failure involves
impairment of the contractile properties of the heart,
which leads to a lower-than-normal cardiac output. Common underlying conditions include coronary atherosclerosis, arterial hypertension, and inflammatory or
degenerative muscle disease.

A number of systemic factors can contribute to the
development and severity of heart failure. Increased
metabolic rate (e.g., fever, coma, thyrotoxicosis),
hypoxia, and anemia require an increased cardiac output to satisfy systemic oxygen demand.

CLINICAL MANIFESTATIONS

1. Increased intravascular volume (dominant feature).
2. Congestion of tissues.
3. Increased pulmonary venous pressure (pulmonary
   edema) manifested by cough and shortness of
   breath.
4. Increased systemic venous pressure as evidenced in
   generalized peripheral edema and weight gain.

5. Diminished cardiac output with accompanying dizziness, confusion, fatigue, exercise or heat intolerance, cool extremities, and oliguria.

LEFT-SIDED CARDIAC FAILURE

1. Most often precedes right-sided cardiac failure.
2. Pulmonary congestion; dyspnea, cough, fatigability; tachycardia with an S_3 heart sound, anxiety, restlessness.
3. Orthopnea and/or proximal nocturnal dyspnea (PND).
4. Cough may be dry and nonproductive, but is most often moist.
5. Large quantities of frothy sputum, which is sometimes blood-tinged, may be produced.

RIGHT-SIDED CARDIAC FAILURE

1. Congestion of the viscera and peripheral tissues is predominant.
2. Edema of the lower extremities (dependent edema), usually pitting edema, weight gain, hepatomegaly.
3. Distended neck veins, ascites, anorexia, and nausea.
4. Nocturia and weakness.

DIAGNOSTIC EVALUATION

Evaluation of the clinical manifestations and hemodynamic monitoring.

MANAGEMENT

The goals of treatment are to promote rest to reduce workload; increase the force and efficiency of myocardial contractions with pharmacologic agents; and eliminate the excessive accumulation of body water by means of diuretic therapy, diet, and rest.

Pharmacologic Therapy

1. Cardiac glycosides.
2. Diuretic therapy.
3. Vasodilator therapy.

Dietary Support

Sodium restriction to prevent, control, or eliminate edema.

NURSING PROCESS

Assessment

The focus of the nursing assessment for the patient with cardiac failure is directed toward observing for signs and symptoms of pulmonary and systemic fluid overload. All untoward signs are recorded and reported.

1. Respiratory: auscultate at frequent intervals to determine presence or absence of crackles and wheezes. Note rate and depth of respirations.
2. Cardiac: auscultate for the presence of an S_3 or S_4 heart sound, may mean pump is beginning to fail.
3. Sensorium/level of consciousness.
4. Periphery: assess dependent parts of the patient's body for edema and the liver for hepatojugular reflux (HJR) and jugular vein distention (JVD).
5. Urinary output: measure frequently.

Major Nursing Diagnosis

1. Activity intolerance related to fatigue and dyspnea secondary to decreased cardiac output.
2. Anxiety related to breathlessness and restlessness secondary to inadequate oxygenation.
3. Altered peripheral tissue perfusion related to venostasis.
4. Knowledge deficit of self-care program related to nonacceptance of necessary lifestyle changes.

Collaborative Problems

1. Phlebothrombosis.
2. Pulmonary embolism.
3. Cardiogenic shock.

Planning and Implementation

The major goals may include promotion of rest, relief of anxiety, attainment of normal tissue perfusion, and knowledge of self-care program.

Interventions

POSITIONING

1. Elevate head of bed on 20–30 cm (8–10 inch) blocks or place patient in a comfortable armchair.
2. Support lower arms with pillows to eliminate fatigue.

RELIEVING ANXIETY

1. Raise the head of the bed and keep a night light on.
2. Provide for the presence of a family member for reassurance.
3. Administer oxygen during the acute stage.

ADMINISTERING MEDICATIONS WITH CAUTION

1. Note that patients with hepatic congestion are unable to detoxify drugs within a normal time frame.
2. Assess for digitalis toxicity (i.e., anorexia, nausea, and vomiting, which are early effects).
3. Diuretics should be administered in the early morning; observe for side effects, i.e., hyponatremia, hypokalemia.
4. Vasodilator therapy (sodium nitroprusside); monitor pulmonary artery pressures and cardiac output.

AVOIDING STRESS

Promote physical comfort and avoid situations that tend to cause anxiety and agitation.

PROMOTING NORMAL TISSUE PERFUSION

1. Encourage moderate daily exercise to enhance blood flow to peripheral tissues.
2. Provide for adequate oxygenation and appropriate diuresis.
3. Promote adequate rest (physical and emotional).

✎ **PATIENT EDUCATION AND HEALTH MAINTENANCE: CARE IN THE HOME AND COMMUNITY**

C

1. Plan activities of daily living to minimize breathlessness and fatigue.
2. Teach patient to live within the limits of the cardiac reserve, i.e., obtain adequate rest, take prescribed medications on time, and understand side effects and precautions.
3. Limit sodium as directed; avoid straying from dietary restrictions.
4. Review activity program with patient, i.e., any activity that produces symptoms must be curtailed.
5. Encourage adequate medical follow-up.
6. Teach patient to avoid noxious agents that may contribute to cardiac failure, e.g., coffee, tobacco, unregulated or excessive exercise.

For more information see Chapter 28 in Smeltzer and Bare: *Brunner and Suddarth's Textbook of Medical–Surgical Nursing,* 8th Edition. Philadelphia: Lippincott–Raven, 1996.

CARDIAC TAMPONADE

Cardiac tamponade is a life-threatening compression of the heart as a result of fluid within the pericardial sac. It is usually caused by blunt or penetrating trauma to the chest; may also follow invasive diagnostic cardiac procedures, certain disease processes, and high-dose radiation to the chest.

CLINICAL MANIFESTATIONS

1. Falling blood pressure, rising venous pressure (distended neck veins), and distant (muffled) heart sounds.
2. Pulsus paradoxus.
3. Anxious, confused, and restless.

4. Dyspnea, tachypnea, and precordial pain.
5. Central venous pressure (CVP) elevated.

MANAGEMENT

1. Thoracotomy for penetrating cardiac injuries.
2. Pericardiocentesis.

For more information see Chapter 28 in Smeltzer and Bare: *Brunner and Suddarth's Textbook of Medical–Surgical Nursing,* 8th Edition. Philadelphia: Lippincott–Raven, 1996.

CARDIOGENIC SHOCK

See Shock, Cardiogenic

CARDIOMYOPATHIES

Myopathy is a disease of muscle. The cardiomyopathies are a group of diseases that affect the structure and function of the myocardium. Cardiomyopathies are categorized by pathologic, physiologic, and clinical signs. They are defined as (1) dilated or congestive cardiomyopathy; (2) hypertrophic cardiomyopathy; (3) restrictive cardiomyopathy. These diseases lead to severe heart failure and often death. Cardiomyopathy is a series of progressive events that culminates in impaired pumping of the left ventricle. It enlarges to accommodate the demands and eventually fails. Failure of the right ventricle usually accompanies this process.

CLINICAL MANIFESTATIONS

1. May occur at any age and affects both men and women.
2. Present initially with signs and symptoms of heart failure.

3. Dyspnea on exertion, proximal nocturnal dyspnea (PND), cough, and easy fatigability are early symptoms.
4. Systemic venous congestion, jugular vein distention, pitting edema of dependent body parts, hepatic engorgement, and tachycardia with physical examination.

DIAGNOSTIC EVALUATION

1. Patient history and ruling out other causes of failure.
2. ECG, echocardiogram, and cardiac catheterization.

MANAGEMENT

Medical management is directed toward correcting the heart failure. When heart failure has progressed beyond being medically responsive, heart transplant is the patient's only hope for survival. In some cases, ventricular assist devices are necessary to support the failing heart until a suitable donor becomes available.

NURSING PROCESS

Assessment

1. Take detailed history of presenting signs and symptoms.
2. Careful psychosocial history: identify family support system and involve in patient management.
3. Physical assessment directed toward signs and symptoms of congestive heart failure. Evaluate fluid volume status, vital signs (pulse pressure), and auscultation for an S_3.
4. Use cardiac monitor if dysrhythmia is a significant problem.

Major Nursing Diagnosis

1. Potential ineffective breathing pattern related to myocardial failure.
2. Activity intolerance related to excessive fluid volume.

3. Anxiety related to the disease process.
4. Potential noncompliance with the self-care program.

Collaborative Problems

Cardiac failure.

Planning and Implementation

The major goals include absence of respiratory difficulties, increased activity tolerance, reduction of anxiety, and compliance with the self-care program.

Interventions

RELIEVING RESPIRATORY DIFFICULTIES

1. Administer prescribed medications on time.
2. Document patient's response carefully.
3. Administer oxygen per nasal cannula as indicated.
4. Allow patient to rest at the bedside in a chair for most comfort.
5. Keep patient warm and change positions frequently to stimulate circulation and reduce skin breakdown.
6. Maintain environment free of dust, lint, flowers, and perfumes.

INCREASING ACTIVITY TOLERANCE

1. Plan nursing care so that activities are of short duration.
2. Avoid activities that deplete the patient's energy.

REDUCING ANXIETY

1. Provide the patient with appropriate information about signs and symptoms.
2. Provide an atmosphere in which the patient feels free to verbalize fears.
3. Provide time for the patient to discuss concerns if facing death or awaiting transplant surgery.
4. Give spiritual, psychological, and emotional support.

PATIENT EDUCATION AND HEALTH MAINTENANCE: CARE IN THE HOME AND COMMUNITY

C

1. Teach patient what self-care activities are necessary and how to perform them at home.
2. Maintain attention to a medication program to prevent cardiac failure.
3. Assist in review of lifestyle and work to incorporate therapeutic activities.
4. Establish trust with patient and provide realistic hope to reduce anxiety while awaiting a donor heart.
5. Allow patient and significant others the freedom to begin the grieving process when they can no longer be helped by any therapeutic technique.

For more information see Chapter 29 in Smeltzer and Bare: *Brunner and Suddarth's Textbook of Medical–Surgical Nursing,* 8th Edition. Philadelphia: Lippincott–Raven, 1996.

CATARACTS

A cataract is an opacification of the normally clear, transparent crystalline lens. It is usually a result of aging but may be present at birth. It may also be associated with blunt or penetrating trauma, long-term corticosteroid use, systemic disease such as diabetes mellitus, hypoparathyroidism, radiation exposure, exposure to long hours or bright sunlight (ultraviolet light), or other eye disorders.

CLINICAL MANIFESTATIONS

1. Diminished visual acuity, disabling glare, dimmed or blurred vision with distortion of images, poor night vision.
2. The pupil may appear yellowish, gray, or white; develops gradually over a period of years, and as

the cataract worsens, stronger glasses no longer improve sight.

DIAGNOSTIC EVALUATION

Primarily by subjective symptoms.
1. Usual eye tests.
2. Keratometry.
3. Slit-lamp and ophthalmic examination.
4. A-scan ultrasound.
5. Endothelial cell counter.

MANAGEMENT

There is no medical treatment for cataracts, although two surgical techniques are available: intracapsular cataract extraction (ICCE) and extracapsular cataract extraction (ECCE).

1. Indications for surgery are loss of vision that interferes with normal activities or a cataract that is causing glaucoma.
2. Cataracts are removed under local anesthesia on an outpatient basis.
3. Severe visual loss and eventual blindness will occur unless surgery is performed.

✎ PATIENT EDUCATION AND HEALTH MAINTENANCE: CARE IN THE HOME AND COMMUNITY

1. Provide postoperative discharge teaching concerning eye medications, cleansing and protection, activity level and restrictions, diet, pain control, positioning, office appointments, expected postoperative course, and symptoms to report immediately to the surgeon.
2. Instruct patient to make arrangements for transportation home, care during that evening, and a follow-up visit to the surgeon the next day.
3. Restrict bending and lifting heavy objects.
4. Instruct to wear eye shield at night and eyeglasses

(sunglasses in bright light) during the day for 2 weeks.

For more information see Chapter 56 in Smeltzer and Bare: *Brunner and Suddarth's Textbook of Medical–Surgical Nursing*, 8th Edition. Philadelphia: Lippincott–Raven, 1996.

CEREBRAL ANEURYSM

See Aneurysm, Intracranial

CEREBRAL VASCULAR ACCIDENT (CVA)(STROKE)

A stroke is a sudden loss of brain function resulting from a disruption of the blood supply to a part of the brain. Stroke is the primary neurologic problem in the United States and in the world. Causes of strokes are usually one of four events: (1) thrombosis, (2) cerebral embolism, (3) ischemia, (4) cerebral hemorrhage. The result is an interruption in the blood supply to the brain, causing temporary or permanent loss of movement, thought, memory, speech, or sensation.

RISK FACTORS AND PREVENTION

1. Hypertension is the major risk factor.
2. Cardiovascular disease (cerebral embolism may originate in the heart).
3. High normal hematocrit level (related to cerebral infarction).
4. Diabetes (accelerated atherogenesis).
5. Oral contraceptives, enhanced by coexisting hypertension, age over 35 years, cigarette smoking, and high estrogen levels.
6. Excessive or prolonged fall of blood pressure may cause general cerebral ischemia.

7. Drug abuse, particularly in adolescents and young adults.
8. Counsel younger persons to control blood lipids (cholesterol), blood pressure, cigarette smoking, and obesity.
9. There may be a link between alcohol consumption and stroke.

CLINICAL MANIFESTATIONS

Motor Loss

1. Hemiplegia, hemiparesis.
2. Flaccid paralysis and loss or decrease in the deep tendon reflexes (initial clinical feature).

Communication Loss

1. Dysarthria.
2. Dysphasia or aphasia.
3. Apraxia.

Perceptual Disturbances

1. Homonymous hemianopia (loss of half of the visual field).
2. Disturbances in visual-spatial relationships (frequently seen in patients with left hemiplegia).
3. Sensory losses: slight impairment of touch or more severe with loss of proprioception, difficulty in interrupting visual, tactile, and auditory stimuli.

Impairment of Mental Activity and Psychological Effects

1. Frontal lobe damage: learning capacity, memory, or other higher cortical intellectual functions may be impaired. Such dysfunction may be reflected in a limited attention span, difficulties in comprehension, forgetfulness, and lack of motivation.
2. Depression, other psychological problems: emotional liability, hostility, frustration, resentment, and lack of cooperation.

Bladder Dysfunction

1. Transient urinary incontinence.
2. Persistent urinary incontinence or urinary retention (may be symptomatic of bilateral brain damage).
3. Continuing bladder and bowel incontinence (may reflect extensive neurologic damage).

MANAGEMENT OF THE ACUTE PHASE OF A PATIENT WITH STROKE

1. The acute phase usually lasts 48 to 72 hours.
2. Maintain the airway and adequate ventilation.
3. Place patient in a lateral or semiprone position with head of bed slightly elevated.
4. Endotracheal intubation and mechanical ventilation.
5. Monitor for pulmonary complications (aspiration, atelectasis, pneumonia).
6. Examine heart for abnormalities in size, rhythm, and signs of congestive heart failure.

Medical Management

1. Diuretics.
2. Anticoagulants.
3. Antiplatelet drugs.

NURSING PROCESS

Assessment

Maintain a neurologic flow sheet to reflect the following nursing assessment parameters:

1. A change in the level of responsiveness.
2. Presence or absence of voluntary or involuntary movements of the extremities: muscle tone, body posture, and head position.
3. Stiffness or flaccidity of the neck.
4. Eye opening, comparative size of the pupils and pupillary reactions to light, and ocular position.
5. Color of the face and extremities; temperature and moisture of the skin.

6. Quality and rates of pulse and respiration; arterial blood gases, body temperature, and arterial pressure.
7. Ability to speak.
8. Volume of fluids ingested or administered and volume of urine excreted per 24 hours.
9. Orient to time and place at frequent intervals to reduce anxiety and offer reassurance when beginning to regain consciousness.

AFTER ACUTE PHASE

Assess the following functions:

1. Mental status (memory, attention span, perception, orientation, affect, speech/language).
2. Sensation/perception (usually patient has decreased awareness of pain and temperature).
3. Motor control (upper and lower extremity movement); bladder function.
4. Continue focusing nursing assessment on the impairment of function in the patient's daily activities.

Major Nursing Diagnosis

1. Impaired physical mobility related to hemiparesis, loss of balance and coordination, spasticity, and brain injury.
2. Self-care deficits (hygiene, toileting, transfers, feeding) related to stroke sequela.
3. Incontinence related to flaccid bladder, detrusor instability, confusion, difficulty in communicating.
4. Altered thought processes related to brain damage, confusion, inability to follow instruction.
5. Impaired verbal communication related to brain damage.
6. Altered family processes related to catastrophic illness and caregiving burdens.

Collaborative Problems

1. Decreased cerebral blood flow.
2. Inadequate oxygen delivery to the brain.

Planning and Implementation: Rehabilitation Phase

The major goals may include improvement of mobility, avoidance of shoulder pain, achievement of self-care, attainment of bladder control, improvement of thought processes, achievement of some form of communication, maintenance of skin integrity, restoration of family functioning, and absence of complications.

Interventions

MONITORING AND MANAGING POTENTIAL COMPLICATIONS

1. Assess vital signs and oxygenation status for adequate blood flow to the brain and tissues.
2. Improve respiratory gas exchange with supplemental oxygen, suctioning, and chest physiotherapy.
3. Maintain adequate cardiac output by medications and fluid administration.

IMPROVING MOBILITY AND PREVENTING DEFORMITIES

1. Position to prevent contractures; use measures to relieve pressure, assist in maintaining good body alignment, prevent compressive neuropathies.
2. Keep patient flat in bed except when engaged in activities of daily living (ADL).
3. Prevent foot drop and heel cords from shortening by using a foot board at intervals during the flaccid period.
4. Use a bed cradle to keep bedding off extremities as soon as spasticity develops.
5. Apply a posterior splint at night to prevent flexion of the affected extremity.
6. Prevent external rotation of hip joint with a trochanter roll.
7. Prevent adduction of the affected shoulder with a pillow placed in the axilla.
8. Elevate the affected arm to prevent edema and fibrosis.
9. Position fingers so they are barely flexed; place hand in slight supination.

10. Use a volar resting splint to support the wrist and hand.
11. Change position every 2 hours; place patient in a prone position for 15–30 minutes several times a day.

RETRAINING THE AFFECTED EXTREMITIES

1. Exercise: provide full range of motion four or five times a day to maintain joint mobility and prevent contracture.
2. Observe for signs of shortness of breath, chest pain, cyanosis, and increasing pulse rate during the exercise period.

PREPARING FOR AMBULATION

1. Start an active rehabilitation program when consciousness returns.
2. Assist patient in learning to maintain balance in a sitting position before learning to balance in standing position.
3. Begin patient walking as soon as standing balance is achieved.
4. Keep training periods for ambulation short and frequent.

ACHIEVING SELF-CARE

1. Encourage patient to assist in personal hygiene.
2. Help to set realistic goals and add a new task daily.
3. Encourage to carry out all self-care activities on the unaffected side as the first step of setting goals.
4. Make sure patient does not neglect affected side.
5. Improve morale by making sure patient is fully dressed during ambulatory activities.
6. Assist with dressing activities, e.g., clothing fitted with Velcro closures; put garment on the affected side first.
7. Give emotional support to prevent overfatigue and discouragement.

ATTAINING BLADDER CONTROL

Analyze voiding pattern and offer urinal/bedpan on this schedule.

IMPROVING THOUGHT PROCESSES

1. Structure a training program using cognitive-perceptual retraining, visual imagery, reality orientation, and cueing procedures to compensate for losses.
2. Give positive feedback, and convey an attitude of confidence and hopefulness.

ACHIEVING COMMUNICATION

1. Tailor an individualized program.
2. Establish goals and expect the patient to take an active part.
3. Make the atmosphere conducive to communication.
4. Lend strong moral support and understanding to ally anxiety.
5. Be consistent in schedule, routines, and repetitions.
6. Surround patient with familiar objects and caring people.
7. Maintain the patient's attention, speak slowly, and give one instruction at a time; allow patient time to process.

IMPROVING FAMILY COPING THROUGH HEALTH TEACHING

1. Provide counseling and support to family.
2. Ease the burden of the family in providing continuous 24-hour care with respite care and/or adult day care center.
3. Involve others in the patient's care, stress management techniques, and maintenance of personal health for family coping.
4. Give family information about the expected outcome of the stroke and counsel them to avoid doing things that the patient can do.
5. Develop attainable goals for the patient at home by involving the total health care team, patient, and family.

6. Explain to the family that emotional lability usually improves with time.

REGAINING SEXUAL FUNCTION

Encourage sexual counseling about alternative approaches to sexual expression.

 ## PATIENT EDUCATION AND HEALTH MAINTENANCE: CARE IN THE HOME AND COMMUNITY

Planning Care

Advise patient and family that rehabilitation may be prolonged, requiring patience and perseverance.

Emotional Aspects

1. Provide a speech therapist to come to the home and allow the family to be involved and give them practical instructions to help the patient between speech therapy sessions.
2. Advise family that the patient will tire easily, will become irritable and upset by small events, and is likely to show less interest in things.
3. Discuss patient's depression with the physician in relation to antidepressant therapy.
4. Encourage family to support the patient and give positive reinforcement.

Home Modifications

Have occupational therapist make a home assessment and recommendations to help the patient become more independent.

Supportive Resources

1. Encourage to attend community-based stroke clubs to give a feeling of belonging and fellowship with others.
2. Encourage to continue with hobbies, recreational and leisure interests, and contact with friends to prevent social isolation.

✪ Gerontologic Considerations

Do not let patient's age be a reason for failure to initiate a full rehabilitation program.

For more information see Chapter 59 in Smeltzer and Bare: *Brunner and Suddarth's Textbook of Medical–Surgical Nursing,* 8th Edition. Philadelphia: Lippincott–Raven, 1996.

CERVICAL CANCER

See Cancer of the Cervix

CHEST PAIN

See Angina Pectoris

CHF

See Cardiac Failure

CHOLECYSTITIS

The gallbladder may be the site of an acute infection causing pain, tenderness, and rigidity of the upper right abdomen; cholecystitis is associated with nausea and vomiting. Most patients with acute cholecystitis have calculous cholecystitis (i.e., gallbladder stones obstructing bile outflow). Acalculous cholecystitis describes gallbladder inflammation in the absence of obstruction by gallstones. It occurs after major surgical procedures, severe trauma, or burns.

For more information see Chapter 38 in Smeltzer and Bare: *Brunner and Suddarth's Textbook of Medical–Surgical Nursing,* 8th Edition. Philadelphia: Lippincott–Raven, 1996.

CHOLELITHIASIS

Cholelithiasis (calculi or gallstones) usually form in the gallbladder from solid constituents of bile and vary greatly in size, shape, and composition. There are two major types of gallstones: pigment stones, which contain an excess of unconjugated pigments in the bile, and cholesterol stones, which are the most common. Risk factors for pigment stones include cirrhosis, hemolysis, and infections of the biliary tree. These stones cannot be dissolved and must be removed surgically. Risk factors for cholesterol stones include oral contraceptives, estrogens, and clofibrate. Women are four times more likely to develop cholesterol stones and gallbladder disease; usually over 40, multiparous, and obese.

CLINICAL MANIFESTATIONS

1. May be silent, producing no pain and only mild gastrointestinal symptoms.
2. May be acute or chronic with epigastric distress (fullness, abdominal distention, and vague upper right quadrant pain) following a high-fat meal.
3. If the cystic duct is obstructed, the gallbladder becomes distended and eventually infected; fever and palpable abdominal mass may be felt. Biliary colic with excruciating upper right abdominal pain, radiating to back or right shoulder, nausea and vomiting several hours after a heavy meal.
4. Jaundice occurs with obstruction of the common bile duct.
5. Very dark urine; clay-colored stool.
6. Vitamin deficiencies of A, D, E, and K (fat-soluble vitamins).
7. Abscess, necrosis, and perforation with peritonitis may result if the gallstone continues to obstruct the duct.

DIAGNOSTIC EVALUATION

1. Abdominal x-ray, ultrasonography, radionuclide imaging, or cholescintography.
2. Endoscopic retrograde cholangiopancreatography (ERCP).
3. Percutaneous transhepatic cholangiography (PTC).

NONSURGICAL MANAGEMENT

Major objectives of medical therapy are to reduce the incidence of acute attacks of gallbladder pain and cholecystitis by supportive and dietary management, and, if possible, to remove the cause by pharmacotherapy, endoscopic procedures, or surgical intervention.

1. Dissolve gallstones by infusion of a solvent into the gallbladder.
2. Remove stones through ERCP endoscope.

Supportive and Dietary Management

1. Achieve remission with rest, IV fluids, nasogastric (NG) suction, analgesia, and antibiotics.
2. Diet immediately after an attack is usually low-fat liquids.

Pharmacotherapy

1. Analgesics such as meperidine may be required; avoid the use of morphine as it increases spasm of the sphincter of Oddi.
2. Chenodeoxycholic acid (chenodiol or CDCA) is effective in dissolving primarily cholesterol stones.
3. Long-term follow-up and monitoring of liver enzymes are indicated.

Lithotripsy

1. Extracorporeal shock-wave lithotripsy: repeated shock waves directed at the gallstone located in the gallbladder or common bile duct to fragment the stones.

2. Intracorporeal shock-wave lithotripsy: stones may be fragmented by ultrasound, pulsed laser, or hydraulic lithotripsy applied through an endoscope directly to the stones.

SURGICAL MANAGEMENT

1. Cholecystectomy: gallbladder is removed after ligation of the cystic duct and artery.
2. Minicholecystectomy: gallbladder is removed through a 4 cm incision.
3. Laparoscopic cholecystectomy: performed through a small incision or puncture made through the abdominal wall in the umbilicus.

NURSING PROCESS FOR PATIENT UNDERGOING SURGERY FOR GALLBLADDER DISEASE

Assessment

1. Assess health history with focus on occurrence of abdominal pain and discomfort and factors precipitating discomfort.
2. Assess respiratory status.

Major Nursing Diagnosis

1. Pain and discomfort related to surgical incision.
2. Altered nutrition related to inadequate bile secretion.
3. Knowledge deficit about self-care activities after discharge.

Collaborative Problems

1. Bleeding.
2. Gastrointestinal symptoms.

Planning and Implementation

Goals include relief of pain, absence of respiratory complications, absence of complications of altered biliary drainage related to surgical intervention, improved nutritional intake, and understanding of self-care routines.

Postoperative Nursing Interventions

Provide water and other fluids and soft diet, after bowel sounds return.

RELIEVING PAIN

Administer analgesics as ordered.

IMPROVING RESPIRATORY STATUS

Teach patient to expand lungs fully to prevent atelectasis; promote early ambulation.

IMPROVING NUTRITIONAL STATUS

Advise patient at time of discharge to maintain a nutritious diet and avoid excessive fats; fat restriction is usually lifted in 4–6 weeks.

MONITORING AND MANAGING COMPLICATIONS

1. Bleeding: assess periodically for increased tenderness and rigidity of the abdomen and report; instruct patient and family to report change in color of stools.
2. Gastrointestinal symptoms: assess for loss of appetite, vomiting, pain, distention of the abdomen, and temperature elevation; report promptly.

✎ PATIENT EDUCATION AND HEALTH MAINTENANCE: CARE IN THE HOME AND COMMUNITY

1. Instruct patient in proper care of drainage tubes and to report to physician promptly changes in the amount or characteristics of drainage.
2. Instruct about which medications are required and their actions.
3. Instruct to report to the physician symptoms of jaundice, dark urine, pale-colored stools, pruritus or signs of inflammation and infection, i.e., pain or fever.

After laparoscopy procedure

1. Provide written and verbal instructions to patient and family about management of postoperative pain, and signs and symptoms of intra-abdominal complications that should be reported. These include loss of appetite, vomiting, pain, distention of abdomen, and temperature elevation.
2. Make arrangements for assistance at home during the first 24–48 hours because of drowsiness.

✪ GERONTOLOGIC CONSIDERATIONS

Surgical intervention for disease of the biliary tract is the most common operative procedure performed in the elderly.

Biliary disease may be accompanied or preceded by symptoms of septic shock: oliguria, hypotension, mental changes, tachycardia, and tachypnea.

Mortality from serious complications is high. Risk of complications and shorter hospital stays make it essential that older patients and their family members receive specific information about signs and symptoms of complications and measures to prevent them.

Cholecystectomy is usually well tolerated and low risk if expert assessment and care are provided before, during, and after surgery.

For more information see Chapter 38 in Smeltzer and Bare: *Brunner and Suddarth's Textbook of Medical–Surgical Nursing,* 8th Edition. Philadelphia: Lippincott–Raven, 1996.

CHROMOPHOBIC TUMORS

See Pituitary Tumors

C

CHRONIC BRONCHITIS

See Bronchitis, Chronic

CHRONIC GLOMERULONEPHRITIS

See Glomerulonephritis, Chronic

CHRONIC INTERSTITIAL NEPHRITIS

See Pyelonephritis, Chronic

CHRONIC LYMPHOCYTIC LEUKEMIA

See Leukemia, Lymphocytic, Chronic

CHRONIC MYELOGENOUS LEUKEMIA

See Leukemia, Myelogenous, Chronic

CHRONIC OBSTRUCTIVE PULMONARY DISEASE (COPD)

COPD is a broad classification of disorders, including chronic bronchitis, bronchiectasis, emphysema, and asthma. It is an irreversible condition associated with dyspnea on exertion and reduced airflow. Cigarette smoking, air pollution, and occupational exposure (coal, cotton, grain) are important risk factors that contribute to its development, which may occur over a 20- to 30-year span.

CLINICAL MANIFESTATIONS

See Asthma; Bronchiectasis; Bronchitis, Chronic; and Emphysema.

MANAGEMENT

See Asthma; Bronchiectasis; Bronchitis, Chronic; and Emphysema.

NURSING PROCESS

Assessment

OBTAIN A HISTORY ABOUT CURRENT RESPIRATORY SYMPTOMS AND PREVIOUS DISEASE MANIFESTATIONS

1. Duration of respiratory difficulty.
2. Dyspnea, shortness of breath, wheezing, exercise tolerance, fatigue.
3. Effect on eating and sleeping habits.

ADDITIONAL DATA OBTAINED THROUGH OBSERVATION AND EXAMINATION

1. Pulse, respiratory rate, and rhythm.
2. Contraction of abdominal muscles during inspiration.
3. Use of accessory muscles to breathe; prolonged expiration.
4. Cyanosis, neck vein engorgement.
5. Peripheral edema.
6. Cough, color, amount and consistency of sputum.
7. Status of patient's sensorium, increasing stupor, apprehension.

Major Nursing Diagnosis

1. Impaired gas exchange related to ventilation-perfusion inequality.
2. Ineffective airway clearance related to bronchial constriction, increased mucus production, ineffective cough, and bronchopulmonary infection.

3. Ineffective individual coping related to less socialization, anxiety, depression, lower activity level, and the inability to work.
4. Knowledge deficit of self-care procedures to be performed at home.

Collaborative Problems

1. Respiratory insufficiency/failure.
2. Atelectasis.
3. Pneumonia.
4. Pneumothorax.
5. Pulmonary hypertension.

Planning and Implementation

The major goals include improvement of gas exchange, achievement of airway clearance, improvement in coping ability, and adherence to therapeutic program and home care.

Interventions

IMPROVING GAS EXCHANGE

1. Monitor dyspnea and hypoxia.
2. Administer medications and be alert for potential side effects.
3. Monitor prescribed oxygen effectiveness, i.e., arterial blood gases (ABGs).

REMOVING BRONCHIAL SECRETIONS

1. Encourage high fluid intake to liquify secretions.
2. Provide small-volume nebulizer treatments.
3. Provide postural drainage.
4. Instruct in effective breathing techniques.

PREVENTING BRONCHOPULMONARY INFECTIONS

1. Instruct patient to report if sputum becomes discolored and/or any worsening of respiratory symptoms.
2. Instruct to avoid outdoor exposure when pollen count is high or significant air pollution; may increase bronchospasm.

3. Instruct to avoid high climate temperatures and humidity.
4. Encourage immunization against *Haemophilus influenzae* and *Streptococcus pneumoniae.*

BREATHING EXERCISES AND RETRAINING

Teach breathing techniques, including diaphragmatic, pursed-lip breathing, inspiratory muscle training, and energy conservation.

COPING MEASURES

1. Encourage the patient to remain active up to level of symptom tolerance.
2. Place emphasis on controlling symptoms and increasing self-esteem, sense of mastery and of well-being.
3. Direct patient to support groups.

✎ PATIENT EDUCATION AND HEALTH MAINTENANCE: CARE IN THE HOME AND COMMUNITYY

1. Educate patient about disease process, including health hazard of smoking.
2. Help to accept realistic short-term and long-range goals.
3. Increase exercise tolerance in milder disease process.
4. Preserve present pulmonary function and relieve symptoms as much as possible (severely disabled).
5. Instruct in proper use of oxygen and caution family about the dangers of increasing oxygen flow rate.
6. Reassure that oxygen is not "addicting" and explain precautions in using oxygen (no smoking).
7. Avoid stressful situations that might trigger a coughing episode or emotional disturbance.
8. Direct patient to community resources, i.e., pulmonary rehabilitation programs, smoking cessation programs, senior citizen social groups, and other programs to help improve coping skills.

Monitor and Manage Potential Complications

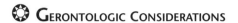

1. Teach patient and family to observe carefully for signs and symptoms of complications.
2. Emphasize if condition worsens to the point of acute respiratory failure that intubation and mechanical ventilation will be necessary.

✪ GERONTOLOGIC CONSIDERATIONS

COPD accentuates many of the physiologic changes associated with aging and is manifested in airway obstruction (in bronchitis) and excessive loss of elastic lung recoil (in emphysema). Additional changes in ventilation-perfusion ratios occur.

For more information see Chapter 24 in Smeltzer and Bare: *Brunner and Suddarth's Textbook of Medical–Surgical Nursing*, 8th Edition. Philadelphia: Lippincott–Raven, 1996.

CHRONIC OTITIS MEDIA

See Otitis Media, Chronic

CHRONIC PANCREATITIS

See Pancreatitis, Chronic

CHRONIC PHARYNGITIS

See Pharyngitis, Chronic

CHRONIC PRIMARY ADRENOCORTICOL INSUFFICIENCY (ADDISON'S DISEASE)

Addison's disease is caused by a deficiency of cortical hormones. It results when the adrenal cortex function is inadequate to meet the patient's need for cortical hormones. Autoimmune or idiopathic atrophy of the adrenal glands is responsible for 75% of the cases. Other causes include surgical removal of both adrenal glands or infection (tuberculosis or histoplasmosis) of the adrenal glands. Inadequate secretion of ACTH from the primary pituitary gland results in adrenal insufficiency. Symptoms may also result from sudden cessation of exogenous adrenocortical hormonal therapy.

CLINICAL MANIFESTATIONS

1. Chief clinical manifestations include muscular weakness, anorexia, gastrointestinal symptoms, fatigue, emaciation, dark pigmentation of the skin, hypotension, low blood glucose, low serum sodium, and high serum potassium.
2. In severe cases, disturbance of sodium and potassium may be marked by depletion of sodium and water and severe, chronic dehydration.

Addisonian Crisis

This medical emergency develops as the disease progresses.

1. Cyanosis, fever, and classic signs of shock: pallor, apprehension, rapid weak pulse, rapid respirations, and low blood pressure.
2. Complaints of headache, nausea, abdominal pain, diarrhea, signs of confusion, and restlessness.
3. Slight overexertion, exposure to cold, and acute infections decrease salt intake and may lead to circulatory collapse.

4. Stress of surgery or dehydration from preparation for diagnostic tests or surgery may precipitate Addisonian or hypotensive crisis.

DIAGNOSTIC EVALUATION

Definitive diagnosis is confirmed by low levels of adreno-cortical hormones in blood or urine.

MANAGEMENT

Immediate treatment is directed toward combating shock.

1. Restore blood circulation, administer fluids, monitor vital signs, and place patient in a recumbent position with legs elevated.
2. Administer hydrocortisone IV, followed by 5% dextrose in normal saline.
3. Vasopressor amines may be required if hypotension persists.
4. Antibiotics may be prescribed for infection.
5. Oral intake may be initiated as soon as tolerated.
6. If the adrenal gland does not regain function, life-long replacement of corticosteroids and mineralcorticoids will be required.
7. Dietary intake will need to be supplemented with salt during times of gastrointestinal losses of fluids through vomiting and diarrhea.

NURSING PROCESS

Assessment

FOCUSING ON FLUID IMBALANCE AND STRESS

1. Check blood pressure from a lying to standing position.
2. Assess skin color and turgor.
3. Assess history of weight changes, muscle weakness, and fatigue.
4. Ask patient and family members about onset of illness or increased stress that may have precipitated crisis.

Major Nursing Diagnosis

1. Fluid volume deficit related to inadequate fluid intake and to fluid loss secondary to inadequate adrenal hormone secretion.
2. Knowledge deficit about the need for hormone replacement and dietary modification.

Collaborative Problems

Addisonian crisis.

Planning and Implementation

Goals may include improving fluid balance, improving response to activity and decreasing stress, increasing knowledge about the need for hormone replacement and dietary modifications, and absence of complications.

Interventions

RESTORING FLUID BALANCE

1. Record weight changes daily.
2. Assess skin turgor and mucous membranes.
3. Instruct patient to report increased thirst.
4. Monitor lying, sitting, and standing blood pressures frequently.
5. Encourage to consume food and fluids that assist in restoring and maintaining fluid and electrolyte balance, i.e., foods high in sodium during gastrointestinal disturbances and very hot weather.
6. Assist patient in learning to administer hormone replacement and to modify dosage during illness and stress.
7. Provide patient with written and verbal instructions about steroid therapy.

IMPROVING ACTIVITY TOLERANCE

1. Take precautions to avoid unnecessary activities that might be stressful and could precipitate a hypotensive episode.

2. Detect signs of infection or presence of stressors that may have triggered the crisis.
3. Provide a quiet, nonstressful environment during acute crises, i.e., all activities are carried out for the patients.
4. Explain all procedures to reduce fear and anxiety.
5. Explain to the family the rationale for minimizing stress during acute crisis.

MONITORING AND MANAGING COMPLICATIONS (ADDISONIAN CRISIS)

1. Assess for signs and symptoms of crisis: circulatory collapse and shock.
2. Avoid physical and psychological stress, i.e., exposure to cold, overexertion, infection, and emotional distress.
3. Initiate immediate treatment with IV fluid, glucose, and electrolytes, especially sodium; corticosteroid supplements; and vasopressors.
4. Avoid patient exertion; anticipate and take measures to meet patient's needs.
5. Monitor symptoms, vital signs, weight, fluid and electrolyte balance to evaluate patient's progress to precrisis state.
6. Identify factors that led to crisis episode.

✎ PATIENT EDUCATION AND HEALTH MAINTENANCE: CARE IN THE HOME AND COMMUNITY

Give patient and family members explicit verbal and written instructions about the rationale for replacement therapy and proper dosage.

1. Teach how to modify the drug dosage and increase salt in times of illness and stressful situations.
2. Provide the patient and family with a syringe and vial of injectable steroid (Solu-Cortef) for emergency use and instruct how to use.

3. Advise patient to inform health care providers of receiving steroids, and wear a Medic Alert bracelet.
4. Teach patient and family the signs of excessive or insufficient hormone replacement.
5. Instruct patient regarding modification of diet (sodium) for illness and hot weather to maintain fluid and electrolyte balance.
6. Encourage patients to weigh themselves daily and detect significant changes in weight that indicate fluid loss or retention due to too much or too little hormone.
7. If the patient is unable to return to work and family responsibilities after hospital discharge, refer to community health nurse.
8. Assess recovery, monitor hormone replacement, and assess stress in the home.
9. Assess patient's plans for follow-up visits to the clinic or a physician's office.

For more information see Chapter 40 in Smeltzer and Bare: *Brunner and Suddarth's Textbook of Medical–Surgical Nursing*, 8th Edition. Philadelphia: Lippincott–Raven, 1996.

CHRONIC PYELONEPHRITIS

See Pyelonephritis, Chronic

CHRONIC RENAL FAILURE

See Renal Failure, Chronic

CIRRHOSIS, HEPATIC

Cirrhosis or scarring of the liver is divided into three types: Laënnec's portal cirrhosis (alcoholic, nutritional), most frequently due to chronic alcoholism and the most common type of cirrhosis; postnecrotic cirrhosis, a late result of a previous acute viral hepatitis; and biliary cirrhosis, a result of chronic biliary obstruction and infection, incidence lower than that of Laënnec's and postnecrotic cirrhosis.

CLINICAL MANIFESTATIONS

1. Liver enlargement early in the course (fatty liver); later in course liver size decreases from scar tissue.
2. Portal obstruction and ascites: chronic dyspepsia, constipation or diarrhea, splenomegaly; spider telangiectases may be observed.
3. Gastrointestinal varices: distended abdominal blood vessels; varices or hemorrhoids; small hematemesis; profuse hemorrhage from the stomach, and esophageal varices in about 25% of patients.
4. Edema.
5. Vitamin deficiency (A, C, and K) and anemia.
6. Mental deterioration with impending hepatic encephalopathy and hepatic coma.

DIAGNOSTIC EVALUATION

1. Liver function tests, laparoscopy, in conjunction with biopsy.
2. Ultrasound scanning.
3. Computed tomography (CT) scan.
4. Magnetic resonance imaging (MRI).
5. Radioisotopic liver scans.

MANAGEMENT

Based on presenting symptoms.

1. Antacids, vitamins, and nutritional supplements, potassium-sparing diuretics, avoidance of alcohol.
2. Colchicine may increase the length of survival in patients with mild to moderate cirrhosis.

NURSING PROCESS

Assessment

1. Focus on diet intake, onset of symptoms, history of precipitating factors, i.e., long-term alcohol abuse.
2. Assess mental status through interview and interaction with the patient; note orientation to time, place, person.
3. Note relationships with family, friends, and coworkers regarding incapacitation secondary to alcohol abuse and cirrhosis.
4. Note abdominal distention and bloating, gastrointestinal bleeding, bruising, and weight changes.
5. Document exposure to toxic agents; hepatotoxic medications.

MAJOR NURSING DIAGNOSIS

1. Activity intolerance related to fatigue, general debility, muscle wasting, and discomfort.
2. Risk for infection related to increased susceptibility from weakened condition.
3. Altered nutrition related to chronic gastritis, decreased gastrointestinal motility, and anorexia.
4. Impaired skin integrity related to compromised immunologic status.
5. Risk for injury related to altered clotting mechanisms and portal hypertension.

Collaborative Problems

1. Bleeding and hemorrhage.
2. Hepatic encephalopathy.

Planning and Implementation

Goals may include independence in activities, improvement of nutritional status, improvement of skin integrity, decreased potential for injury, improvement of mental status, and absence of complications.

Interventions

PROVIDING REST AND PREVENTING INFECTION

1. Position bed for maximal respiratory efficiency; provide oxygen if needed.
2. Initiate efforts to prevent respiratory, circulatory, and vascular disturbances.

IMPROVING NUTRITIONAL STATUS

1. Provide a nutritious, high-protein diet supplemented by B complex vitamins and others including A, C, and K and folic acid if there is no indication of impending coma.
2. Provide small, frequent meals and encourage patient to eat.
3. Provide nutrients by feeding tube or total parenteral nutrition (TPN).
4. Provide patients with fatty stools (steatorrhea) with water-soluble forms of fat-soluble vitamins A, D, and E and give folic acid and iron to prevent anemia.
5. Provide a low-protein diet temporarily if patient shows signs of impending or advancing coma; restore protein intake to normal or above when patient's condition permits.

PROVIDING SKIN CARE

1. Change position frequently.
2. Avoid using irritating soaps and adhesive tape.
3. Provide lotion to soothe the irritated skin; take measures to prevent the patient's scratching of the skin.

REDUCING RISK OF INJURY

1. Use padded side rails if patient becomes agitated or restless.
2. Orient to time, place, and procedures to minimize agitation.
3. Instruct patient to ask for assistance to get out of bed.
4. Provide safety measures to prevent cuts (electric razor).

MONITORING AND MANAGING COMPLICATIONS

Preventing bleeding due to decreased production of pro-thrombin and monitoring for hepatic encephalopathy are the primary concerns.

1. Observe for melena and check stools for blood.
2. Use appropriate dietary modification and stool soft-eners to assist in preventing straining during defe-cation.
3. Monitor closely for GI bleeding.
4. Keep equipment to treat hemorrhage from esophageal varices readily available, i.e., IV fluids, medications, Sengstaken-Blakemore tube.
5. Monitor closely to identify early evidence of condi-tion. See section on hepatic encephalopathy.

✎ PATIENT EDUCATION AND HEALTH MAINTENANCE: CARE IN THE HOME AND COMMUNITY

Prepare for discharge by providing dietary instruction including exclusion of alcohol.

1. Refer to Alcoholics Anonymous if necessary.
2. Continue sodium restriction.
3. Provide necessary written instruction, teaching, and reinforcement.
4. Encourage rest and possibility of change in lifestyle.
5. Instruct family about the symptoms of impending encephalopathy and possibility of bleeding tenden-cies and infection.
6. Refer patient to a community health nurse to visit the patient in the home after discharge and assist in transition from hospital to home.

For more information see Chapter 38 in Smeltzer and Bare: *Brunner and Suddarth's Textbook of Medical–Surgical Nursing,* 8th Edition. Philadelphia: Lippincott–Raven, 1996.

CLL

See Leukemia, Lymphocytic, Chronic

C

COLORECTAL CANCER

See Cancer of the Large Intestine (Colon and Rectum)

COMA

See Unconscious Patient

CONGESTIVE HEART DISEASE

See Cardiac Failure

CONGESTIVE HEART FAILURE

See Cardiac Failure

CONSTIPATION

Constipation refers to an abnormal infrequency of defecation, and also to abnormal hardening of stools that make their passage difficult and sometimes painful. This type is referred to as colonic constipation. It can be caused by certain medications and a variety of disease conditions. Other causative factors include weakness, immobility, debility, fatigue, and inability to increase intra-abdominal pressure to facilitate the passage of stools. Constipation develops when people do not take the time to defecate or as the result of dietary habits (low consumption of fiber and inadequate fluid intake, lack of regular exercise, and a stress-filled life). Perceived constipation is a subjective problem that occurs when an individual's bowel elimination pattern is not consistent with what he or she perceives as normal. Chronic laxative use contributes to this problem.

CLINICAL MANIFESTATIONS

1. Abdominal distention, borborygmus (intestinal rumbling), pain, and pressure.
2. Decreased appetite, headache, fatigue, indigestion, sensation of incomplete emptying.
3. Straining at stool; elimination of small-volume, hard, dry stool.

DIAGNOSTIC EVALUATION

Diagnosis is based on barium enema, sigmoidoscopy, stool for occult blood, anorectal pressure studies, defecography, and bowel transit studies.

MANAGEMENT

Treatment should be aimed at the underlying cause of constipation.

1. Discontinue abusive laxative use; increase fluid intake; include fiber in diet, biofeedback, and an exercise routine to strengthen abdominal muscles.
2. If laxative is necessary, use bulk-forming agents, saline and osmotic agents, lubricants, stimulants, or fecal softeners.
3. Specific drug therapy to increase intrinsic motor function (prokinetic agents, i.e., Cisapride).

Nursing Process

ASSESSMENT

Use tact and respect with patient when talking about bowel habits and obtaining health history.

1. Onset and duration of constipation, current and past elimination patterns, patient's expectation of normal bowel elimination, lifestyle, and occupation.

2. History of laxative/enema use.
3. Current drug therapy, past medical history.
4. Presence of any of the following: rectal pressure/fullness, abdominal pain, straining at defecation, watery diarrhea, and flatus.

Physical Assessment

1. Inspect stool for color, odor, consistency, size, shape, and components.
2. Auscultate abdomen for bowel sounds; presence and character.
3. Note abdominal distention.
4. Inspect perianal area for hemorrhoids, fissures, and skin irritation.

Major Nursing Diagnosis

1. Colonic constipation or fecal impaction related to health habits or the effect of immobility on peristalsis.
2. Knowledge deficit about health maintenance practices to prevent constipation.

Collaborative Problems

1. Arterial hypertension.
2. Fecal impaction.
3. Anorectal disease (hemorrhoids, anal fissures).
4. Megacolon.

Planning and Implementation

The major goals may include restoration/maintenance of a regular pattern of normal bowel elimination, adequate intake of fluids and high-fiber foods, understanding of methods for avoiding constipation, relief of anxiety about bowel elimination patterns, and the absence of potential complications.

Interventions

MAINTAINING ELIMINATION

1. Assist to assume the normal position for defecation (semisquatting).
2. Assist patient to a bedside commode whenever possible.
3. Place a small support under the lumbosacral curve to minimize strain and increase comfort while using the bedpan.
4. Monitor frequency and consistency of stool, and document.
5. Set up a routine schedule for bowel elimination.

MONITORING AND MANAGING COMPLICATIONS

1. Monitor closely for evidence of arterial hypertension related to Valsalva maneuver or anorectal disease; administer stool softeners to decrease straining.
2. Prescribe mineral oil and saline enemas if fecal impaction is present; manual extraction may be needed.
3. Provide for emergency colectomy if signs and symptoms of megacolon or perforation are present.

✎ PATIENT EDUCATION AND HEALTH MAINTENANCE: CARE IN THE HOME AND COMMUNITY

1. Carefully assess the patient to determine if constipation is a problem.
2. Design a specific teaching program to prevent constipation; include information about the causes of constipation, dietary practices, and exercise activity that promote healthy bowel habits.
3. Explain the physiology of defecation and emphasize heeding promptly the urge to defecate.
4. Instruct patient to have a regular time for defecation and provide adequate time (after breakfast).
5. Educate patient about what constitutes the prescribed diet (high residue, high fiber).

6. Teach patient to add bran daily and gradually increase amount used; emphasize increased fluid intake.
7. Recommend frequent ambulation and abdominal muscle toning exercises.
8. Encourage patient confined to bed to perform range-of-motion exercises, turn frequently from side-to-side, and lie prone (if not contraindicated) for 30 minutes every 4 hours.

✪ GERONTOLOGIC CONSIDERATIONS

Elderly persons report problems with constipation five times more frequently than younger people. Contributing factors are loose-fitting dentures, loss of teeth, and difficulty chewing; they eat soft, processed foods that are low in fiber (convenience foods). Reduced fluid intake thus decreases bulk and makes passage of stool more difficult.

Lack of exercise and prolonged bed rest also contribute by decreasing abdominal muscle tone, intestinal and anal sphincter tone, and motility. Dulled nerve impulses contribute to decreased sensation to defecate. Overuse of laxatives in an attempt to have a daily bowel movement promotes dependency.

For more information see Chapter 37 in Smeltzer and Bare: *Brunner and Suddarth's Textbook of Medical–Surgical Nursing,* 8th Edition. Philadelphia: Lippincott–Raven, 1996.

CONTACT DERMATITIS

Contact dermatitis is an inflammatory reaction of the skin to physical, chemical, or biologic agents. It may be of the primary irritant type, or it may be allergic (allergic contact dermatitis). The epidermis is damaged by repeated physical and chemical irritations. Common causes of irritant dermatitis are soaps, detergents, scouring compounds, and industrial chemicals. Predisposing factors include extremes of heat and cold, frequent soap and water, and a preexisting skin disease.

CLINICAL MANIFESTATIONS

Eruptions begin when the causative agent contacts the skin.

1. Itching, burning, and erythema; followed by edema, papules, vesicles, and oozing or weeping.
2. In the subacute phase, the vesicular changes are less marked and alternate with crusting, drying, fissuring, and peeling.
3. If repeated reactions occur or the patient continually scratches the skin, lichenification and coloration occur; secondary bacterial invasion may follow.

MANAGEMENT

1. Rest the involved skin and protect it from further damage.
2. Differentiate between allergic type and irritant type.
3. Identify the offending irritant and remove.
4. Use bland, unmedicated lotions for small patches of erythema; apply cool wet dressings over small areas of vesicular dermatitis.
5. In widespread conditions, a short course of systemic steroids may be prescribed.

✎ PATIENT EDUCATION AND HEALTH MAINTENANCE: CARE IN THE HOME AND COMMUNITY

Instruct the patient to adhere to the following instructions for at least 4 months, until the skin appears completely healed:

1. Think about what may have caused the problem.
2. Avoid contact with irritants.
3. Avoid heat, soap, and rubbing the skin.
4. Avoid topical medications except when prescribed.

5. Wash the skin thoroughly, immediately after exposure to irritants or antigens.
6. Wear cotton-lined gloves for washing dishes, not more than 15–20 minutes at a time.

For more information see Chapter 54 in Smeltzer and Bare: *Brunner and Suddarth's Textbook of Medical–Surgical Nursing,* 8th Edition. Philadelphia: Lippincott–Raven, 1996.

C

CORONARY ARTERY DISEASE

Coronary artery disease (CAD) is a major threat to the health and well-being of the American population. Although the major focus of heart disease has been focused on men, women (especially postmenopausal women) have been shown to have mortality rates from coronary artery disease similar to those of men. Because CAD is so prevalent in the United States, nurses need to be familiar with the various types of cardiac problems and methods for assessing and possibly preventing these disorders. The anatomic structure of the coronary arteries makes them particularly susceptible to the development of atheromatous plaques because of the many angles and curves. The three major coronary arteries most susceptible to atheroma development are the right coronary artery, the left anterior descending artery, and the left circumflex artery. Clinical problems related to CAD disease described in this book can be found under Angina Pectoris; Cardiac Failure; Coronary Atherosclerosis; and Myocardial Infarction.

For more information see Chapter 28 in Smeltzer and Bare: *Brunner and Suddarth's Textbook of Medical–Surgical Nursing,* 8th Edition. Philadelphia: Lippincott–Raven, 1996.

COPD

See Chronic Obsructive Pulmonary Disease

COR PULMONALE

See Pulmonary Heart Disease

CORONARY ATHEROSCLEROSIS

Coronary atherosclerosis (a form of arteriosclerosis) is characterized by an abnormal accumulation of lipid substances and fibrous tissue in the vessel wall. This leads to changes in arterial structure and function, and reduction of blood flow to the myocardium. Causes probably involve alterations in lipid metabolism, blood coagulation, and the biophysical and biochemical properties of the arterial walls. Atherosclerosis is a progressive disease. Progress can be curtailed and in some cases reversed.

CLINICAL MANIFESTATIONS

Result from narrowing of the arterial lumen and obstruction of blood flow to myocardium.

1. Chest pain.
2. Angina pectoris.
3. Myocardial infarction.
4. ECG changes, ventricular aneurysms.
5. Dysrhythmias, sudden death.

MODIFIABLE RISK FACTORS

1. Cigarette smoking.
2. Elevated blood pressure.
3. High blood cholesterol (hyperlipidemia).
4. Hyperglycemia (diabetes mellitus).
5. Obesity.
6. Physical inactivity.
7. Use of oral contraceptives.
8. Behavior patterns (stress, aggressiveness, hostility).
9. Geography: higher incidence in industrialized regions.

NONMODIFIABLE RISK FACTORS

1. Positive family history.
2. Increasing age.
3. Gender: occurs three times more often in men than in women.
4. Race: higher incidence in blacks than in whites.

 ### Gerontologic Considerations

Aging produces changes in the integrity of the lining of the walls of arteries (arteriosclerosis), impeding blood flow, and tissue nutrition. These changes are often sufficient to diminish oxygenation and increase myocardial oxygen consumption (MVO^2). The result can be debilitating angina pectoris and eventually congestive heart failure.

For more information see Chapter 28 in Smeltzer and Bare: *Brunner and Suddarth's Textbook of Medical–Surgical Nursing,* 8th Edition. Philadelphia: Lippincott–Raven, 1996.

COUGH, PRODUCTIVE

See Bronchitis, Chronic

CROHN'S DISEASE

See Regional Enteritis

CUSHING'S SYNDROME

Cushing's syndrome results from excessive adrenocortical activity. It may result from excessive administration of cortisone or ACTH or from hyperplasia of the adrenal cortex. It may be caused by several mechanisms including a tumor of the pituitary gland that produces ACTH.

Administration of cortisone or ACTH may also produce Cushing's syndrome. Regardless of the cause, the normal feedback mechanisms that control the function of the adrenal cortex become ineffective.

CLINICAL MANIFESTATIONS

1. Growth arrest, obesity, musculoskeletal changes, and glucose intolerance.
2. The classic picture of an adult with Cushing's syndrome shows a central type obesity, with a fatty "buffalo hump" in the neck and supraclavicular areas, a heavy trunk, and relatively thin extremities. Skin is thinned, fragile, easily traumatized; ecchymosis and striae develop.
3. Weakness and lassitude; sleep is disturbed because of altered diurnal secretion of cortisol.
4. Excessive protein catabolism with muscle wasting and osteoporosis; kyphosis, backache, and compression fractures of the vertebrae.
5. Retention of sodium and water occurs, contributing to hypertension and congestive heart failure.
6. "Moon-faced" appearance and oiliness of the skin and acne.
7. Increased susceptibility to infection.
8. Hyperglycemia or overt diabetes.
9. Weight gain, slow healing of minor cuts and bruises.
10. In females of all ages virilization may occur from excess androgens: appearance of masculine traits and recession of feminine traits; excessive hair on face, breasts atrophy, menses cease, clitoris enlarges, and voice deepens. Libido is lost in males and females.
11. Changes occur in mood and mental activity; psychosis may develop.
12. If Cushing's syndrome is the result of pituitary tumor, visual disturbances may occur because of pressure on the optic chiasm.

DIAGNOSTIC EVALUATION

1. 24-hour urine collection for levels of 17-hydroxycorticosteroids and 17-ketosteroids (urinary metabolites of cortisol and androgens). Elevated in Cushing's syndrome.
2. Dexamethasone suppression test.
3. CT scan or MRI may localize adrenal tissue and detect adrenal tumors.

MANAGEMENT

Treatment is usually directed at the pituitary gland because the majority of cases are due to pituitary tumors rather than tumors of the adrenal cortex.

1. Surgical removal of the tumor is the primary treatment of choice.
2. Implantation of needle containing radioactive isotopes into the pituitary gland.
3. Adrenalectomy in patients with primary adrenal hypertrophy.
4. Postoperatively, temporary replacement therapy with hydrocortisone may be necessary until the adrenal glands begin to respond normally (may be several months).
5. If bilateral adrenalectomy was performed, lifetime replacement of adrenal cortex hormones is necessary.
6. If Cushing's syndrome is a result of exogenous corticosteroids, reduce the drug to the minimum level to treat the underlying disease.

NURSING PROCESS

Assessment

Focus on the effects on the body of high concentrations of adrenal cortex hormones.

1. Obtain information about the patient's level of activity and ability to carry out routine and self-care activities.

2. Observe skin for trauma, infection, breakdown, bruising, and edema.
3. Note changes in physical appearance.
4. Assess patient's mental function.

Major Nursing Diagnosis

1. Impaired skin integrity related to edema, impaired healing, and thin and fragile skin.
2. Risk for injury and infection related to weakness and altered protein metabolism and inflammatory response.
3. Body image disturbance related to altered physical appearance, impaired sexual functioning, and decrease in activity level.
4. Altered thought processes related to mood swings, irritability, and depression.

Collaborative Problems

1. Addisonian crisis.
2. Adverse effects of adrenocortical activity.

Planning and Implementation

The major goals include increased ability to carry out self-care activities, improved skin integrity, decreased risk of injury and infection, improved body image, improved mental function, and absence of complications.

Interventions

1. Monitor fluid and electrolyte status.
2. Weigh daily.
3. Monitor and report blood glucose.

DECREASING RISK OF INJURY AND INFECTION

1. Provide a protective environment to prevent falls, fractures, and other injuries to bones and soft tissues.
2. Avoid unnecessary exposure to people with infections.
3. Assess frequently for subtle signs of infections (corticosteroids mask signs of inflammation and infection).

4. Recommend foods high in protein, calcium, and vitamin D to minimize muscle wasting and osteoporosis.

ENCOURAGING REST AND ACTIVITY

1. Encourage moderate activity to prevent complications of immobility and promote increased self-esteem.
2. Plan rest periods throughout the day.
3. Promote a relaxing, quiet environment.

PROMOTING SKIN CARE

1. Use meticulous skin care to avoid traumatizing fragile skin.
2. Avoid adhesive tape that can tear and irritate the skin.
3. Assess bony prominences frequently.
4. Encourage patient to change positions frequently.

IMPROVING BODY IMAGE

1. Major physical changes will disappear in time if the cause of Cushing's syndrome can be treated successfully.
2. Weight gain and edema may be modified by a low-carbohydrate, low-sodium diet.

IMPROVING THOUGHT PROCESSES

1. Explain to the patient and family the cause of emotional instability and help them cope with mood swings, irritability, and depression that may occur.
2. Report any psychotic behavior.
3. Encourage patient and family members to verbalize feelings.

MONITORING AND MANAGING COMPLICATIONS

1. Adrenal hypofunction and addisonian crisis: monitor for hypotension, rapid, weak pulse, rapid respiratory rate, pallor, and extreme weakness; administer intravenous fluid and electrolytes and corticosteroids as needed.

2. Monitor for circulatory collapse and shock present in addisonian crisis.
3. Identify factors that may have led to crisis.

For more information see Chapter 40 in Smeltzer and Bare: *Brunner and Suddarth's Textbook of Medical–Surgical Nursing,* 8th Edition. Philadelphia: Lippincott–Raven, 1996.

CVA

See Cerebral Vascular Accident

CYSTITIS (LOWER URINARY TRACT INFECTION)

Cystitis is an inflammation of the urinary bladder that is most often caused by an ascending infection from the urethra. Other causes may be urine flowing back from the urethra into the bladder (ureterovesical reflux), fecal contamination, or the use of a catheter or cystoscope. Cystitis occurs more often in women; usually caused by *Escherichia coli.* The onset of sexual activity is associated with an increased frequency of urinary tract infections in women, particularly those who fail to void after intercourse. Infection is also associated with diaphragm-spermicide contraception because it may cause a partial urethral obstruction and prevent complete emptying of the bladder. Cystitis in men is secondary to some other factor (i.e., infected prostate, epididymitis, or bladder stones).

CLINICAL MANIFESTATIONS

1. Urgency, frequency, burning, and pain on urination.
2. Nocturia, pain or spasm in bladder region and suprapubic area.
3. Pyuria, bacteria, and hematuria.

MANAGEMENT

1. Ideal treatment is an antibacterial agent that effectively eradicates bacteria from the urinary tract with minimal effects on fecal and vaginal flora.
2. Sulfisoxazole (Gantrisin), trimethoprimsulfamethoxazole (TMP/SMZ, Bactrim or Septra), nitrofurantoin (Macrodantin).
3. Uncomplicated lower urinary tract infections in women: include single-dose administration, short-course (3–4 days) medication regimes, or 7- to 10-day courses.

RECURRENCE

1. About 20% of women treated for uncomplicated urinary tract infections (UTIs) experience a recurrence.
2. Repeated infections at close intervals suggest a cause for referral to a urologist to investigate and correct abnormalities.
3. Recurrence in men is usually due to persistence of the same organism; further evaluation and treatment are indicated.
4. Reinfection of women with new bacteria is more common than persistence of the initial bacteria.
5. If diagnostic evaluation reveals no structural abnormalities, patient may be instructed to begin treatment on own, whenever symptoms occur, and contact health care provider only with persistence of symptoms, the occurrence of fever, or if the number of treatment episodes exceeds four in a 6-month period.
6. Long-term use of antimicrobial agents decreases risk of reinfection.

NURSING PROCESS

Assessment

1. History of urinary signs and symptoms.
2. Presence of pain, frequency, urgency, and hesitancy and changes in urine.

3. Usual pattern of voiding, to detect factors that may predispose the patient.
4. Infrequent emptying of the bladder, association of symptoms of urinary tract infections with sexual intercourse, contraceptive practices, and personal hygiene.
5. Check urine for volume, color, concentration, cloudiness, and odor.

Major Nursing Diagnosis

1. Pain and discomfort related to inflammation and infection of the urethra, bladder, and other urinary tract structures.
2. Knowledge deficit regarding factors predisposing to infection and recurrence, detection and prevention of recurrence, and pharmacologic therapy.

Collaborative Problems

1. Renal failure due to extensive damage of kidney.
2. Sepsis.

Planning and Implementation

Major goals may include relief of pain and discomfort; relief from frequency, urgency, and hesitancy; increased knowledge of preventive measures and treatment modalities; and absence of potential complications.

Interventions

RELIEVING PAIN AND DISCOMFORT

1. Use antispasmodic drugs to relieve bladder irritability and pain.
2. Relieve urgency, discomfort, and spasm with aspirin, heat to the perineum, and hot tub baths.

RELIEVING FREQUENCY, URGENCY, AND HESITANCY

1. Encourage to drink liberal amounts of fluid to promote renal blood flow and to flush bacteria from the urinary tract.

2. Avoid fluids that may be irritating to the bladder (e.g., coffee, tea, colas).
3. Encourage frequent voiding (every 2–3 hours) to empty the bladder completely.

C

MONITORING AND MANAGING COMPLICATIONS

1. Recognize signs and symptoms of UTIs early; initiate prompt treatment.
2. Manage UTIs with appropriate antimicrobial therapy, liberalization of fluids, frequent voiding, and hygienic measures.
3. Notify physician if fatigue, nausea, vomiting, or pruritus occurs.
4. Provide for periodic monitoring of renal function.
5. Avoid indwelling catheters if possible; remove at earliest opportunity.
6. Provide strict aseptic technique if an indwelling catheter is necessary.
7. Check vital signs and level of consciousness for impending sepsis.
8. Report positive blood cultures and elevated WBC counts.

✎ PATIENT EDUCATION AND HEALTH MAINTENANCE: CARE IN THE HOME AND COMMUNITY

1. Reduce concentrations of pathogens of the vaginal opening by hygienic measures: shower rather than bathe; cleanse around the perineum and urethral meatus after each bowel movement with front-to-back motion.
2. Drink liberal amounts of fluid during the day to flush out bacteria, avoiding coffee, tea, colas, and alcohol.
3. Void every 2–3 hours during the day and completely empty the bladder.
4. If sexual intercourse is the initiating event for development of bacteriuria, void immediately after sexual intercourse and take prescribed single-dose oral antimicrobial agent.

5. Instruct to take medication after emptying bladder before going to bed to ensure adequate concentration of the drug during the night.
6. Monitor and test urine for bacteria with dip slides (Microstix).
7. See health care provider regularly for follow-up, recurrence of symptoms, and infection that is non-responsive to treatment.

For more information see Chapter 43 in Smeltzer and Bare: *Brunner and Suddarth's Textbook of Medical–Surgical Nursing,* 8th Edition. Philadelphia: Lippincott–Raven, 1996.

DERMATITIS, CONTACT

See Contact Dermatitis

DERMATITIS, EXFOLIATIVE

See Exfoliative Dermatitis

DERMATOSES, SEBORRHEIC

See Seborrheic Dermatoses

DIABETES INSIPIDUS

Diabetes insipidus is a disorder of the posterior lobe of the pituitary gland due to a deficiency of vasopressin, the antidiuretic hormone (ADH). It is characterized by polydipsia and polyuria. Causes of diabetes insipidus may be (1) secondary related to head trauma, brain tumor, or surgical ablation or irradiation of the pituitary gland, also infections of the central nervous system or metastatic tumors (lung or breast); (2) nephrogenic related to failure of the renal tubules to respond to ADH; (3) drug-related nephrogenic caused by a variety of medications (e.g., lithium, demeclocyclin); (4) primary, hereditary, with symptoms possibly beginning at birth (defect in pituitary gland). The disease cannot be controlled by limiting the intake of fluids, because loss of high volumes of urine continues even without fluid replacement. Attempts to restrict fluids cause the patient to experience an insatiable craving for fluid and to develop hypernatremia and severe dehydration.

CLINICAL MANIFESTATIONS

1. Polyuria: enormous daily output of very dilute urine; specific gravity 1.001 to 1.005; usually has abrupt onset, but may be insidious in adults.
2. Polydipsia: intense thirst, 4 to 40 liters of fluid daily, special craving for cold water.

DIAGNOSTIC EVALUATION

Fluid deprivation test, fluids are withheld for 8 to 12 hours until 3% to 5% of the body weight is lost. Inability to increase specific gravity and osmolality of the urine during test is characteristic of diabetes insipidus.

MANAGEMENT

The objectives of therapy are to assure adequate fluid replacement, to replace vasopressin, and to search for and correct the underlying intracranial pathology.

Vasopressin Replacement

1. Desmopressin (DDAVP), administered intranasally, two administrations daily to control symptoms.
2. Intramuscular administration of ADH (vasopressin tannate in oil) every 24 to 96 hours to reduce urinary volume; rotation of injection sites to prevent lipodystrophy.
3. Lypressin (DIAPID) absorbed through nasal mucosa into blood; duration may be short for patients with severe disease.

Fluid Conservation

1. Clofibrate, a hypolipidemic agent, has an antidiuretic effect on patients who have some residual hypothalamic vasopressin.
2. Chlorpropamide (Diabinese) and thiazide diuretics used in mild forms to potentiate the action of vasopressin; may cause hypoglycemic reactions.

Nephrogenic Origin

1. Thiazide diuretics, mild salt depletion, and prostaglandin inhibitors (e.g., ibuprofen, endomethacin).

Nursing Interventions

1. Encourage and support patient while undergoing studies for possible cranial lesion.
2. Instruct patient and family members about follow-up care and emergency measures.
3. Advise patient to wear a Medic Alert bracelet and to carry medication information about this disorder at all times.
4. Use caution with administration of vasopressin if coronary artery disease is present because of vaso-constriction.

For more information see Chapter 40 in Smeltzer and Bare: *Brunner and Suddarth's Textbook of Medical–Surgical Nursing,* 8th Edition. Philadelphia: Lippincott–Raven, 1996.

DIABETES MELLITUS

Diabetes mellitus is a group of disorders characterized by elevated levels of blood glucose (hyperglycemia). There may be a decrease in the body's ability to respond to insulin and/or a decrease or absence of insulin produced by the pancreas. This leads to hyperglycemia, which may lead to acute metabolic complications such as diabetic ketoacidosis and hyperglycemic hyperosmolar nonketotic (HHNK) syndrome. Long-term hyperglycemia may contribute to chronic microvascular complications (kidney and eye disease) and neuropathic complications. Diabetes is also associated with an increased occurrence of macrovascular diseases, including myocardial infarction, strokes, and peripheral vascular disease.

TYPES OF DIABETES

Type I: Insulin-Dependent Diabetes Mellitus (IDDM)

1. 5% to 10% of diabetics have Type I. Beta cells of the pancreas that normally produce insulin are destroyed by an autoimmune process. Insulin injections are needed to control the blood glucose levels.
2. Sudden onset usually before the age of 30 years.

Type II: Non-Insulin-Dependent Diabetes Mellitus (NIDDM)

1. 90% to 95% of diabetics have Type II. It results from a decreased sensitivity to insulin (insulin resistance) or from a decreased amount of insulin production.
2. First treated with diet and exercise; if elevated glucose levels persist, supplement with oral hypoglycemic agents (insulin injections are required if oral agents will not control hyperglycemia).
3. Occurs most frequently in those over 30 years of age and in the obese.

Other Conditions or Syndromes

1. Gestational diabetes mellitus (GDM): onset during pregnancy (second or third trimester).
2. Impaired glucose tolerance: blood glucose level between normal and that of diabetes; 25% eventually develop diabetes.
3. Previous abnormality of glucose tolerance (PrevAGT): current normal glucose metabolism; previous history of hyperglycemia.
4. Potential abnormality of glucose tolerance (PotAGT): no history of glucose intolerance; encourage ideal body weight; increased risk of diabetes if positive family history, obesity, mothers of babies over 9 pounds.
5. Pancreatic diseases.
6. Hormonal abnormalities.

7. Drugs (glucocorticoids and estrogen-containing preparations).

CLINICAL MANIFESTATIONS

Type I Diabetes

1. Fasting hyperglycemia.
2. Glucosuria, osmotic diuresis, polyuria, polydipsia, and polyphagia.
3. Other symptoms include fatigue and weakness.
4. Diabetic ketoacidosis (DKA) causes signs and symptoms of abdominal pain, nausea, vomiting, hyperventilation, fruity odor of breath; if untreated, altered level of consciousness, coma, and death.

Type II Diabetes

1. Slow (over years), progressive glucose intolerance.
2. Symptoms are frequently mild and may include fatigue, irritability, polyuria, polydipsia, skin wounds that heal poorly, vaginal infections, or blurred vision (if glucose levels are very high).
3. Long-term complications if diabetes goes undetected for many years (e.g., eye disease, peripheral neuropathy, peripheral vascular disease), which may have developed before the actual diagnosis is made.

DIAGNOSTIC EVALUATION

1. Presence of abnormally high blood glucose levels: fasting plasma glucose levels above 140 mg/dl or random plasma glucose levels over 200 mg/dl on more than one occasion.
2. Oral glucose tolerance test (OGTT).

MANAGEMENT

The main goal of treatment is to try to normalize insulin activity and blood glucose levels to reduce the development of vascular and neuropathic complications. The therapeutic goal within each type of diabetes is to achieve normal blood glucose levels (euglycemia) without hypoglycemia and without seriously disrupting the patient's usual activities. There are five components of management for diabetes: diet, exercise, monitoring, medication (as needed), and education.

1. Primary treatment of Type I diabetes is insulin.
2. Primary treatment of Type II diabetes is weight loss.
3. Exercise is important in enhancing the effectiveness of insulin.
4. Use oral hypoglycemia agents if diet and exercise are not successful in controlling blood glucose levels.
5. Since treatment varies throughout course because of changes in lifestyle, physical and emotional status, as well as advances in therapy, constantly assess and modify treatment plan as well as daily adjustments in therapy. Also, it is essential to provide education to both patient and family.

DIETARY MANAGEMENT

1. Provision of all the essential food constituents (e.g., vitamins, minerals).
2. Achievement and maintenance of ideal weight; meeting energy needs.
3. Prevention of wide daily fluctuations in blood glucose levels; keep as close to normal as is safe and practical.
4. Decrease of blood lipid levels, if elevated.
5. Patients who require insulin to help control blood glucose levels should maintain consistency in the number of calories and carbohydrates eaten at different mealtimes.
6. For obese patients (especially Type II diabetes) weight loss is the key to the treatment and the major preventive factor for the development of diabetes.

Caloric Requirements

1. Determine basic caloric requirements, taking into consideration age, sex, body weight, and degree of activity.
2. Long-term weight reduction can be achieved with diet caloric levels between 1000 and 1200 calories; more realistic recommendations may be 1200 to 1500 calories.
3. The American Diabetes and American Dietetic Associations recommend that for all levels of caloric intake, 50% to 60% of calories be derived from carbohydrates, 20% to 30% from fat, and the remaining 12% to 20% from protein.

D

COMPLICATIONS OF DIABETES

Complications associated with both types of diabetes are classified as acute or chronic.

Acute Complications

Acute complications occur from short-term imbalances in blood glucose.

1. Hypoglycemia.
2. Diabetic ketoacidosis (DKA).
3. Hyperglycemic hyperosmolar nonketotic (HHNK) syndrome.

Chronic Complications

Generally occur 10 to 15 years after onset.

1. Macrovascular (large vessel disease): affects coronary, peripheral vascular, and cerebral vascular circulations.
2. Microvascular (small vessel disease): affects the eyes (retinopathy) and kidneys (neuropathy). Control blood glucose levels to delay or avoid onset of both microvascular and macrovascular complications.
3. Neuropathic diseases: affect sensory motor and autonomic nerves and contribute to such problems as impotence and foot ulcers.

NURSING PROCESS FOR THE PATIENT WITH NEWLY DIAGNOSED DIABETES MELLITUS

Assessment

1. Focus on signs and symptoms of prolonged hyperglycemia and physical, social, and emotional factors that affect ability to learn and perform diabetes self-care activities.
2. Ask for a description of symptoms that preceded the diagnosis, i.e., polyuria, polydipsia, polyphagia, skin dryness, blurred vision, weight loss, vaginal itching, and nonhealing ulcers.
3. Assess for signs of DKA including ketonuria, Kussmaul respirations, orthostatic hypotension, and lethargy.
4. Question regarding DKA symptoms of nausea, vomiting, and abdominal pain.
5. Monitor laboratory signs for metabolic acidosis (decreased pH, decreased bicarbonate) and for signs of electrolyte imbalance.
6. Assess Type II diabetics for signs of HHNK syndrome: hypotension, altered sensorium, seizures, decreased skin turgor, hyperosmolarity, and electrolyte imbalance.
7. Assess physical factors that impair ability to learn or perform self-care skills, i.e., visual defects, motor coordination defects, neurologic defects.
8. Evaluate patient's social situation for factors that influence diabetic treatment and education plan such as decreased literacy; limited financial resources/lack of health insurance; presence or absence of family support; typical daily schedule, e.g., work, meals, exercise, travel plans.
9. Assess emotional status through observation of general demeanor.
10. Assess coping skills by asking how the patient has dealt with difficult situations in the past.

Major Nursing Diagnosis

1. Risk for fluid volume deficit related to polyuria and dehydration.
2. Altered nutrition related to imbalance of insulin, food, and physical activity.
3. Knowledge deficit about diabetes self-care skills/information.
4. Potential self-care deficit related to physical impairments or social factors.
5. Anxiety related to loss of control, fear of inability to manage diabetes, misinformation related to diabetes, fear of diabetes complications.

Collaborative Problems

1. Fluid overload, pulmonary edema, congestive heart failure.
2. Hypokalemia.
3. Hyperglycemia and ketoacidosis.
4. Hypoglycemia.
5. Cerebral edema.

Planning and Implementation

The major goals may include attainment of fluid and electrolyte balance, optimal control of blood glucose, regaining weight lost, ability to perform basic (survival) diabetes skills and self-care activities, reduction in anxiety, and absence of complications.

Interventions

MAINTAINING FLUID AND ELECTROLYTE BALANCE

1. Measure intake and output.
2. Administer IV fluids and electrolytes as ordered.
3. Encourage fluid intake.
4. Measure serum electrolytes and monitor.
5. Monitor vital signs to detect dehydration: tachycardia, orthostatic hypotension.

IMPROVING NUTRITIONAL INTAKE

1. Plan the diet with glucose control as the primary goal.
2. Take into consideration the patient's lifestyle, cultural background, activity level, and food preferences.
3. Encourage to eat full meals and snacks as ordered.
4. Make arrangements for extra snacks before increased physical activity.
5. Ensure that insulin orders are altered as needed for delays in eating due to diagnostic and other procedures.

REDUCING ANXIETY

1. Provide emotional support.
2. Clear up misconceptions patient or family may have regarding diabetes.
3. Encourage patient and family to focus on learning self-care behaviors.
4. Encourage patient to perform the skills feared most, i.e., self-injection or finger stick for glucose monitoring.
5. Give positive enforcement for self-care behaviors attempted.

MONITORING AND MANAGING POTENTIAL COMPLICATIONS

1. Fluid overload: measure vital signs and monitor hemodynamic status at frequent intervals; assess cardiac rate and rhythm, breath sounds, venous distention, skin turgor, and urine output; monitor IV fluid and other fluid intake.
2. Hypokalemia: replace potassium cautiously, ensure that kidneys are functioning prior to administration; monitor cardiac rate, rhythm, ECG, and serum potassium levels.
3. Hyperglycemia and ketoacidosis: monitor blood glucose levels and urine ketones; administer medications (insulin, oral hypoglycemic agents); monitor for signs and symptoms of impending hyper-

glycemia and ketoacidosis, administering insulin and IV fluids to correct.

4. Hypoglycemia: treat with juice or glucose tablets; encourage to eat full meals or snacks as prescribed; review with patients signs and symptoms, possible causes, and measures to prevent and treat.

5. Cerebral edema: prevent by gradual reduction in the blood glucose level; monitor blood glucose level, serum electrolyte levels, urine output, mental status, and neurological signs; minimize activities that increase intracranial pressure.

✎ Patient Education and Health Maintenance: Care in the Home and Community

1. Teach patient survival skills, including simple pathophysiology, treatment modalities, recognition and prevention of acute complications, and pragmatic information (where to obtain supplies, when to call physician).
2. Teach preventive behaviors for long-term diabetic complications.

Specialized Patient Education and Home Health Care

1. Provide special equipment for instruction of diabetes such as magnifying glass for insulin preparation or injection aid device for insulin injection
2. Tailor information according to patient's ability to understand.
3. Instruct family to assist in diabetes management.
4. Recommend follow-up education with home health nurse or outpatient diabetic education center.
5. Assist in identifying community resources for education and supplies, giving consideration to financial limitations and physical limitations.

Health Teaching About Diet

1. Initial education addresses the importance of consistency in eating habits, the relationship of food

and insulin, and provision of individualized meal plan.

2. Follow-up education focuses on more in-depth management skills, such as restaurant eating, food labels, adjusting meals for exercise, illness, and special occasions.
3. Determine if patient is able to learn and use the exchange system.
4. Simplify information and provide many opportunities for practice and repetition.
5. Teach patients to read labels of "health" foods because they often contain sugar products (i.e., honey, brown sugar, and corn syrup) and may contain saturated vegetable fats, hydrogenated vegetable fats, or animal fats that may be contraindicated with elevated blood lipids.

Exercise

1. Exercise is extremely important because of its effects on lowering blood glucose and reducing cardiovascular risk factors.
2. Effects of exercise are useful in losing weight, easing stress, and maintaining a feeling of well-being.
3. Exercise alters blood lipids, increasing levels of high-density lipoproteins (HDL) and decreasing total cholesterol and triglyceride levels.
4. Teach patient with blood glucose levels over 250 mg/dl not to begin exercising until the urine ketone test is negative and blood glucose levels are closer to normal. (High blood glucose levels stimulate secretion of glucagon, growth hormone, and catecholamines, resulting in release of more glucose from the liver and increase in blood glucose.)
5. Teach patient to eat a 15-gram carbohydrate snack (fruit exchange) or a snack of complex carbohydrates with protein before moderate exercise to prevent hypoglycemia.
6. Be aware of postexercise hypoglycemia that occurs many hours after exercise.

7. Test blood glucose before, during, and after exercise and eat carbohydrate snacks as needed to maintain blood glucose; reduce dosage of insulin that peaks at the time of exercise if necessary.
8. Exercise and dietary management improves glucose metabolism and enhances loss of body fat in persons with Type II diabetes.
9. Exercise coupled with weight loss improves insulin sensitivity and may decrease need for insulin or oral agents in Type II diabetes.
10. Encourage regular daily exercise rather than sporadic exercise.
11. All persons with diabetes should discuss an exercise program with their physician.

Self-Monitoring of Blood Glucose (SMBG)

1. SMBG allows adjustment in treatment regimen for optimal blood glucose.
2. Allows for detection and prevention of hypo- and hyperglycemia, which possibly reduces long-term diabetic complications.
3. SMBG is recommended for all people with diabetes and highly recommended for patients with unstable diabetes and those with complications.
4. SMBG is helpful for monitoring the effectiveness of exercise, diet, and oral agents if patients are not taking insulin.

Glycosylated Hemoglobin

1. A blood test that reflects average blood glucose levels over a period of approximately 2–3 months.
2. Normal values range from 4% to 8% (may differ slightly from test to test).

Urine Testing for Ketones (Acetone)

1. Urine testing should be performed whenever patients with Type I diabetes have glucosuria or unexplained elevated blood glucose levels (over 250 mg/dl), and during illness and pregnancy.

Insulin Therapy

1. Insulin preparations vary according to four main characteristics: time course of action, concentration, species (source), and manufacturer.
2. Time course: insulins may be grouped into three categories based on onset, peak, and duration of action.
3. Short-acting insulin includes regular insulin (marked "R" on the bottle), also known as crystalline zinc insulin (CZI); it is clear in appearance. Onset of regular insulin is ½ to 1 hour; peak 2–4 hours; duration 6–8 hours.
4. Intermediate-acting insulins include NPH insulin and Lente ("L") insulin and are white and milky in appearance.
5. Onset of intermediate-acting insulins is 3–4 hours; peak 4–12 hours; duration 16–20 hours.
6. Long-acting insulin includes Ultralente ("UL") insulin, which has a long, slow, sustained action with an onset of 6–8 hours; peak 12–16 hours; duration 20–30 hours.
7. U-100 is the most common concentration of insulin in the United States (100 units of insulin per 1 cubic centimeter [cc]).

Problems with Insulin

1. Local allergic reactions may occur in the form of redness, swelling, tenderness, and induration up to 1–2 hours after the injection is given.
2. Systemic allergic reactions are rare and occasionally associated with generalized edema or anaphylaxis.
3. Insulin lipodystrophy is a localized disturbance of fat metabolism, prevented by rotation of injection sites and avoiding injecting insulin into the hypertrophied areas.
4. Clinical insulin resistance may occur because immune antibodies develop and bind the insulin,

decreasing availability for use; treat by administering a purer insulin preparation and occasionally prednisone to block the production of antibodies.

Oral Hypoglycemic Agents

1. Oral hypoglycemic agents may be effective for Type II diabetic patients who cannot be treated by diet management alone. A functioning pancreas is necessary for these agents to be effective and they cannot be used in the treatment of Type I diabetics and patients prone to ketoacidosis.
2. Hypoglycemia may occur when an excessive dose of an oral hypoglycemic is used or meals are omitted or food intake is decreased.
3. Avoid ingestion of alcohol because disulfiram (Antabuse) type reaction may occur.
4. Oral hypoglycemic drugs may be discontinued temporarily when insulin is needed if the patient develops hyperglycemia due to infection, trauma, or surgery.

Promoting Compliance

1. Avoid the use of "scare" tactics (blindness or amputation) if patient does not comply with the treatment plan.
2. Do not judge the patient; it only promotes feelings of guilt and low self-esteem.
3. Distinguish among problems of compliance, knowledge deficit, and self-care deficit and do not assume that problems with diabetes are related to nonadherence.
4. Recognize that physical (e.g., visual acuity) and emotional factors may impair the patient's ability to perform self-care skills.
5. Assess for signs of infection or emotional stress that lead to elevated glucose levels despite adherence to treatment regimen.

GERONTOLOGIC CONSIDERATIONS

Elevation of blood glucose increases in frequency with advancing age.

Physical activity that is consistent and realistic is beneficial to the elderly with diabetes.

Advantages of exercise include a decrease in hyperglycemia, general sense of well-being, utilization of ingested calories, and weight reduction. Consider physical impairment from other chronic diseases when planning an exercise regimen.

For more information see Chapter 39 in Smeltzer and Bare: *Brunner and Suddarth's Textbook of Medical–Surgical Nursing,* 8th Edition. Philadelphia: Lippincott–Raven, 1996.

DIABETIC KETOACIDOSIS

Diabetic ketoacidosis (DKA) is caused by an absence or inadequate amount of insulin. This results in disorders in the metabolism of carbohydrates, protein, and fat. The three main clinical features of DKA are (1) dehydration, (2) electrolyte loss, and (3) acidosis. When insulin is lacking, the amount of glucose entering the cells is reduced; there is increased production of glucose by the liver. Both of these factors lead to hyperglycemia followed by polyuria, which leads to dehydration and electrolyte loss. Patients with severe DKA may lose an average of 6.5 liters of water and up to 400–500 mEq each of sodium, potassium, and chloride over 24 hours. In DKA there is also an excess production of ketone bodies because of the lack of insulin that would normally prevent this from occurring. Three main causes of DKA are (1) decreased or missed dose of insulin, (2) illness or infection, and (3) initial manifestation of undiagnosed or untreated diabetes.

CLINICAL MANIFESTATIONS

1. Polyuria and polydipsia (increased thirst).
2. Blurred vision, weakness, and headache.

3. Orthostatic hypotension in patients with volume depletion.
4. Weak, rapid pulse may occur.
5. Gastrointestinal symptoms such as anorexia, nausea, and abdominal pain (may be severe).
6. Acetone breath (fruity odor).
7. Kussmaul respirations, hyperventilation with very deep, but not labored, respirations.
8. Mental status changes vary widely from patient to patient. Some may be alert, whereas others are lethargic, or comatose.

D

Laboratory Values

1. Blood glucose from 300–800 mg/dl (may be lower or higher).
2. Low serum bicarbonate (0–15 mEq/L).
3. Low pH (6.8–7.3), low pCO_2 (10–30 mm Hg).
4. Sodium and potassium levels may be low, normal, or high depending on amount of water loss (dehydration).
5. Elevated creatinine, blood urea nitrogen (BUN), hemoglobin, and hematocrit may be seen with dehydration.

MANAGEMENT

Treatment of DKA is aimed at correction of the three main problems: dehydration, electrolyte loss, and acidosis.

Dehydration

1. Patients may need up to 6–10 liters of IV fluid to replace fluid loss caused by polyuria, hyperventilation, diarrhea, and vomiting.
2. Initially 0.9% normal saline is administered at a high rate of 0.5–1 L/hr for 2–3 hours (hypotonic normal saline of 0.45% may be used for hypertension or hypernatremia or congestive heart failure).
3. 0.45% normal saline is fluid of choice after the first few hours provided blood pressure is stable and sodium level is not low.

4. Monitor fluid volume status (including checking for orthostatic changes of blood pressure and heart rate), lung assessment, and intake and output.
5. Initial urine output will lag behind IV fluid intake due to dehydration.
6. Use plasma expanders for correction of severe hypotension that does not respond to IV fluid treatment.
7. Monitor for signs of fluid overload in the older patient or those at risk for congestive heart failure.

Electrolyte Loss

1. Potassium is the main electrolyte of concern in treating DKA.
2. Cautious replacement of potassium is vital for avoidance of severe cardiac dysrhythmias that occur with hypokalemia.
3. Observe for signs of hyperkalemia, i.e., tall, peaked T waves on the ECG, and obtain frequent potassium values during first 8 hours of treatment.
4. Withhold potassium only if hyperkalemia is present and patient is not urinating.

Acidosis

1. Acidosis of DKA is reversed with insulin, which inhibits the fat breakdown.
2. Infuse insulin at a slow, continuous rate, e.g., 5 units per hour.
3. Monitor blood glucose values hourly.
4. Add dextrose to IV fluids when blood glucose reaches 250–300 mg/dl to avoid too rapid a drop in blood glucose.
5. IV mixtures of regular insulin only may be used.
6. IV insulin must be infused continuously until subcutaneous administration of insulin is resumed.
7. IV insulin must be continued until the serum bicarbonate improves and patient can eat; normalized blood glucose levels are not an indication that acidosis has resolved.

PREVENTION AND EDUCATION

Sick-Day Rules

1. Teach patient not to eliminate insulin doses when sick and nausea and vomiting occur.
2. Teach patients to take their usual insulin dose or previously prescribed "sick-day" doses and attempt to consume frequent small portions of carbohydrates.
3. Teach to drink fluid every hour including broth for avoidance of dehydration.
4. Check blood glucose every 3–4 hours.
5. Notify physician if unable to take fluids without vomiting or elevated glucose persists.
6. Teach patients how to contact their physician 24 hours a day.

Self-Management Skills

1. Insulin administration.
2. Blood glucose testing.
3. Assess skills to ensure that accidental error in insulin administration or blood glucose testing did not occur.

Recommend Psychologic Counseling

For patient and family if intentional alteration in insulin dosing was the cause of DKA.

For more information see Chapter 39 in Smeltzer and Bare: *Brunner and Suddarth's Textbook of Medical–Surgical Nursing*, 8th Edition. Philadelphia: Lippincott–Raven, 1996.

DIARRHEA

Diarrhea is a condition in which there is an unusual frequency of bowel movements (more than 3/day), as well as changes in the amount and the consistency (liquid stool). It is usually associated with urgency, perianal discomfort, incontinence, or a combination of these factors.

Three factors determine its severity: intestinal secretions, altered mucosal absorption, and increased motility. Diarrhea can be acute or chronic. It is classified as high volume, low volume, secretory, osmotic, or mixed. It can be caused by certain medications, tube feedings, metabolic and endocrine disorders, and viral/bacterial infections. Other causes are nutritional and malabsorptive disorders, anal sphincter deficit, Zollinger-Ellison syndrome, paralytic ileus, and intestinal obstruction.

CLINICAL MANIFESTATIONS

1. Increased frequency and fluid content of the stool.
2. Abdominal cramps, distention, intestinal rumbling (borborygmus), anorexia, and thirst.
3. Painful spasmodic contractions of the anus and ineffectual straining (tenesmus) may occur with each defecation.
4. May be explosive or gradual in nature and onset. Associated symptoms are dehydration and weakness.
5. Watery stools may indicate small-bowel disease.
6. Loose, semisolid stools are associated with disorders of the colon.
7. Voluminous greasy stools suggest intestinal malabsorption.
8. Mucus and pus in the stools denote inflammatory enteritis or colitis.
9. Oil droplets on the toilet water are diagnostic of pancreatic insufficiency.
10. Nocturnal diarrhea may be a manifestation of diabetic neuropathy.

DIAGNOSTIC EVALUATION

When cause is unknown: stool exam, i.e., infectious or parasitic organisms, proctosigmoidoscopy, and barium enema.

MANAGEMENT

Primary medical management is directed at controlling or curing the underlying disease.

1. For mild diarrhea, increase oral fluids; oral glucose and electrolyte solution may be prescribed.
2. For moderate diarrhea, nonspecific drugs, diphenoxylate (Lomotil) and loperamide (Imodium) to decrease motility from a noninfectious source.
3. Antimicrobials are prescribed when the infectious agent has been identified or diarrhea is severe.
4. Intravenous therapy for rapid hydration, especially for the very young or elderly.

NURSING PROCESS

Assessment

1. Complete health history to identify onset and pattern of diarrhea, and presence of the following: any related signs and symptoms; current drug therapy; daily dietary intake; past related medical history; and recent travel to another geographic area.
2. Observe and perform a complete physical assessment paying special attention to characteristic bowel sounds, inspection of stool, and blood pressure (postural hypotension).
3. Inspect mucous membranes and skin to determine hydration status; inspect perianal skin for irritation; note intake and output, weight.

Major Nursing Diagnosis

1. Diarrhea related to infection, ingestion of irritating foods, or disorder of the bowel
2. Risk for fluid volume deficit related to frequent passage of stools and insufficient fluid intake.
3. Anxiety related to frequent, uncontrolled elimination.
4. Risk for impaired skin integrity related to frequent, loose stools.

Collaborative Problems

1. Dehydration.
2. Fluid and electrolyte imbalance.
3. Cardiac dysrhythmias.

Planning and Implementation

The major goals may include regaining normal bowel patterns, avoidance of fluid and electrolyte deficit, reduction of anxiety, maintenance of perianal skin integrity, and absence of potential complication.

Interventions

CONTROLLING DIARRHEA.

1. Encourage bed rest, liquids, and foods low in bulk until acute period subsides.
2. Recommend bland diet when food intake is tolerated.
3. Limit caffeine (stimulates intestinal motility). Avoid very hot/cold foods.
4. Restrict milk products, fat, whole grain products, fresh fruits, and vegetables for several days.
5. Administer antidiarrheal drugs as prescribed.

MAINTAINING FLUID BALANCE

1. Assess for dehydration (decreased skin turgor, tachycardia, decreased pulse volume, decreased serum sodium, thirst).
2. Keep an accurate record of intake and output; weigh daily.
3. Encourage oral fluid replacement in the form of water, juices, bouillon, and commercial preparations such as Gatorade; give parenteral fluids as ordered.

REDUCING ANXIETY

1. Provide opportunity for patient to express fears/worry about being embarrassed by lack of control over bowel elimination.
2. Assist to identify any factors that precipitate diar-

rhea. Teach patient to be sensitive to body clues; use absorbent underwear; and take prescribed antianxiety medications.

PROVIDING SKIN CARE

Instruct patient to follow a perianal care routine such as wipe or pat area dry after defecation, cleanse with mild soap and warm water, pat dry immediately with cotton balls, and apply lotion or ointment as a skin barrier.

PREVENTING INFECTION

1. Treat all patients with diarrhea as potentially infectious.
2. Use universal precautions to prevent the spread of the disease.

MONITORING AND MANAGING POTENTIAL COMPLICATIONS

1. Monitor serum electrolyte levels, vital signs, changes in tendon reflexes and muscle strength; administer electrolyte replacements as prescribed.
2. Report evidence of dysrhythmias or a change in the level of consciousness.

✪ GERONTOLOGIC CONSIDERATIONS

Older persons can quickly become dehydrated and suffer from low potassium (hypokalemia) as a result of diarrhea.

Instruct those taking digitalis to be aware of the signs of dehydration and hypokalemia because low levels of potassium intensify the action of digitalis and lead to digitalis toxicity.

Skin in the elderly is sensitive to rapid perianal excoriation because of decreased turgor and reduced subcutaneous fat layers.

For more information see Chapter 37 in Smeltzer and Bare: *Brunner and Suddarth's Textbook of Medical–Surgical Nursing*, 8th Edition. Philadelphia: Lippincott–Raven, 1996.

DIC

See Disseminated Intravascular Coagulopathy

DISC, HERNIATED

See Herniation or Rupture of an Intervertebral Disc

DISC, RUPTURED

See Herniation or Rupture of an Intervertebral Disc

DISSEMINATED INTRAVASCULAR COAGULOPATHY (DIC)

DIC is a bleeding disorder characterized by low fibrinogen, prolonged prothrombin time, and partial thromboplastin time, thrombocytopenia, and elevated fibrin split products. Widespread clotting in small vessels of the body may occur, causing clotting factors and platelets to be used up. Such patients may bleed from mucous membranes, venipuncture sites, and the gastrointestinal and urinary tracts. Bleeding can range from minimal occult internal bleeding to profuse hemorrhaging from all orifices. Patients may also develop organ necrosis, such as renal failure, pulmonary and multifocal central nervous system infarctions due to micro- and macrothromboses. Illnesses predisposing to DIC include:

1. Septicemia.
2. Premature separation of the placenta in pregnant women.
3. Metastatic malignancies.
4. Hemolytic transfusion reactions.
5. Massive tissue trauma and shock.

CLINICAL MANIFESTATIONS

DIC should be suspected in any patient with a predisposing cause who develops purpura, a bleeding tendency, tissue hypoxemia, and signs of renal damage.

D

MANAGEMENT

The goals of management include controlling hemorrhage and clotting, and restoring acid-base balance and homeostasis. The best treatment is correction of the underlying disease.

Serious hemorrhage requires replacement therapy.

1. Packed red cells, platelet concentrates, and volume expanders without clotting proteins (e.g., albumin), plasma protein fraction, and hydroxyethyl starch.
2. If blood products with clotting factors are used, administer heparin prior to transfusion to reduce intravascular clotting.

For more information see Chapter 16 in Smeltzer and Bare: *Brunner and Suddarth's Textbook of Medical–Surgical Nursing,* 8th Edition. Philadelphia: Lippincott–Raven, 1996.

DIVERTICULAR DISORDERS

A diverticulum is an outpouching or herniation of the mucous membrane lining of the bowel through a defect in the muscle layer. Diverticula may occur anywhere along the gastrointestinal tract. Diverticulosis exists when multiple diverticula are present without inflammation or symptoms. Diverticulitis results when food and bacteria retained in the diverticulum produce infection and inflammation that can impede draining and lead to perforation or abscess. Diverticulitis is more common in the sigmoid colon, and in those over 60. A congenital predisposition is likely when the disorder is present in those under 40 years of age. A low intake of dietary fiber is considered a major cause. It may occur in acute attacks or persist as a long-continued, smoldering infection.

CLINICAL MANIFESTATIONS

Diverticulosis

1. Constipation from spastic colon syndrome often precedes development.
2. Bowel irregularity and diarrhea.
3. Crampy pain in the left lower quadrant.
4. Low-grade fever.
5. Nausea and anorexia.

Diverticulitis

1. Narrowing of the large bowel with fibrotic stricture.
2. Cramps.
3. Narrow stools.
4. Increased constipation.
5. Occult bleeding.
6. Weakness.
7. Fatigue.

DIAGNOSTIC EVALUATION

1. Radiographic studies (barium enema).
2. Sigmoidoscopy.
3. Colonoscopy.
4. CT scan.
5. WBC and sedimentation rate elevated.

MANAGEMENT

1. Diverticulosis: a high-fiber diet is prescribed to prevent constipation.
2. Diverticulitis: the bowel is rested; withhold oral fluids, administer IV fluids, institute NG suctioning; broad-spectrum antibiotics and analgesics are prescribed. A low-fiber diet may be necessary until signs of infection decrease. For spastic pain, antispasmodics are taken before meals and at bedtime;

sedatives and tranquilizers and bowel antimicrobials may be required.

3. Normal stools can be achieved by bulk preparations (Metamucil), stool softeners, warm oil enemas, and evacuant suppositories.

4. Surgery is usually necessary only if severe hemorrhage occurs; recurrence of diverticula is common. Type of surgery performed varies according to the extent of complications found during surgery.

NURSING PROCESS

Assessment

1. Assess health history including onset and duration of pain, dietary habits, and elimination patterns.

2. Physical assessment should include auscultation for bowel sounds, tenderness over left lower quadrant, palpation of sigmoid for masses, inspection of stool for pus, mucus, and blood, elevation of temperature and pulse rate.

Major Nursing Diagnosis

1. Constipation related to narrowing of the colon secondary to thickened muscular segments and strictures.

2. Pain related to inflammation and infection.

3. Altered gastrointestinal tissue perfusion related to the infectious process.

Collaborative Problems

1. Peritonitis.
2. Abscess formation.
3. Bleeding.

Planning and Implementation

The major goals may include attainment and maintenance of normal elimination, reduction in pain, improvement in gastrointestinal tissue perfusion, and absence of potential complications.

Interventions

MAINTAINING NORMAL ELIMINATION PATTERNS

1. Increase fluid intake to 2 L/day within limits of patient's cardiac reserve.
2. Promote foods that are soft but have increased fiber diet.
3. Encourage individualized exercise program to improve abdominal muscle tone.
4. Review patient's routine to establish a set time for meals and defecation.
5. Increase daily intake of bulk laxatives, i.e., Metamucil, stool softeners, or oil-retention enemas.

RELIEVING PAIN

1. Administer analgesics for pain and antispasmodics.

IMPROVING GASTROINTESTINAL TISSUE PERFUSION

1. Monitor vital signs and urine output.
2. Administer IV fluids.

MONITORING AND MANAGING POTENTIAL COMPLICATIONS

1. Identify persons at risk.
2. Assess for indicators of perforations: tender, rigid abdomen; elevated WBC count; elevated sedimentation rate; increased temperature; tachycardia and hypotension.
3. Perforation constitutes a surgical emergency.

✪ GERONTOLOGIC CONSIDERATIONS

Incidence of diverticular disease increases with age because of degeneration and structural changes in the circular muscle layers of the colon, and cellular hypertrophy.

Symptoms are less pronounced among the elderly, who may not experience abdominal pain until infection occurs. They delay reporting symptoms because they fear surgery or cancer.

Blood in stool may frequently be overlooked because of failure to examine the stool or inability to see changes because of diminished vision.

For more information see Chapter 37 in Smeltzer and Bare: *Brunner and Suddarth's Textbook of Medical–Surgical Nursing,* 8th Edition. Philadelphia: Lippincott–Raven, 1996.

DKA

See Diabetic Ketoacidosis

ELEPHANTIASIS

See Lymphedema and Elephantiasis

EMBOLISM, ARTERIAL

See Arterial Embolism

EMPHYSEMA, PULMONARY

Pulmonary emphysema is defined as a nonuniform pattern of abnormal, permanent distention of the air spaces with destruction of the alveolar walls. It appears to be an end-stage process that has progressed slowly for many years. In a small percentage of patients there is a familial predisposition associated with a plasma protein abnormality (deficiency of α_1-antitrypsin).

Emphysema is classified as:

1. Panlobular (panacinar): characterized by destruction of the respiratory bronchiole, alveolar duct, and alveoli; air spaces within the lobule are more or less enlarged, with little inflammatory disease. Often referred to as a "pink puffer."
2. Centrilobular (centriacinar): causes pathologic changes in the bronchioles, producing chronic hypoxia, hypercapnia, polycythemia, and episodes of right-sided heart failure. Often referred to as a "blue bloater" (both types of emphysema can occur together).

CLINICAL MANIFESTATIONS

Dyspnea with Insidious Onset

1. History of cigarette smoking, chronic cough, wheezing, shortness of breath, and tachypnea, exacerbated by respiratory infection.
2. Slight exertion produces dyspnea and fatigue.
3. On inspection, "barrel chest" due to air trapping, muscle wasting, and pursed-lip breathing.
4. On auscultation, diminished breath sounds with crackles, rhonchi, and prolonged expiration.
5. Hyperresonance with percussion, and a decrease in fremitus.
6. Anorexia, weight loss, and weakness.
7. Hypoxemia and hypercapnia in advanced stages.
8. Inflammatory reactions and infections from pooled secretions.

DIAGNOSTIC EVALUATION

Primarily chest films, pulmonary function tests, blood gases.

MANAGEMENT

The major goals are to improve quality of life, slow progression of the disease, and treatment of obstructed airways to relieve hypoxia.

1. Treatment to improve ventilation and decrease work of breathing.
2. Prevention and prompt treatment of infection.
3. Physical therapy to conserve and increase pulmonary ventilation.
4. Proper environmental conditions to facilitate breathing.
5. Supportive and psychological care.
6. Ongoing program of patient education and rehabilitation.
7. Bronchodilators or aerosol therapy (dispensing particles in a fine mist).

E

8. Treatment of infection (antimicrobial therapy at the first sign of respiratory infection).
9. Corticosteroids remain controversial; used after maximum bronchodilator and bronchial hygiene measures unsuccessful.
10. Oxygenation in low concentrations for severe hypoxemia.

For Nursing Management and Patient Education, see Chronic Obstructive Pulmonary Disease, Nursing Process.

For more information see Chapter 24 in Smeltzer and Bare: *Brunner and Suddarth's Textbook of Medical–Surgical Nursing,* 8th Edition. Philadelphia: Lippincott–Raven, 1996.

EMPYEMA

Empyema is a collection of infected liquid or pus in the pleural cavity. At first pleural fluid is thin, progresses to a fibropurulent stage, then to a stage where it encloses the lung with a thick exudative membrane.

CLINICAL MANIFESTATIONS

1. Fever, night sweats, pleural pain, dyspnea, anorexia, and weight loss.
2. Absence of breath sounds; flatness to chest percussion; decreased fremitus.

DIAGNOSTIC EVALUATION

Chest films and thoracentesis.

MANAGEMENT

The objectives of management are to drain the pleural cavity and to achieve full expansion of the lung; accomplished by adequate drainage, antibiotics (large doses), and/or streptokinase. Drainage of the pleural fluid or pus depends on the stage of the disease and is accomplished by:

1. Needle aspiration (thoracentesis) if fluid is not too thick.
2. Closed chest drainage.
3. Open chest drainage to remove thickened pleura, pus, and debris and resect the underlying diseased pulmonary tissue.
4. Decortication, if inflammation has been longstanding.

E

Nursing Interventions

1. Help patient cope with condition, instruct in breathing exercises (pursed lip and diaphragmatic breathing).
2. Provide care specific to method of drainage of pleural fluid.

For more information see Chapter 24 in Smeltzer and Bare: *Brunner and Suddarth's Textbook of Medical–Surgical Nursing*, 8th Edition. Philadelphia: Lippincott–Raven, 1996.

END-STAGE RENAL DISEASE

See Renal Failure, Chronic

ENDOCARDITIS, INFECTIVE

Infective endocarditis (bacterial endocarditis) is an infection of the valves and the endothelial surface of the heart. It is caused by direct invasion of bacteria or other organisms leading to deformity of the valve leaflets. Causative organisms include many bacterial types, e.g., *streptococci, pneumococci, staphylococci,* and fungi. Risk factors include valvular heart disease, rheumatic heart disease, mitral valve prolapse, or prosthetic valve surgery. It is more common in older persons, probably because of decreased immunologic response to infection, metabolic changes from the aging process, and increased invasive diagnostic procedures, especially in genitourinary disease. There is a high incidence of staphylococcal endocarditis among IV drug users. Hospital-acquired endocarditis occurs most often in patients with debilitating disease, indwelling catheters, and those on prolonged IV or antibiotic therapy. Patients on immunosuppressive medications or steroids may develop fungal endocarditis.

CLINICAL MANIFESTATIONS

1. Insidious onset; signs and symptoms develop from toxicity of infection, destruction of heart valves, and embolization of fragments of vegetative growths on the heart.
2. General manifestations include vague complaints of malaise, anorexia, weight loss, and back and joint pain.
3. Fever is intermittent; may be absent in patients who are receiving antibiotics or corticosteroids, the elderly, or those who have congestive heart failure or renal failure.
4. Splinter hemorrhages under the fingernails and toenails, and petechiae in the conjunctiva and mucous membranes.
5. Hemorrhages with pale centers (Roth's spots) in the fundi of the eyes.
6. Cardiac manifestations include heart enlargement, congestive heart failure, and heart murmurs (may be absent initially); changing murmurs indicate valvular damage.
7. Central nervous system manifestations include headache, transient cerebral ischemia, focal neurologic lesions, and strokes.
8. Emboli involving other organ systems manifest in the lung (recurrent pneumonia; pulmonary abscesses), kidney (hematuria; renal failure), spleen (left upper quadrant pain), heart (myocardial infarction), brain (stroke), and peripheral vessels.

MANAGEMENT

The objective of treatment is total eradication of the invading organism through adequate doses of an appropriate antimicrobial agent.

1. Isolate causative organism through serial blood cultures. Blood cultures are taken to monitor the course of therapy.
2. After recovery from the infectious process, seriously damaged valves may require replacement.
3. Patient's temperature is monitored for treatment effectiveness.

E

COMPLICATIONS

Complications include congestive heart failure, cerebral vascular complications, valve stenosis or regurgitation, myocardial damage, and mycotic aneurysms.

SURGERY

Surgical valve replacement is required for development of congestive heart failure; more than one serious systemic embolic episode; uncontrolled infection, recurrent infection, or fungal endocarditis.

PREVENTION

Antibiotic prophylaxis is recommended for persons at risk undergoing invasive procedures.

For more information see Chapter 29 in Smeltzer and Bare: *Brunner and Suddarth's Textbook of Medical–Surgical Nursing*, 8th Edition. Philadelphia: Lippincott–Raven, 1996.

ENDOCARDITIS, RHEUMATIC

Rheumatic endocarditis is directly attributed to rheumatic fever caused by group A streptococcal infection. Rheumatic fever affects all bony joints, producing a polyarthritis. The most serious damage occurs in the heart. Rheumatic endocarditis manifests itself by tiny, translucent vegetations that resemble beads about the size of a pinhead, arranged in a row along the free margins of the valve flaps. The flaps gradually become shorter and thicker than normal, which prevents them from closing the valve orifice completely. The result is valvular regurgitation (leakage); most common is mitral regurgitation. Valvular stenosis may also occur. A small percentage of patients become critically ill with intractable heart failure, serious dysrhythmias, and rheumatic pneumonia. Eventually the heart murmurs characteristic of valvular stenosis, regurgitation, or both become audible on auscultation; "thrills" may be detectable upon palpation. The myocardium can compensate for these valvular defects very well for a time. Sooner or later decompensation occurs and is manifested by congestive heart failure.

CLINICAL MANIFESTATIONS

Cardiac symptoms depend on which side of the heart is involved. Severity of symptoms depends on size and location of the lesion. Mitral valve is most often affected, producing symptoms of left-sided heart failure: shortness of breath, crackles, and wheezes.

MANAGEMENT

1. The goals of medical management are aggressive eradication of the causative organism and prevention of additional complications such as a thromboembolic event.
2. Long-term antibiotic therapy is the treatment of choice. Parenteral penicillin remains the medication of choice.
3. If valve function is faulty, the disease is quiet; no therapy is required as long as the heart pumps effectively.

PREVENTION

1. Prevention through early and adequate treatment of streptococcal infection in all persons.
2. A first-line approach is to recognize streptococcal infections, treat them adequately, and control community epidemics. A throat culture is the only

method by which accuracy of diagnosis can be determined.
3. Susceptible patients may require long-term oral antibiotic therapy. May be required to take prophylactic antibiotics before procedures, i.e., dental checkups or cystoscopy.

For more information see Chapter 29 in Smeltzer and Bare: *Brunner and Suddarth's Textbook of Medical–Surgical Nursing,* 8th Edition. Philadelphia: Lippincott–Raven, 1996.

E

ENDOMETRIAL CANCER

See Cancer of the Endometrium

ENDOMETRIOSIS

Endometriosis is a benign lesion with cells similar to those lining the uterus growing aberrantly in the pelvic cavity outside the uterus. There is a high incidence among patients who bear children later, and have fewer children. It is usually found in the young, nulliparous woman aged 25 to 35. There appears to be a familial predisposition to endometriosis. In mild to moderate endometriosis, the use of hormonal or surgical treatment relieves pain and enhances the chance of pregnancy. For women over age 35 or those not concerned with reproduction, definitive surgery (total hysterectomy) provides another alternative.

CLINICAL MANIFESTATIONS

1. Symptoms vary with the location of endometrial tissue.
2. Chief symptom is a type of dysmenorrhea: deep-seated aching in the lower abdomen, vagina, posterior pelvis, and back, occurring 1 or 2 days before menstrual cycle and lasting 2 or 3 days.

3. Some patients have no pain.
4. Abnormal uterine bleeding and dyspareunia (painful intercourse).
5. Nausea and diarrhea.

DIAGNOSTIC EVALUATION

Laparoscopy confirms the diagnosis and helps to stage the disease.

MANAGEMENT

Treatment depends on patient's symptoms, desire for pregnancy, and extent of the disease. If the woman is asymptomatic, observation every 6 months may be all that is required. Palliative measures, i.e., analgesics, prostaglandin inhibitors, and pregnancy; pregnancy alleviates symptoms because no menstruation occurs.

Hormonal therapy

1. Oral contraceptives for 6–9 months to suppress menstruation and relieve menstrual pain.
2. Synthetic androgen, danazol (Danocrine), causes atrophy of the endometrium and subsequent amenorrhea (expensive and may cause troublesome side effects, i.e., fatigue, depression, weight gain, oily skin, decreased breast size, mild acne, hot flashes, and atrophy of the vagina).
3. Gonadotropin-releasing hormone (GnRH) agonist or GnRH blocker called Synarel results in decreased estrogen production and subsequent amenorrhea. Administered by nasal spray twice a day for 6 months. Side effects related to low estrogen levels.

Surgery

1. Laparoscopy performed to fulgurate endometrial implants and to lyse adhesions.
2. Laser surgery to vaporize endometrial implants or to coagulate the implant and destroy the endometriosis.

3. Other surgical procedures may include laparotomy, uterine suspension, abdominal hysterectomy, bilateral salpingo-oophorectomy, and appendectomy.

Nursing Interventions

1. Obtain health history and physical examination concentrating on identifying length of specific symptoms and defining woman's reproductive desires.
2. Assess for pain and evaluate techniques and prescribed medications that provide relief.
3. Explain various diagnostic procedures to alleviate anxiety.
4. Provide emotional support to the woman and her partner who wish to have children.
5. Respect and address psychosocial impact of realization that pregnancy is not easily possible.
6. Discuss alternatives such as in vitro fertilization (IVF) or adoption and offer referrals.
7. Encourage to seek care of dysmenorrhea or abnormal bleeding patterns.
8. Direct to the Endometriosis Association for more information and support.

For more information see Chapter 45 in Smeltzer and Bare: *Brunner and Suddarth's Textbook of Medical–Surgical Nursing,* 8th Edition. Philadelphia: Lippincott–Raven, 1996.

EOSINOPHILIC TUMORS

See Pituitary Tumors

EPIDIDYMITIS

Epididymitis is an infection of the epididymis that usually results from an infected prostate. It may also develop as a complication of gonorrhea. In men under 35 years of age, the major cause is *Chlamydia trachomatis.*

CLINICAL MANIFESTATIONS

1. Unilateral pain and soreness in the inguinal canal along the course of the vas deferens.
2. Pain and swelling in the scrotum and groin.
3. Extremely painful and swollen epididymis; temperature elevated.
4. Pyuria and bacteriuria with resulting chills and fever.

MANAGEMENT

1. If seen within first 24 hours after onset of pain, spermatic cord may be infiltrated with a local anesthetic agent for relief.
2. If chlamydial in origin, patient and patient's sexual partners must be treated with antibiotics.
3. Observe for abscess formation.
4. If no improvement within 2 weeks, underlying testicular tumor should be considered.
5. Epididymectomy (excision of the epididymis from the testes) for recurrent, incapacitating episodes or chronic, painful conditions.

Nursing Interventions

1. Place on bed rest with scrotum elevated with a scrotal bridge or folded towel to prevent traction on spermatic cord and improve venous drainage and relieve pain.
2. Give antimicrobials as prescribed.
3. Provide intermittent cold compresses to scrotum to help ease pain; later, local heat or sitz baths may hasten resolution of inflammatory process.
4. Give analgesics as prescribed for pain relief.

✎ PATIENT EDUCATION AND HEALTH MAINTENANCE: CARE IN THE HOME AND COMMUNITY

1. Patient should avoid straining, lifting, and sexual excitement until the infection is under control.

2. Instruct to continue with analgesics and antibiotics as prescribed and to use ice packs as necessary for discomfort.
3. It may take 4 weeks or longer for the epididymis to return to normal.

For more information see Chapter 47 in Smeltzer and Bare: *Brunner and Suddarth's Textbook of Medical–Surgical Nursing*, 8th Edition. Philadelphia: Lippincott–Raven, 1996.

E

EPILEPSIES

The epilepsies are a symptom-complex of several disorders of brain function characterized by recurring seizures. There may be associated loss of consciousness, excess movement, or loss of muscle tone or movement, and disturbances of behavior, mood, sensation, and perception. The basic problem is thought to be an electrical disturbance (dysrhythmia) in the nerve cells in one section of the brain, causing them to emit abnormal, recurring, uncontrolled electrical discharges. The characteristic epileptic seizure is a manifestation of this excessive neuronal discharge. In most cases the cause is unknown (idiopathic). There is evidence that susceptibility to some types may be inherited. Epilepsies often follow many medical disorders, traumas, and drug or alcohol intoxication. They are also associated with brain tumors, abscesses, and congenital malformations. Epilepsy begins before the age of 20 in over 75% of patients. Epilepsy is not synonymous with mental retardation or illness.

CLINICAL MANIFESTATIONS

Seizures range from simple staring spells to prolonged convulsive movements with loss of consciousness. Seizures are classified as partial, generalized, and unclassified according to the area of brain involved. Aura, a premonitory or warning sensation, occurs before seizure (e.g., seeing a flashing light, hearing a sound).

Simple Partial Seizures

Only a finger or hand may shake; or mouth jerks uncontrollably; talks unintelligibly; may be dizzy; may experience unusual or unpleasant sights, sounds, odors, or taste—all without loss of consciousness.

Complex Partial Seizures

Remains motionless or moves automatically but inappropriately for time and place; may experience excessive emotions of fear, anger, elation, or irritability; does not remember episode when it is over.

Generalized Seizures (Grand Mal Seizures)

Involve both hemispheres of the brain, intense rigidity of entire body followed by jerky alternations of muscle relaxation and contraction (generalized tonic-clonic contraction).

1. Simultaneous contractions of diaphragm and chest muscles produce characteristic epileptic cry.
2. Tongue is chewed, incontinent of urine and stool.
3. Convulsive movements last 1 or 2 minutes.
4. Relaxes and lies in deep coma, breathing noisily.

Postictal State

After the seizure, patient is often confused and hard to arouse, may sleep for hours. Many complain of headache or sore muscles.

DIAGNOSTIC EVALUATION

1. CT imaging to detect lesions, focal abnormalities, cerebral vascular abnormalities, and cerebral degenerative changes.
2. Electroencephalogram (EEG) aids in classifying the type of seizure.

MANAGEMENT

The management of epilepsy is planned according to a long-range program and tailored to meet the special needs of each patient.

The goals of treatment are to stop the seizures as quickly as possible, to ensure adequate cerebral oxygenation, and to maintain the patient in a seizure-free state.

E

1. Establish an airway and adequate oxygenation (intubate if necessary); establish an IV line for medications and blood work.
2. Give intravenous diazepam slowly in an attempt to halt seizures.
3. Give other anticonvulsant medications (phenytoin, phenobarbital) as prescribed after the diazepam to maintain a seizure-free state.
4. Monitor vital signs and neurologic signs continuously.
5. Monitor EEG to determine the nature of epileptogenic activity.
6. Use general anesthesia with a short-acting barbiturate, if initial treatment is unsuccessful.
7. Measure serum concentration of the anticonvulsant medication patient was taking.
8. Patient may die from cardiac involvement or respiratory depression.
9. Assess potential for postictal cerebral swelling.

Medication Therapy

MEDICATION THERAPY IS USED TO ACHIEVE SEIZURE CONTROL.

1. Usual treatment is single drug therapy.
2. Major anticonvulsant medications include carbamazepine, primidone, phenytoin, phenobarbital, ethosuximide, and valproate.
3. Perform periodic physical examinations and laboratory tests for patients receiving medications known to have toxic side effects.

4. Prevent or control gingival hyperplasia with thorough oral hygiene, regular dental care, and regular gum massage for patients taking phenytoin (Dilantin).

Surgery

1. Indicated when epilepsy results from intracranial tumors, abscess, cysts, or vascular anomalies.
2. Surgical removal of the epileptogenic focus is done for seizures that originate in a well-circumcised area of the brain that can be excised without producing significant neurologic defects.

NURSING PROCESS

Assessment

1. Obtain a complete seizure history; ask about factors or events that may precipitate the seizures; document alcohol intake.
2. Assess effects of epilepsy on lifestyle.
3. Observation and neurologic nursing assessment during and after a seizure.

Major Nursing Diagnosis

1. Fear related to the ever-present possibility of having seizures.
2. Ineffective coping related to stresses imposed by epilepsy.
3. Knowledge deficit about epilepsy and its control.

Collaborative Problems

Status epilepticus.

Planning and Implementation

The major goals may include maintenance control of seizures, achievement of a satisfactory psychosocial adjustment, and acquisition of knowledge, understanding about the condition, and absence of complications of epilepsy.

Interventions

1. Provide ongoing assessment and monitoring of respiratory and cardiac function.
2. Monitor the seizure type and general condition of the patient.
3. Turn patient to side-lying position to assist in draining pharyngeal secretions.
4. Have suction equipment available for danger of aspiration.
5. Monitor IV line closely for dislodgement during seizures.
6. Protect patient from injury during seizures with padded side rails and keep under constant observation.
7. Do not restrain patient's movements during seizure activity.

CONTROLLING SEIZURES

1. Reduce fear that a seizure may occur unexpectedly by patient's compliance to prescribed treatment.
2. Emphasize that the prescribed anticonvulsant medication must be taken on a continuing basis and is not habit forming.
3. Assess lifestyle and environment to determine factors that precipitate seizures, e.g., emotional disturbances, new environmental stressors, onset of menstruation in female patients, or fever.
4. Encourage to follow a regular and moderate routine in lifestyle, diet (avoiding excessive stimulants), exercise, and rest.
5. Avoid photic stimulation (i.e., bright flickering lights, television viewing); dark glasses or covering one eye may help.
6. Provide classes in stress management.
7. Restrict alcoholic beverages.

IMPROVING COPING MECHANISMS

1. Understand that epilepsy imposes feelings of fear, alienation, depression, and uncertainty.

2. Provide counseling to the individual and family to understand the condition and limitations imposed.
3. Provide social and recreational opportunities.
4. Provide comprehensive mental health services to patients who exhibit symptoms of schizophrenia, impulsive or irritable behavior.

MONITORING AND MANAGING COMPLICATIONS (STATUS EPILEPTICUS)

Status epilepticus (acute prolonged seizure activity) is a series of generalized convulsions that occur without full recovery of consciousness between attacks.

1. Continuous clinical or electrical seizures lasting at least 30 minutes, even without impairment of consciousness.
2. Considered a major medical emergency.
3. Repeated episodes of cerebral anoxia and swelling may lead to irreversible and fatal brain damage.
4. Common factors that precipitate status epilepticus include withdrawal of anticonvulsant medication, fever, and intercurrent infection.

✎ PATIENT EDUCATION AND HEALTH MAINTENANCE: CARE IN THE HOME AND COMMUNITY

Mental Outlook

1. Modify the attitudes of the patient and family toward the disease itself; provide factual information concerning epilepsy.
2. Instruct patient to carry an emergency medical identification card or wear an identification bracelet.

Genetic Counseling

Provide genetic counseling if desired (heredity transmission of epilepsy has not been proved).

Financial Considerations

The Epilepsy Foundation of America offers a mail-order program for medications at minimum cost and access to life insurance.

Vocational Rehabilitation

The State Vocational Rehabilitation Agency, Epilepsy Foundation of America, Veterans Administration, the U.S. Civil Service Commission.

General Information

The Commission for the Control of Epilepsy and Its Consequences makes recommendations covering all aspects of the problem of epilepsy in the United States.

For more information see Chapter 60 in Smeltzer and Bare: *Brunner and Suddarth's Textbook of Medical–Surgical Nursing,* 8th Edition. Philadelphia: Lippincott–Raven, 1996.

EPISTAXIS (NOSEBLEED)

Epistaxis is a hemorrhage from the nose caused by the rupture of tiny, distended vessels in the mucous membrane. The anterior septum is the most common site. Causes include trauma, infection, drugs, cardiovascular diseases, blood dyscrasias, nasal tumors, low humidity, foreign body, and a deviated nasal septum. Vigorous nose blowing and nose picking are additional causes.

MANAGEMENT

Dependent on Bleeding Site

1. Nasal speculum or headlight used to determine site.
2. Apply direct pressure.
3. Sit patient upright with the head tilted forward to prevent swallowing and aspiration of blood.
4. Compress the soft outer portion of the nose against the midline septum for 5 or 10 minutes continuously.

Additional Treatment If Indicated

1. Anterior nosebleeds, cauterization by chemical agents, i.e., silver nitrate and Gelfoam, or electro-cautery; topical vasoconstrictors, i.e., adrenalin (1:1000), cocaine (0.5%), phenylephrine.
2. Posterior nosebleeds, drug-moistened cotton pledgets inserted into nostril to reduce blood flow; suction to remove excess blood and clots from the field of inspection.
3. Pack nose with petrolatum impregnated gauze when origin of bleed cannot be identified. Keep packing in place for 48 hours or up to 5 or 6 days if necessary to control bleeding.

Nursing Interventions

1. Monitor vital signs and assist in control of bleeding.
2. Provide tissues and an emesis basin for expectoration of blood.
3. Reassure bleeding can be controlled.
4. Maintain a calm, kind, efficient manner.

DISCHARGE TEACHING

1. Review ways to prevent epistaxis including avoiding forceful nose blowing, straining, high altitudes, and nasal trauma (including nose picking).
2. Provide adequate humidification to prevent drying of nasal passages.
3. Instruct patient how to apply direct pressure to nose with thumb and index finger for 15 minutes if recurrent nosebleed.
4. Instruct to seek medical attention if recurrent bleeding cannot be stopped.

For more information see Chapter 23 in Smeltzer and Bare: *Brunner and Suddarth's Textbook of Medical–Surgical Nursing,* 8th Edition. Philadelphia: Lippincott–Raven, 1996.

ESOPHAGEAL CANCER

See Cancer of the Esophagus

ESOPHAGEAL VARICES, BLEEDING

E

Bleeding or hemorrhage from esophageal varices is one of the major causes of death in patients with cirrhosis. Esophageal varices are dilated torturous veins usually found in the submucosa of the lower esophagus; they may develop higher in the esophagus or extend into the stomach. The condition nearly always is caused by portal hypertension. Risk factors for hemorrhage include muscular strain from heavy lifting; straining at stool, sneezing, coughing, or vomiting; esophagitis, or irritation of vessels; salicylates and any drug that erodes the esophageal mucosa.

CLINICAL MANIFESTATIONS

1. Hematemesis and melena, mainly in those who have abused alcohol.
2. Dilated veins usually cause no symptoms unless portal pressure increases and mucosa becomes thin (then massive hemorrhage takes place).

DIAGNOSTIC EVALUATION

1. Endoscopy, barium swallow, ultrasound, CT scan, and angiography.
2. Neurologic and portal hypertension assessment.
3. Liver function tests.

MANAGEMENT

The goals of management are aggressive medical care and expert nursing care.

1. Evaluate extent of bleeding and monitor vital signs continuously when hematemesis and melena are present.

2. Note signs of potential hypovolemia.
3. Monitor blood volume with central venous pressure or arterial catheter.
4. Give oxygen to prevent hypoxia and to maintain adequate blood oxygenation.
5. Provide intravenous fluids and volume expanders to restore fluid volume and replace electrolytes.
6. Assess for need of blood transfusion.
7. Monitor intake and output.

Nonsurgical Management

Nonsurgical treatment is preferable because of high mortality of emergency surgery for control of bleeding of esophageal varices and because of poor physical condition of the patient with severe liver dysfunction.

1. Pharmacologic therapy: vasopressin (Pitressin), propranolol (Inderal), somatostatin.
2. Balloon tamponade, saline lavage, endoscopic sclerotherapy.
3. Transjugular intrahepatic portosystemic shunting (TIPS).

Surgical Management

1. Surgical bypass procedures, i.e., portacaval anastomosis, splenorenal shunt, mesocaval shunt.
2. Devascularization and transection.

Nursing Interventions

Provide support before and during examination by endoscopy to relieve stress.

1. Monitor carefully to detect early signs of cardiac dysrhythmias, perforation, and hemorrhage.
2. Do not give fluids after the examination until the gag reflex returns.
3. Use lozenges and gargles to relieve throat discomfort.
4. No oral intake is permitted if patient is actively bleeding.

Postoperative Nursing Interventions

1. Provide support and explanations regarding care and procedures.
2. Give postoperative care similar to that for any abdominal operation.
3. Assess closely for complications, including hypovolemic or hemorrhagic shock, hepatic encephalopathy, electrolyte imbalance, metabolic and respiratory alkalosis, alcohol withdrawal syndrome, and seizures.
4. Monitor closely to prevent accidental removal or displacement of tube, subsequent airway obstruction, and aspiration related to balloon tamponade.
5. Explain procedure to patient briefly to obtain cooperation with insertion and maintenance.
6. Provide frequent oral hygiene.
7. Ensure patency of nasogastric tube to prevent aspiration. Observe gastric aspirate for blood and cessation of bleeding.
8. Observe for aspiration, perforation of esophagus, and recurrence of bleeding related to endoscopic sclerotherapy.
9. Observe for development of portal systemic encephalopathy.
10. Observe for rebleeding related to esophageal transection and devascularization.

✪ GERONTOLOGIC CONSIDERATIONS

Bleeding esophageal varices can quickly lead to hemorrhagic shock and should be considered an emergency.

For more information see Chapter 38 in Smeltzer and Bare: *Brunner and Suddarth's Textbook of Medical–Surgical Nursing,* 8th Edition. Philadelphia: Lippincott–Raven, 1996.

ESRD

See Renal Failure, Chronic

EXFOLIATIVE DERMATITIS

Exfoliative dermatitis is a serious condition characterized by a progressive inflammation in which erythema
and scaling occur in a more or less generalized distribution. This condition starts acutely as either a patchy
or a generalized erythematous eruption. Exfoliative dermatitis has a variety of causes. It is considered to be a
secondary or reactive process to an underlying skin or
systemic disease. It may appear as a part of the lymphoma group of diseases and may precede the appearance of lymphoma. Preexisting skin disorders implicated
as a cause include psoriasis, atopic dermatitis, and contact dermatitis. It also appears as a severe drug reaction,
including penicillin and phenylbutazone. The etiology is
unknown in approximately 25% of cases.

CLINICAL MANIFESTATIONS

1. Chills, fever, prostration, severe toxicity, and an
   itchy scaling of the skin.
2. Profound loss of stratum corneum (outermost layer
   of the skin), e.g., capillary leakage, hypoproteinemia, negative nitrogen balance.
3. Widespread dilation of cutaneous vessels resulting
   in large amounts of body heat loss.
4. Skin color changes from pink to dark red; after a
   week, exfoliation (scaling) begins in the form of thin
   flakes that leave the underlying skin smooth and
   red, with new scales forming as the older ones
   come off.
5. Possible hair loss.
6. Relapses are common.
7. Systemic effects: high-output congestive heart failure, intestinal disturbances, gynecomastia, hyperuricemia, and temperature disturbances.

MANAGEMENT

Goals of management are to maintain fluid and electrolyte balance and to prevent infection. Treatment is individualized and supportive and started as soon as condition is diagnosed.

1. Hospitalize patients and place on bed rest.
2. Discontinue all medications that may be implicated.
3. Maintain a comfortable room temperature because of patient's abnormal thermoregulatory control.
4. Maintain fluid and electrolyte balance, e.g., considerable water and protein loss from the skin surface.
5. Give plasma expanders as indicated.
6. Carry out continual nursing assessment to detect infection.
7. Administer prescribed antibiotics on the basis of culture and sensitivity.
8. Observe for signs and symptoms of congestive heart failure.
9. Assess for hypothermia because of increased skin blood flow coupled with increased water.
10. Use topical therapy to give symptomatic relief.
11. Use soothing baths, compresses, and lubrication with emollients to treat extensive dermatitis.
12. Give prescribed oral or parenteral steroids when disease is not controlled by more conservative therapy.
13. Advise to avoid all irritants, particularly medications.

For more information see Chapter 54 in Smeltzer and Bare: *Brunner and Suddarth's Textbook of Medical–Surgical Nursing*, 8th Edition. Philadelphia: Lippincott–Raven, 1996.

FACIAL PARALYSIS

See Bell's Palsy

FLU

See Influenza

FOLIC ACID DEFICIENCY

See Anemia, Megaloblastic

FULMINANT HEPATIC FAILURE

See Hepatic Failure, Fulminant

GALLBLADDER

See Cholecystitis

GALLSTONES

See Cholelithiasis

GASTRIC CANCER

See Cancer of the Stomach

GASTRINOMA

See Zollinger-Ellison Syndrome

GASTRITIS

ACUTE GASTRITIS

Gastritis (inflammation of the stomach mucosa) is most often due to dietary indiscretion, i.e., eating too much, too rapidly, food that is too highly seasoned, or food that is infected. Other causes include alcohol, aspirin, bile reflux, or radiation therapy. Gastritis may also be the first sign of acute systemic infection. A more severe form of acute gastritis is caused by strong acids or alkalies, which may cause the mucosa to become gangrenous or to perforate.

CLINICAL MANIFESTATIONS

1. Superficial ulceration may occur and can lead to hemorrhage.
2. Abdominal discomfort with headache, lassitude, nausea, and anorexia. Vomiting and hiccuping may occur.
3. Some patients are asymptomatic.
4. Colic and diarrhea may result if irritating food is not vomited, but reaches the bowel.
5. The patient usually recovers in about a day, although appetite may be diminished for 2 to 3 days.

CHRONIC GASTRITIS

Prolonged inflammation of the stomach caused by either benign or malignant ulcers of the stomach, or by the bacteria *Helicobacter pylori.* Chronic gastritis may be classified as type A or B. Type A is associated with autoimmune diseases, i.e., pernicious anemia. It occurs in the fundus or body of the stomach. Type B *(H. pylori)* affects the antrum and pylorus. It may be associated with *H. pylori* bacteria, dietary factors such as hot drinks, spices, drug use, alcohol, smoking, or reflux of intestinal contents into the stomach.

CLINICAL MANIFESTATIONS

1. Type A gastritis: essentially asymptomatic except for symptoms of B_{12} deficiency.
2. Type B gastritis: patients complain of anorexia, heartburn after eating, belching, sour taste in mouth, or nausea and vomiting.

DIAGNOSTIC EVALUATION

1. Type A associated with absence or low levels of hydrochloric acid.
2. Type B associated with hyperchlorhydria.
3. Gastroscopy, upper gastrointestinal, x-ray series, and histologic examination.

MANAGEMENT

Acute Gastritis

1. Refrain from alcohol and eating until symptoms subside; progress to nonirritating diet.
2. If symptoms persist, IV fluids may be necessary.
3. If bleeding is present, management is similar to that of upper gastrointestinal tract hemorrhage.
4. If gastritis is due to ingestion of strong acids or alkalies, dilute and neutralize the acid with common antacids, e.g., aluminum hydroxide.
5. If gastritis is due to ingestion of strong alkali, use diluted lemon juice or diluted vinegar.
6. If corrosion is severe, avoid emetics and lavage because of danger of perforation.

Chronic Gastritis

1. Diet modification, rest, stress reduction, and pharmacotherapy.
2. *H. pylori* may be treated with antibiotics (i.e., tetracycline or amoxicillin) and bismuth salts (Pepto Bismol).

NURSING PROCESS

Assessment

1. Ask about presenting signs and symptoms; heartburn, indigestion, nausea, vomiting; when do symptoms occur; are symptoms related to anxiety, stress, allergies, eating or drinking too much or too quickly?
2. How are symptoms relieved?
3. Inquire as to whether others in the patient's environment have similar symptoms; whether blood has been vomited or any caustic element has been swallowed.
4. Perform complete physical assessment. Note abdominal tenderness, dehydration, and evidence of systemic disorder that may be responsible for symptoms.

Major Nursing Diagnosis

1. Anxiety related to treatment.
2. Altered nutrition, less than body requirements, related to inadequate intake of nutrients.
3. Risk for fluid volume deficit related to insufficient fluid intake and excessive fluid loss subsequent to vomiting.
4. Knowledge deficit about dietary management and disease process.
5. Pain related to irritated stomach mucosa.

Collaborative Problems

1. Perforation.
2. Hemorrhage.
3. Pyloric obstruction.

Planning and Implementation

The major goals may be to reduce anxiety, avoid irritating foods and assure adequate intake of nutrients, maintain fluid balance, increase awareness of dietary management, and relieve pain.

Interventions

REDUCING ANXIETY

1. Carry out emergency measures for ingestion of acids or alkalies.
2. Offer support therapy to patient and family during treatment and after the ingested acid or alkali has been neutralized or diluted.
3. Prepare patient for additional diagnostic studies (endoscopy) or surgery.
4. Use a calm approach and answer questions as completely as possible; explain all procedures and treatments.

PROMOTING NUTRITION

1. Provide physical and emotional support for patients with acute gastritis.

2. Avoid foods and fluids by mouth for hours or days until acute symptoms subside.
3. Provide IV therapy as necessary and monitor serum electrolyte values daily.
4. Offer ice chips and clear liquids when symptoms subside.
5. Encourage patient to report any symptoms suggesting a repeat episode of gastritis as food is introduced.
6. Discourage caffeinated beverages (caffeine increases gastric activity and pepsin secretion).

7. Discourage alcohol and cigarette smoking (nicotine inhibits neutralization of gastric acid in the duodenum).
8. Teach that nicotine increases muscular activity in the bowel, leading to nausea and vomiting (parasympathetic stimulation).

PROMOTING FLUID BALANCE

1. Monitor daily intake and output for dehydration.
2. Assess electrolyte values every 24 hours for fluid imbalance.
3. Be alert for indicators of hemorrhagic gastritis (hematemesis, tachycardia, hypotension) and notify physician.

RELIEVING PAIN

1. Instruct to avoid foods and beverages that may be irritating to the gastric mucosa.
2. Assess level of pain and attainment of comfort through use of medications and avoidance of irritating substances.

✎ PATIENT EDUCATION AND HEALTH MAINTENANCE: CARE IN THE HOME AND COMMUNITY

1. Assess knowledge about gastritis and develop an individualized teaching plan.
2. Take into account daily caloric needs and food preferences.

3. Provide a list of substances to avoid (caffeine, nicotine, spicy foods, irritating or highly seasoned foods, alcohol).
4. Educate about antibiotics, antacids, bismuth salts, sedatives, or anticholinergics that may be prescribed.
5. Give patients with pernicious anemia instructions regarding need for long-term vitamin B_{12} injections.

For more information see Chapter 36 in Smeltzer and Bare: *Brunner and Suddarth's Textbook of Medical–Surgical Nursing,* 8th Edition. Philadelphia: Lippincott–Raven, 1996.

GLAUCOMA

Glaucoma refers to a group of diseases that differ in their pathophysiology, clinical presentation, and treatment. They are generally characterized by visual field loss caused by damage to the optic nerve. Damage is related to the level of intraocular pressure (IOP), which is too high for proper functioning of the optic nerve. Glaucoma is one of the leading causes of blindness in Western society. When it is diagnosed early and managed properly, blindness is almost always preventable. Most cases are asymptomatic until extensive and irreversible damage has occurred. Routine eye examinations and screening clinics are vital to the detection of this disease. Glaucoma affects people of all ages but is more prevalent with increasing age. Others at risk are diabetics, African Americans, those with a family history of glaucoma, and people with previous eye trauma or surgery or who have had long-term steroid treatment.

CLASSIFICATION

There are two categories of glaucoma: open angle and angle closure. The categories are further divided into:

1. Primary glaucomas: cause unknown; usually bilateral and thought to have a hereditary component.
2. Secondary glaucomas: cause known; often unilateral.

Causes of Secondary Open-Angle Glaucoma

1. Long-term corticosteroid use.
2. Intraocular tumors.
3. Uveitis from diseases such as herpes simplex and herpes zoster.
4. Trabecular meshwork blockage by lens material, viscoelastic substance (used in cataract surgery), blood, or pigment.

Causes of Normal-Tension Glaucoma and Ocular Hypertension

IOP pressures in the normal range may be too high for continued optic nerve health.

Combined-Mechanism Glaucoma

1. Combination of two or more forms of disease.
2. Open-angle glaucoma complicated by angle-closure glaucoma is the most common form.

DIAGNOSTIC EVALUATION

Examination of the eye, diagnostic tests, and ocular and medical histories.

CLINICAL MANIFESTATIONS

Primary Open-Angle Glaucoma

1. Most common type.
2. Difficult to recognize early because it is asymptomatic until late in its course.
3. Insidious in onset, slowly progressive, and small areas of peripheral vision loss may go unnoticed.
4. One eye frequently is involved earlier and more severely than the other.

Acute Angle-Closure Glaucoma

1. Symptoms include pain, halo vision, blurred vision, redness, and change in the eye's appearance.

2. Ocular pain caused by rapid rise in IOP by inflammation or medication-induced side effects.
3. Severe ocular pain accompanied by nausea, vomiting, sweating, or bradycardia.

MANAGEMENT

The objective of treatment is to lower the IOP to a level consistent with retaining vision. Treatment varies depending on classification of the disease and response to therapy. Medication therapy, laser surgery, and conventional surgery may be used to control progressive damage.

Pharmacotherapy

1. Pharmacotherapy is the initial and principal treatment for primary open-angle glaucoma.
2. Acute angle-closure glaucoma is treated with medication to reduce IOP before laser or incisional iridectomy.
3. Secondary glaucomas are treated with anti-inflammatory agents for uveitis; antiviral agents, cycloplegics, and topical corticosteroids for herpes simplex and herpes zoster.

Other Pharmacologic Agents

1. Beta-adrenergic antagonists, most widely used hypotensive agents, effective in many types of glaucoma.
2. Cholinergic agents (topical), used in short-term management of glaucoma with pupillary block.
3. Adrenergic agonists (topical), reduce IOP by increasing aqueous humor outflow.
4. Carbonic anhydrase inhibitor (systemically), lower IOP by reducing aqueous humor formation.
5. Osmotic diuretics reduce IOP by increasing the osmolality of the plasma to draw water from the eye into the vascular circulation.

Surgery

1. Ophthalmic laser surgery is indicated as the primary treatment for glaucoma or required when medication therapy is poorly tolerated or ineffective in lowering IOP.
2. Conventional surgery procedures performed when laser techniques are unsuccessful or when the patient is not a good candidate for laser surgery (e.g., a patient who is unable to sit still or follow instructions).

G

✎ Patient Education and Health Maintenance: Care in the Home and Community

1. Teach that optimum reduction of IOP and control of glaucomatous damage depend on adherence to medication regimen and attendance at follow-up examinations, which are necessary to determine efficacy of treatment. Monitor IOP and assess visual field and optic disc. Frequency of follow-up visits depends on level and stability of IOP and extent of damage.
2. Give written instructions that identify name of medications, description of containers, frequency and times of administration. Check for understanding of the expected action and possible side effects. Stress importance of making medication administration a part of daily routine so doses are not missed. Stress that medication is to be continued even when IOP is under control.
3. Make patient aware that responsibilities include good eye care, maintenance of good physical health, and a lifestyle consistent with low levels of stress. Eye care involves keeping the eyes clean and free of irritants; avoiding rubbing; using nonallergenic cosmetics; and wearing goggles while swimming and protective glasses while playing sports or working in the yard or other potentially hazardous areas.

4. Teach patient to note how the eyes look and feel and report unusual changes to the physician: excessive irritation, watering, blurring, cloudy vision, discharge, rainbows around lights at night, flashes of light, and floating objects in the field of vision.
5. Reinforce that treatment of glaucoma is control rather than cure; it involves lifelong management.
6. Encourage maintaining good health and limiting stress: proper nutrition, salt restriction, avoiding excessive fluid intake, maintaining appropriate weight level, exercising, and taking time for fun and relaxation.
7. Encourage sharing feelings and concerns with family and friends or talking with other patients with glaucoma.

✪ Gerontologic Considerations

Most patients with glaucoma are in the older age group. Often dimming vision is accepted as part of aging and medical assistance is not sought. For people over age 35, tonometry is recommended and periodic checking of eye pressure thereafter.

Help the elderly patient to understand that eyedrops must be continued to keep glaucoma from worsening. Discontinuation of the medication allows glaucoma to continue insidiously until blindness occurs.

Recognize when caring for the elderly patient with glaucoma other problems must be considered, i.e., arthritis, depression, potential for falling, and accidents.

For more information see Chapter 56 in Smeltzer and Bare: *Brunner and Suddarth's Textbook of Medical–Surgical Nursing,* 8th Edition. Philadelphia: Lippincott–Raven, 1996.

GLOMERULONEPHRITIS, ACUTE

Acute glomerulonephritis refers to a group of kidney diseases in which there is an inflammatory reaction in the glomeruli. It is not an infection of the kidney, but the result of untoward side effects of the defense mechanism of the body. In most cases, the stimulus of the reaction is group A streptococcal infection of the throat, which ordinarily precedes the onset of glomerulonephritis by an interval of 2–3 weeks. The streptococcal product, acting as an antigen, stimulates circulating antibodies producing injury to the kidney. Glomerulonephritis may also follow scarlet fever and impetigo and acute viral infections, i.e., upper respiratory infections, mumps, varicella, Epstein-Barr, hepatitis B, and HIV infections. It is predominantly a disease of youth.

CLINICAL MANIFESTATIONS

1. In the more severe form of the disease, headache, malaise, facial edema, and flank pain occur.
2. Mild to severe hypertension and tenderness of the costovertebral angle (CVA) are common.

DIAGNOSTIC EVALUATION

1. Primary presenting feature is microscopic or gross (macroscopic) hematuria.
2. Proteinuria; increased antistreptolysin-O titer; elevated BUN and serum creatinine; anemia.

MANAGEMENT

The goals of management are to preserve kidney function and to treat complications promptly.

1. Penicillin, for residual streptococcal infection.
2. Diuretics and antihypertensive agents.
3. Plasma exchange (plasmapheresis) and treatment with steroids and cytotoxic drugs to reduce inflammatory response, in rapid progressive disease.

4. Dialysis is occasionally necessary.
5. Bed rest, during the acute phase until the urine clears and BUN, creatinine, and blood pressure return to normal.

Nutrition

1. Dietary protein restricted with elevated BUN.
2. Sodium restricted with hypertension, edema, and congestive heart failure.
3. Carbohydrates for energy and to reduce protein catabolism.
4. Fluids given according to fluid losses and daily body weight; intake and output.

 PATIENT EDUCATION AND HEALTH MAINTENANCE: CARE IN THE HOME AND COMMUNITY

1. Instruct to schedule follow-up evaluations of blood pressure, urinalysis for protein, and BUN and creatinine studies to determine if disease has exacerbated.
2. Instruct to notify the physician if symptoms of renal failure occur, e.g., fatigue, nausea, vomiting, diminishing urinary output.
3. Advise to treat infection promptly.
4. Referral to community health nurse is indicated for assessment and detection of early symptoms.

For more information see Chapter 43 in Smeltzer and Bare: *Brunner and Suddarth's Textbook of Medical–Surgical Nursing,* 8th Edition. Philadelphia: Lippincott–Raven, 1996.

GLOMERULONEPHRITIS, CHRONIC

Chronic glomerulonephritis may have its onset as acute glomerulonephritis or may represent a milder type of antigen-antibody reaction that is overlooked. After repeated occurrences of these reactions, the kidneys are reduced to as little as one-fifth of their normal size and consist largely of fibrous tissue. As chronic glomerulonephritis progresses, the following signs and symptoms of renal insufficiency and chronic renal failure occur. The result is severe glomerular damage that results in end-stage renal disease (ESRD).

CLINICAL MANIFESTATIONS

Symptoms are variable. Some patients with severe disease have no symptoms for a long time.

1. First indications may be sudden, severe nosebleed, stroke, or convulsions.
2. Many patients merely notice that their feet are slightly swollen at night.
3. Other symptoms include loss of weight and strength, increasing irritability, and nocturia.
4. Headaches, dizziness, and digestive disturbances are common.

Signs and Symptoms of Renal Insufficiency and Chronic Renal Failure

1. Patient appears poorly nourished with a yellow-gray pigmentation of the skin; periorbital and peripheral edema.
2. Blood pressure normal or severely elevated.
3. Retinal findings: hemorrhage, exudate, narrowed tortuous arterioles, and papilledema.
4. Pale mucous membranes.
5. Neck veins may be distended from fluid overload.
6. Cardiomegaly, gallop rhythm, and other signs of congestive heart failure may be present.
7. Crackles heard in lungs.
8. Peripheral neuropathy with diminished deep tendon reflexes.
9. Neurosensory changes resulting in confusion and limited attention span.
10. Late findings include pericarditis with pericardial friction rub and pulsus paradoxus.

DIAGNOSTIC EVALUATION

Laboratory Abnormalities

1. Urinalysis reveals fixed specific gravity of 1.010, variable proteinuria, and urinary casts.
2. Blood studies related to renal failure progression show hyperkalemia, metabolic acidosis, anemia, hypoalbuminemia, decreased serum calcium and increased serum phosphorus, hypermagnesemia.
3. Chest films may show cardiac enlargement and pulmonary edema.
4. Electrocardiogram may be normal, or may reflect left ventricular hypertrophy.

MANAGEMENT

The treatment of ambulatory patients is guided by symptoms.

1. If hypertension is present, the blood pressure is lowered with sodium and water restriction.
2. Proteins of high biologic value are provided to support good nutritional status.
3. Treat urinary tract infections promptly.
4. If severe edema develops, place on bed rest with head of bed elevated to promote comfort and diuresis.
5. Monitor weight daily.
6. Administer diuretics to reduce fluid overload.
7. Adjust sodium and fluid intake according to the ability of the patient's kidneys to excrete water and sodium.
8. Dialysis is considered early in the course of disease to keep the patient in optimal physical condition, prevent fluid and electrolyte imbalances, and minimize the risk of complications of renal failure.

Nursing Interventions

1. Give emotional support throughout the course of the disease and treatment by providing opportunity for patient and family to verbalize concerns and

have questions answered and options discussed.
2. Observe for signs of deterioration of renal function; report changes in fluid/electrolyte status and cardiac/neurologic status.

✎ PATIENT EDUCATION AND HEALTH MAINTENANCE: CARE IN THE HOME AND COMMUNITY

1. Educate the patient and family about prescribed treatment plan and the risk of noncompliance. Instructions include explanations and scheduling for follow-up evaluations of blood pressure, urinalysis for protein and casts, blood for BUN, and creatinine.
2. Refer to community health or home care nurse for careful assessment of patient progress and continued education about problems to report to health care provider; recommended diet and fluid modifications, and medication teaching.
3. Give patient and family assistance and support regarding dialysis and long-term implications.

For more information see Chapter 43 in Smeltzer and Bare: *Brunner and Suddarth's Textbook of Medical–Surgical Nursing,* 8th Edition. Philadelphia: Lippincott–Raven, 1996.

GOUT

Gout is a heterogeneous group of conditions related to a genetic defect of purine metabolism (hyperuricemia). There is either an oversecretion of uric acid or a renal defect resulting in decreased excretion of uric acid or a combination of both. Primary hyperuricemia may be due to severe dieting or starvation, excessive intake of foods high in purines (shellfish, organ meats), or heredity. In secondary hyperuricemia, the gout is a minor clinical feature secondary to any of a number of genetic or acquired processes, and an increase in cell breakdown.

CLINICAL MANIFESTATIONS

Four stages of gout can be identified: asymptomatic hyperuricemia, acute gouty arthritis, intercritical gout, and chronic tophaceous gout.

Hyperuricemia

1. Fewer than one in five hyperuricemic individuals will develop clinically apparent urate crystal deposits.
2. Subsequent development of gout is directly related to duration and magnitude of hyperuricemia.

Manifestations of Acute Gouty Arthritis

1. Acute arthritis of gout is the most common early sign.
2. The metatarsophalangeal (MTP) joint of the big toe is the most commonly affected; tarsal area, ankle, or knee may also be targeted.
3. The acute attack may be triggered by trauma, alcohol ingestion, drugs, surgical stress, or illness.
4. Abrupt onset occurs at night, causing severe pain, redness, swelling, and warmth over the affected joint.
5. Early attacks tend to subside spontaneously over 3–10 days without treatment.
6. The next attack may not come for months or years; in time, attacks tend to occur more frequently, involve more joints, and last longer.

Tophi (chalky deposit of sodium urate)

1. Noted an average of 10 years after the onset of gout.
2. Tophi are generally associated with frequent and severe inflammatory episodes.
3. Higher serum concentrations of uric acid are associated with tophus formation.
4. Tophi occur in the synovium, olecranon bursa, subchondral bone, infrapatellar and Achilles' tendons, subcutaneous tissue, and overlying joints.

5. Tophi have also been found in aortic walls, heart valves, nasal and ear cartilage, eyelids, cornea, and sclerae.
6. Joint enlargement may cause loss of motion.

Increased Risk of Urolithiasis

1. Incidence of renal stones is two times higher for patients with secondary gout than those with primary gout.
2. Stone formation is related to increased serum uric acid, acidity of urine, and urinary concentration.

MANAGEMENT

1. Hyperuricemia, tophi, joint destruction, and renal problems are treated after the acute inflammatory process has subsided.
2. Uricosuric agents, i.e., probenecid, correct hyperuricemia, and dissolved deposited urate.
3. Colchicine (oral or parenteral) or a NSAID, i.e., endomethacin to relieve acute attacks.
4. Allopurinol helps prevent attacks by lowering serum uric acid levels.
5. Aspiration and intra-articular corticosteroids for large-joint acute attacks.

For more information see Chapter 52 in Smeltzer and Bare: *Brunner and Suddarth's Textbook of Medical–Surgical Nursing,* 8th Edition. Philadelphia: Lippincott–Raven, 1996.

GRAVE'S DISEASE

See Hyperthryroidism

GUILLAIN-BARRE SYNDROME (POLYRADICULONEURITIS)

Guillain-Barré is a clinical syndrome of unknown cause involving the peripheral and cranial nerves. In most patients, the syndrome is preceded by an infection (respiratory or gastrointestinal) 1 to 4 weeks before the onset of neurologic deficits. In some instances, it has occurred after vaccination or surgery. It may be due to a primary viral infection, immune reaction, some other process, or combination of processes. One hypothesis is that a viral infection induces an autoimmune reaction that attacks the myelin of the peripheral nerves.

CLINICAL MANIFESTATIONS

1. Initial neurologic symptoms are paresthesia (tingling and numbness), and muscle weakness of the legs, which may progress to upper extremities, trunk, and facial muscles. Muscle weakness may be followed quickly by complete paralysis.
2. Cranial nerves are frequently affected, leading to paralysis of the ocular, facial, and oropharyngeal muscles, causing difficulty in talking, chewing, and swallowing.
3. Autonomic dysfunction frequently occurs in the form of overreactivity or underreactivity of the sympathetic or parasympathetic nervous system. It is manifested by disturbances of heart rate, rhythm, blood pressure changes, and a variety of other vasomotor disturbances.
4. There may be severe, persistent pain in the back and calves of the legs.
5. Frequently there is loss of position sense and diminished or absent tendon reflexes.
6. Sensory changes are manifested by paresthesias.
7. Most patients make a full recovery over several months to a year; about 10% have residual disability.

DIAGNOSTIC EVALUATION

1. Spinal fluid shows an increased protein concentration with normal cell count.
2. Electrophysiologic testing shows marked slowing of nerve conduction velocity.

MANAGEMENT

1. Considered a medical emergency and the patient is managed in an intensive care unit.
2. Respiratory problems require mechanical ventilation.
3. Plasmapheresis (plasma exchange) may be used in the severely affected patient to limit deterioration and demyelinization.
4. Continuous ECG monitoring: observe and treat cardiac dysrhythmias. Atropine may be administered to avoid episodes of bradycardia during endotracheal suctioning and physical therapy.

NURSING PROCESS

Assessment

1. Assess for acute respiratory failure, a life-threatening problem.
2. Assess for complications including cardiac dysrhythmias, deep vein thrombosis (DVT), and pulmonary embolism (PE).

Major Nursing Diagnosis

1. Ineffective breathing pattern and gas exchange related to rapidly progressive weakness and impending respiratory failure.
2. Impaired physical mobility related to paralysis.
3. Altered nutrition, less than body requirements, related to inability to swallow, which is secondary to cranial nerve dysfunction.
4. Impaired verbal communication related to cranial nerve dysfunction.
5. Fear related to loss of control and paralysis.

Collaborative Problems

Respiratory failure.

Planning and Implementation

The major goals may include maintenance of respiratory function, achievement of mobility, accomplishment of normal nutrition, achievement of communication, reduction of fear and anxiety, and absence of potential complications.

Interventions

MAINTAINING RESPIRATORY FUNCTION

1. Assess carefully for difficulty in coughing and swallowing, which may cause aspiration of saliva and precipitate acute respiratory failure.
2. Provide chest physical therapy and elevate head of bed to facilitate respirations and promote effective coughing.
3. Suction to maintain a clear airway.

MONITORING FOR RESPIRATORY FAILURE

1. Assess for difficulty in coughing and swallowing, indicating deterioration of respiratory function.
2. Watch for breathlessness while talking, shallow and irregular breathing, increasing pulse rate, use of accessory muscles while breathing, and change in respiratory pattern.

PREVENTING COMPLICATIONS FROM MOBILITY

1. Give passive range-of-motion exercises at least twice daily.
2. Collaborate with physical therapist to prevent contracture deformities.
3. Ensure adequate hydration and administer prescribed anticoagulant regimen to prevent DVT and PE, assist with physical therapy, and use antiembolism stockings.

4. Place padding over elbows and head of the fibula to prevent compression neuropathies of the ulnar and peroneal nerves.
5. Use principles of nursing management of the unconscious patient.
6. Use tilt table to help assume upright posture when recovery begins to prevent orthostatic hypotension.

PROVIDING ADEQUATE NUTRITION

1. Provide adequate nutrition to prevent muscle wasting.
2. Provide intravenous feedings as prescribed and monitor bowel sounds.
3. Provide nasogastric tube feedings if patient is unable to swallow.
4. Resume oral feeding when patient can swallow normally.

IMPROVING COMMUNICATION

1. Establish communication through lip reading, use of picture cards, combined with a system of blinking eyes to indicate yes or no if patient is on ventilator or otherwise unable to speak.
2. Provide diversional therapy, i.e., television, tapes, visits to alleviate some of the frustrations that are encountered.

RELIEVING FEAR AND ANXIETY

1. Involve family and friends with selected patient care activities to reduce sense of isolation.
2. Provide patient with information about condition, emphasizing a positive appraisal of coping resources.
3. Encourage relaxation exercises and distraction techniques, giving positive feedback.
4. Create a positive attitude and atmosphere.
5. Give expert nursing care, explanations and reassurance to help patient gain control over situation.

✎ Patient Education and Health Maintenance: Care in the Home and Community

1. Encourage a home program of physical and occupational therapy.
2. Support patient and family through long recovery phase and promote involvement for return of former abilities.
3. Inform of the Guillain-Barré support group.

For more information see Chapter 60 in Smeltzer and Bare: *Brunner and Suddarth's Textbook of Medical–Surgical Nursing,* 8th Edition. Philadelphia: Lippincott–Raven, 1996.

HEAD INJURY

Injuries to the head involve trauma to the scalp, skull, and brain. Head injuries are among the most frequent and serious neurologic disorders and have reached epidemic proportions as a result of traffic accidents. Detectable blood alcohol levels have been found in more than 50% of head-injured patients treated in emergency departments. At least half of all severely head-injured patients have significant injuries to other parts of the body.

SCALP AND SKULL INJURIES

1. Scalp injury may result in an abrasion (brush wound), contusion, laceration, or avulsion. Because of its many blood vessels, the scalp can bleed profusely when injured. Scalp wounds are a portal entry for intracranial infections.
2. Fractures of the skull are a break in the continuity of the skull caused by trauma. They may occur with or without damage to the brain; classified as open (dura is torn) or closed (dura is not torn).

CLINICAL MANIFESTATIONS

Symptoms depend on the amount and distribution of brain injury.

1. Pain, persistent or localized, usually suggests fracture.
2. Fractures of the cranial vault produce swelling in that region.
3. Fractures of the base of the skull frequently produce hemorrhage from the nose, pharynx, or ears, and blood may appear under the conjunctiva.

4. Ecchymosis may be seen over the mastoid (Battle's sign).
5. Drainage of cerebral spinal fluid (CSF) from the ears and the nose suggests basal skull fracture.
6. Drainage of CSF may cause serious infection, i.e., meningitis through a tear in the dura mater.
7. Bloody spinal fluid suggests brain laceration or contusion.

DIAGNOSTIC EVALUATION

1. Physical examination and evaluation of neurologic status.
2. Computed tomography (CT); magnetic resonance imaging (MRI)

MANAGEMENT OF SCALP AND SKULL INJURIES

1. Nondepressed skull fractures generally do not require surgical treatment; require close observation of the patient.
2. Depressed skull fractures call for surgery.

BRAIN INJURY

Concussion

A cerebral concussion after head injury is a temporary loss of neurologic function with no apparent structural damage.

1. Generally involves a period of unconsciousness lasting from a few seconds to a few minutes.
2. Jarring of the brain may be so slight as to cause only dizziness and spots before the eyes.
3. If frontal lobe is affected, patient may exhibit bizarre irrational behavior.
4. If temporal lobe is affected, patient may exhibit temporary amnesia or disorientation.

MANAGEMENT OF CONCUSSION

Headache, Dizziness, Irritability, and Anxiety

1. Give information, explanations, and encouragement to reduce postconcussion syndrome.
2. Instruct family to look for the following signs and notify physician or clinic: difficulty in awakening, difficulty in speaking, confusion, severe headache, vomiting, or weakness of one side of the body.
3. Advise patient to resume normal activities slowly.

H

Contusion

1. A cerebral contusion is a more severe cerebral injury. The brain is bruised, with possible surface hemorrhage.
2. Patient is unconscious; exhibits symptoms of shock; incontinent of bowel and bladder.
3. Aroused with effort but soon slips back into unconsciousness.
4. In general, persons with widespread injury who have abnormal motor function, abnormal eye movements, and elevated intracranial pressure (ICP) have a poor outcome.
5. Conversely, may recover consciousness completely and perhaps pass into a stage of cerebral irritability, e.g., easily disturbed by any form of stimulation, and may become hyperactive.
6. Recovery is not complete at once and residual headache and vertigo are common; impaired mentality or epilepsy may occur.

INTRACRANIAL HEMORRHAGE

Hematomas that develop within the cranial vault are the most serious results of brain injury. The hematoma is referred to as epidural, subdural, or intracerebral, depending on location. Main effects are frequently delayed until the hematoma is large enough to cause distortion and herniation of the brain and increased ICP.

Epidural Hematoma (Extradural Hematoma or Hemorrhage)

1. Blood collected in the epidural space between the skull and dura mater.
2. Symptoms are caused by the expanding hematoma; usually a momentary loss of consciousness at time of injury, followed by an interval of apparent recovery.
3. Sudden signs of compression may appear, i.e., deterioration of consciousness and signs of focal neurologic deficits (dilation and fixation of a pupil or paralysis of an extremity); patient deteriorates rapidly.

MANAGEMENT OF EPIDURAL HEMATOMA

Extreme Emergency

1. Marked neurologic deficit or cessation of breathing may occur within minutes.
2. Burr holes, removing the clots, and controlling bleeding point.

Subdural Hematoma

1. A collection of blood between the dura and the underlying brain.
2. Most common cause is trauma but it may also occur in various bleeding tendencies and aneurysms.
3. May be acute (major head injury), subacute (sequelae of less severe contusions), or chronic (minor head injuries in the elderly).

Intracerebral Hemorrhage/Hematoma

1. Bleeding into the substance of the brain.
2. Commonly seen when forces are exerted to the head over a small area (missile injuries or bullet wounds; stab injury).
3. May also result from systemic hypertension causing degeneration and rupture of a vessel.

NURSING PROCESS FOR THE PATIENT WITH A HEAD INJURY

Assessment

Obtain health history including the following: time of injury; cause of injury; direction and force of the blow; was there a loss of consciousness? The Glasgow Coma Scale serves as an excellent guide for assessing levels of consciousness based on the three criteria of (1) eye opening, (2) verbal responses, and (3) motor responses to a verbal command or painful stimuli.

H

Monitor Vital Signs

1. Monitor at frequent intervals to assess intracranial status.
2. Assess for increasing ICP including slowing of pulse, increasing systolic pressure, and widening pulse pressure.
3. As brain compression increases, vital signs are reversed, pulse and respirations become rapid, blood pressure may decrease.
4. Keep temperature below 38°C (100.4°F) to avoid increased metabolic demands on the brain.
5. Tachycardia and hypotension may indicate bleeding elsewhere in the body.

MOTOR FUNCTION

1. Observe spontaneous movements; ask patient to raise and lower extremities; compare strength of hand grasp at periodic intervals.
2. Note presence or absence of spontaneous movement of each extremity.
3. Assess responses to painful stimuli in absence of spontaneous movement; abnormal response carries a poorer prognosis.
4. Determine patient's ability to speak; note quality of speech.

EYE SIGNS

1. Evaluate spontaneous eye opening.
2. Evaluate size of pupils and reaction to light (unilaterally dilated and poorly responding pupils may indicate developing hematoma). If both pupils are fixed and dilated, it usually indicates overwhelming injury and poor prognosis.

MONITOR FOR COMPLICATIONS (CEREBRAL EDEMA AND HERNIATION)

1. Deterioration in condition may be due to expanding intracranial hematoma, progressive brain edema, and herniation of the brain.
2. Peak swelling occurs approximately 72 hours after injury with resulting elevation of ICP.
3. Take measures to control ICP: elevate head of bed 30°, maintain head and neck in alignment (no twisting), prevent Valsalva maneuver, use medications to decrease ICP, maintain normal body temperature, hyperventilate on mechanical ventilation, maintain fluid restriction, avoid noxious stimuli (suctioning), administer sedation to reduce metabolic demands.

MONITOR FOR OTHER COMPLICATIONS

1. Other complications include systemic infections or neurosurgical infections, i.e., wound infection, osteomyelitis, or meningitis.
2. After injury some patients develop focal nerve palsies such as anosmia (lack of sense of smell) or eye movement abnormalities and focal neurologic defects such as aphasia (memory defect) and seizures.
3. Patients may be left with organic psychosocial deficits and lack insight into their emotional responses.

Major Nursing Diagnosis

1. Ineffective airway clearance and ventilation related to hypoxia.

2. Fluid volume deficit related to disturbances of consciousness and hormonal dysfunction.
3. Altered nutrition, less than body requirements, related to metabolic changes, fluid restrictions, and inadequate intake.
4. Risk for injury (self-directed and directed to others) related to disorientation, restlessness, and brain damage.
5. Altered thought processes (deficits in intellectual function, communication, memory, information processing) related to results of head injury.
6. Potential for ineffective family coping related to unresponsiveness of patient, unpredictability of outcome, prolonged recovery period, and patient's residual physical and emotional deficit.
7. Knowledge deficit about rehabilitation process.
8. Nursing diagnosis for the unconscious patient and patient with increased ICP also apply.

H

Collaborative Problems

1. Cerebral edema.
2. Herniation.

Planning and Implementation

Goals may include attainment of a patent airway, achievement of fluid and electrolyte balance, achievement of adequate nutritional status, prevention of injury, improvement of cognitive function, effective family coping, increased knowledge about rehabilitation process, and prevention of complications.

Nursing Interventions

MAINTAINING THE AIRWAY

1. Position the unconscious patient to facilitate drainage of secretions; elevate head of bed 30° to decrease intracranial venous pressure.
2. Establish effective suctioning procedures.
3. Guard against aspiration and respiratory insufficiency.

4. Monitor arterial blood gases to assess adequacy of ventilation.
5. Monitor the patient on mechanical ventilation.

MAINTAINING FLUID AND ELECTROLYTE BALANCE

1. Monitor serum electrolyte concentrations, especially in patients receiving osmotic diuretics, those with inappropriate antidiuretic hormone secretion, and posttraumatic diabetes insipidus.
2. Record daily weights.

PROVIDING ADEQUATE NUTRITION

1. Start nasogastric feedings as soon as condition has stabilized unless there is discharge of CSF from the nose.
2. Give small frequent feedings to lessen the possibility of vomiting and diarrhea (continuous-drip infusion or controlling pump to regulate the feeding).

PREVENTING INJURY

1. Observe for restlessness that may be due to hypoxia, fever, pain, or a full bladder.
2. Know that restlessness may also be a sign that the unconscious patient is regaining consciousness.
3. Protect from self-injury (padded side rails, hands wrapped in mitts).
4. Avoid restraints when possible because straining can increase ICP.
5. Avoid narcotics for restlessness because the medications depress respiration, constrict pupils, and alter level of consciousness.
6. Keep environmental stimuli to a minimum.
7. Provide adequate lighting to prevent visual hallucinations.
8. Do not disrupt sleep-wake cycles.
9. Use an external sheath catheter for incontinence because an indwelling catheter may produce infection.

IMPROVING COGNITIVE FUNCTIONING

1. Redevelop the patient's ability to devise new problem-solving strategies through cognitive rehabilitation over time.
2. Be aware that there are fluctuations in the orientation and memory and they are easily distracted.
3. Do not push to a level greater than patient's impaired cortical functioning allows because fatigue headache and stress (headache, dizziness) may occur.

SUPPORTING FAMILY COPING

1. Provide family members with accurate and honest information.
2. Encourage them to continue to set well-defined, mutual, short-term goals.
3. Encourage family counseling to deal with feeling of loss and helplessness and receive guidance in the management of inappropriate behaviors.
4. Refer to support groups that provide a forum for sharing problems, networking, and gaining assistance in maintaining realistic expectations.

✎ PATIENT EDUCATION AND HEALTH MAINTENANCE: CARE IN THE HOME AND COMMUNITY

1. Encourage to continue rehabilitation program after discharge. Improvement may take up to 3 or more years after discharge, during which time the family and their coping skills need frequent assessment.
2. Inform patient and family that posttraumatic seizures occur frequently and anticonvulsives may be prescribed for 1–2 years after injury.
3. Encourage to return to normal activities gradually.

For more information see Chapter 60 in Smeltzer and Bare: *Brunner and Suddarth's Textbook of Medical–Surgical Nursing,* 8th Edition. Philadelphia: Lippincott–Raven, 1996.

HEADACHE

One of the most common of all human physical complaints is headache. Headache is actually a symptom rather than a disease entity and may indicate organic disease (neurologic), a stress response, vasodilation (migraine), skeletal muscle tension (tension headache), or a combination of these factors. Headaches are classified as:

1. Migraine (with and without aura).
2. Tension-type headache.
3. Cluster headache and paroxysmal hemicrania.
4. Miscellaneous headaches associated with structural lesion.
5. Headache associated with head trauma.
6. Headache associated with vascular disorders (e.g., subarachnoid hemorrhage).
7. Headache associated with nonvascular intracranial disorders (e.g., brain tumor).
8. Headache associated with use of chemical substances or their withdrawal.
9. Headache associated with noncephalic infection.
10. Headache associated with metabolic disorder (e.g., hypoglycemia).
11. Headache or facial pain associated with disorder of the head, neck, or their structures (e.g., acute glaucoma).
12. Cranial neuralgias (persistent pain of cranial nerve origin).

MIGRAINE HEADACHE

This symptom-complex is characterized by periodic and recurrent attacks of severe headache. The cause of migraine has not been clearly demonstrated, but is primarily a vascular disturbance that occurs more commonly in women and has strong familial tendencies.

CLINICAL MANIFESTATIONS

The classic migraine attack can be divided into three phases: the aura, the headache, and the recovery.

Aura Phase

1. Lasts for up to 30 minutes.
2. Sensory manifestations, predominantly visual disturbances (light flashes).
3. Numbness and tingling of the face or hands, mild confusion, slight weakness of an extremity, and dizziness.

H

Headache Phase

1. Initial symptoms recede, followed by unilateral and throbbing headache.
2. Severe and incapacitating, often associated with photophobia, nausea, and vomiting.
3. Duration varies, from several hours to a day or longer.

Recovery Phase

1. Period of muscle contraction in the neck and scalp with associated muscle ache and point (localized) tenderness.
2. Exhaustion is common.
3. Any physical exertion exacerbates the headache pain.
4. Patients may sleep for extended periods.

DIAGNOSTIC EVALUATION

1. Neurologic exam and headache history.
2. CT or MRI if abnormalities present on neurologic exam.

MANAGEMENT

Therapy is divided into abortive (symptomatic) and preventive approaches.

1. Abortive/symptomatic approach used for frequent attacks and is aimed at relieving or limiting a headache at onset or while in progress.
2. Preventive approach used for those who have frequent attacks at regular or predictable intervals and may have medical conditions that preclude abortive therapies.

MANAGEMENT OF ACUTE ATTACK

Treatment varies greatly; close monitoring is indicated.
1. Ergotamine preparations may be effective if taken early.
2. Lie quietly in a darkened room with head slightly elevated.
3. Drinking black coffee may be helpful.
4. Sumatriptan (Imitrex) for migraine and cluster headaches; Cafergot to relieve moderate to severe migraines.
5. Symptomatic therapy: analgesics, sedatives, antianxiety agents, and antiemetics.

PREVENTION

Pharmacologic Therapy

1. Beta blockers, i.e., propranolol (Inderal), most widely used.
2. Antidepressants, barbiturates, tranquilizers.

NURSING PROCESS

Assessment

1. Detailed history, and physical assessment of the head and neck including neurologic examination. Data obtained for the health history should reflect the patient's own words.
2. Focus health history on assessment of the headache.

Major Nursing Diagnosis

Pain related to vascular changes.

Planning and Implementation

The goals include treating the acute event of the headache and preventing recurrent episodes.

Interventions

RELIEVING PAIN

1. Attempt to abort headache early.
2. Provide comfort measures, e.g., a quiet, dark environment, and elevation of the head of the bed 30°.

✎ PATIENT EDUCATION AND HEALTH MAINTENANCE: CARE IN THE HOME AND COMMUNITY

Knowledge About Precipitating and Alleviating Factors

1. Teach that migraine headaches are likely to occur when a person is ill, overtired, or feeling stressed.
2. Instruct about the importance of proper diet, adequate rest, and coping strategies.
3. Help patient identify circumstances that precipitate headache.
4. Help patients develop insight into their feelings, behaviors, and conflicts to make necessary lifestyle modifications.
5. Suggest regular periods of exercise and relaxation and avoidance of offending factors.
6. Avoid long intervals between meals.
7. Advise patient to awaken at the same time each day; disruption of normal sleeping pattern provokes a migraine in many patients.
8. Investigate possibility of oral contraceptives as a factor.

CLUSTER HEADACHE

Cluster headaches are another severe form of vascular headache seen most frequently in men. The attacks come in clusters or groups, with excruciating pain localized in the eye and orbit and radiating to the facial and temporal regions. The pain is accompanied by watering of the eye and nasal congestion lasting from 15 minutes to 2 hours and may have a crescendo-decrescendo pattern. Cluster headaches respond to vasoconstricting agents such as ergotamine.

CRANIAL ARTERITIS

Inflammation of the cranial arteries is characterized by a severe headache localized in the region of the temporal artery. The inflammation may be generalized or focal. This is a cause of headache in the older population, particularly over age 70. Clinical manifestations: heat, redness, swelling, tenderness or pain over the involved artery. A tender, swollen or nodular temporal artery may be visible. Visual problems are caused by ischemia of the involved structures. The headache is treated with corticosteroid drugs and analgesic agents.

TENSION HEADACHE
(MUSCLE CONTRACTION HEADACHE)

Emotional or physical stress may cause contraction of the muscles in the neck and scalp, resulting in tension headache. This is characterized by a steady, constant feeling of pressure that usually begins in the forehead, the temple, or the back of the neck. Tension headaches tend to be more chronic than severe and are probably the most common type of headache. Obtain relief by local heat, massage, analgesics, antidepressants, and muscle relaxants.

For more information see Chapter 60 in Smeltzer and Bare: *Brunner and Suddarth's Textbook of Medical–Surgical Nursing,* 8th Edition. Philadelphia: Lippincott–Raven, 1996.

HEART FAILURE

See Cardiac Failure

HEMOPHILIA

There are two hereditary bleeding disorders that are clinically indistinguishable, but can be separated by laboratory tests: hemophilia A and hemophilia B. Hemophilia A is due to a deficiency of factor VIII clotting activity. Hemophilia B stems from a deficiency of factor IX. Factor VIII deficiency is about five times more common. Both types are inherited as X-linked traits. Almost all affected persons are males; their mothers and some sisters are carriers but are asymptomatic. The disease is recognized in early childhood, usually in toddlers.

H

CLINICAL MANIFESTATIONS

1. Large, spreading bruises and bleeding into muscles, joints, and soft tissues after even minimal trauma.
2. Pain in joints may occur before swelling and limitation of motion are apparent.
3. Chronic pain or ankylosis (fixation) of the joint may occur. Many patients are crippled by joint damage before adulthood.
4. Spontaneous hematuria and gastrointestinal bleeding can occur.
5. Some patients have a milder deficiency and bleed only after dental extractions or surgery; such hemorrhages can prove fatal if the cause is not recognized quickly.

MANAGEMENT

1. Factor VIII and IX concentrates are given when active bleeding occurs or as a prophylactic measure before dental extractions or surgery.
2. Families are taught how to administer the concentrate at home, at first sign of bleeding.
3. Avoid aspirin or IM injections.
4. Encourage good dental hygiene as a preventive measure.

5. Use splints or other orthopedic devices in patients who have suffered joint or muscle hemorrhages.

NURSING PROCESS

Assessment

1. Assess for evidence of internal bleeding, muscle hematomas, and hemorrhage into joint spaces.
2. Monitor vital signs and hemodynamic pressure readings for hypovolemia.
3. Assess all joints for swelling, mobility limitation, and pain. Perform range of motion slowly, with care to avoid more damage.
4. Assess surgical sites frequently and carefully for bleeding.
5. Question how patient and family are coping with the condition and any limitations imposed on lifestyle and daily activities.

Major Nursing Diagnosis

1. Pain related to joint hemorrhage and subsequent ankylosis.
2. Altered health maintenance related to ongoing need for preventive health practices and coping with chronic illness.
3. Ineffective coping related to the chronicity of the condition and its effect on lifestyle.

Collaborative Problems

Bleeding.

Planning and Implementation

The major goals may include relief or minimization of pain, compliance with measures to prevent bleeding, coping with chronicity and altered lifestyle, and absence of complications.

Interventions

RELIEVING/MINIMIZING PAIN

1. Give analgesics to alleviate pain.
2. Encourage to move slowly and prevent stress on involved joints.
3. Encourage warm baths to promote relaxation, improved mobility, and lessened pain.
4. Avoid heat during bleeding episodes because it potentiates further bleeding.
5. Use splints, canes, or crutches to shift body weight off painful joints.

MONITORING AND MANAGING COMPLICATIONS

1. Assess frequently for signs and symptoms of hypoxia to vital organs: restlessness, anxiety, confusion, pallor, cool clammy skin, chest pain, and decreased urinary output.
2. Assess for hypotension and tachycardia as a result of volume depletion.
3. Monitor hemodynamic parameters; blood studies.
4. Observe for bleeding from the skin, mucous membranes, wounds, and for internal bleeding.
5. Apply cold compresses to bleeding sites when indicated.
6. Administer parenteral medications with small-gauge needles to decrease trauma and bleeding.
7. Administer blood and blood components as prescribed.
8. Use safety precautions to prevent patient injury.

✎ PATIENT EDUCATION AND HEALTH MAINTENANCE: CARE IN THE HOME AND COMMUNITY

Preventive Bleeding Measures

1. Inform patient and family of risk of bleeding and necessary safety precautions.
2. Encourage to alter the home environment to prevent physical trauma.

3. Encourage electric razor for shaving and soft tooth-brush for oral hygiene.
4. Avoid forceful nose blowing, coughing, and straining at stool; use stool softener as necessary.
5. Avoid aspirin and aspirin-containing drugs.
6. Encourage noncontact sports such as swimming, hiking, and golf, and discourage engagement in contact sports.
7. Encourage regular checkups and laboratory studies.

Coping with Chronicity and Altered Lifestyle

1. Assist in coping with the condition because it is chronic and places restrictions on lifestyle. It is an inherited disorder that can be passed to future generations.
2. Encourage to be self-sufficient and to maintain independence.
3. Encourage working through feelings about condition to accept more responsibility for maintaining optimal health.
4. Support patient's and family's efforts to deal with anger if HIV positive. (The percent of persons with hemophilia who are HIV positive is increasing.) Assist in finding support sources for those who are HIV positive.

For more information see Chapter 32 in Smeltzer and Bare: *Brunner and Suddarth's Textbook of Medical–Surgical Nursing,* 8th Edition. Philadelphia: Lippincott–Raven, 1996.

HEMOTHORAX

See Pneumothorax

HEPATIC ENCEPHALOPATHY AND HEPATIC COMA

Hepatic encephalopathy, a complication of liver disease, occurs with profound liver failure and results from the accumulation of ammonia and other toxic metabolites in the blood. Hepatic coma represents the most advanced stage of hepatic encephalopathy. Ammonia accumulates because the damaged liver cells fail to detoxify and convert the ammonia to urea. The increased ammonia concentration in the blood causes brain dysfunction and damage, resulting in hepatic encephalopathy and hepatic coma. Portal system encephalopathy (PSE) is the most common type of hepatic encephalopathy.

CLINICAL MANIFESTATIONS

1. Earliest symptoms of hepatic encephalopathy include minor mental changes and motor disturbances. Slight confusion and alterations in mood occur; patient becomes unkempt in appearance, experiences altered sleep patterns, and tends to sleep during the day and to experience restlessness and insomnia at night.
2. As coma progresses, patient may be difficult to awaken and asterixis (flapping tremor of the hands) may occur. Simple tasks, such as handwriting, become difficult.
3. In early stages, patient's reflexes are hyperactive; with worsening encephalopathy, reflexes disappear and extremities become flaccid.
4. Electroencephalogram (EEG) shows slowing and increase in amplitude of brain waves.
5. Occasionally fetor hepaticus, a characteristic breath odor like freshly mowed grass, acetone, or old wine, may be noticed.
6. Gross disturbances of consciousness and complete disorientation occur as the disease progresses.

7. With further progression frank coma and seizures occur.

MANAGEMENT

1. Observe frequently to assess neurologic status. Keep daily record of handwriting and performance in arithmetic to monitor mental status.
2. Monitor fluid intake and output and body weight daily; vital signs every 4 hours.
3. Monitor for pulmonary or other infection and report promptly.
4. Monitor serum ammonia level daily.
5. Reduce protein intake or eliminate if signs of impending encephalopathy or coma occur.
6. Give an enema as prescribed to reduce ammonia absorption from the GI tract.
7. Administer nonabsorbable antibiotics (neomycin) as an intestinal antiseptic.
8. Monitor electrolyte status and correct if abnormal.
9. Discontinue medications that may precipitate encephalopathy (i.e., sedatives, tranquilizers, analgesics).
10. Administer lactulose (Cephulac) to reduce blood ammonia. Observe for watery diarrheal stools, which indicate lactulose overdose.
11. Other treatments may include intravenous glucose, vitamins, and oxygen administration.

✎ PATIENT EDUCATION AND HEALTH MAINTENANCE: CARE IN THE HOME AND COMMUNITY

1. Instruct family to observe the patient for subtle signs of recurrent encephalopathy.
2. Emphasize importance of periodic follow-up.
3. The home care nurse assesses the patient's physical and mental status and adherence to the prescribed therapeutic regimen.

For more information see Chapter 38 in Smeltzer and Bare: *Brunner and Suddarth's Textbook of Medical–Surgical Nursing,* 8th Edition. Philadelphia: Lippincott–Raven, 1996.

HEPATIC FAILURE, FULMINANT

Fulminant hepatic failure is characterized by the development of hepatic encephalopathy within 8 weeks of the onset of disease in a patient without prior evidence of hepatic dysfunction. There is rapid clinical deterioration caused by massive hepatocellular injury and necrosis. Mortality is extremely high. Viral hepatitis is the most common cause; other causes include toxic drugs, chemicals, metabolic disturbances, and structural changes.

CLINICAL MANIFESTATIONS

1. Jaundice and profound anorexia.
2. Often accompanied by coagulation defects, renal failure, electrolyte disturbances, infection, hypoglycemia, encephalopathy, and cerebral edema.

MANAGEMENT

1. Blood or plasma exchanges, charcoal hemoperfusion, and corticosteroids.
2. Liver transplantation, treatment of choice.

For more information see Chapter 38 in Smeltzer and Bare: *Brunner and Suddarth's Textbook of Medical–Surgical Nursing,* 8th Edition. Philadelphia: Lippincott–Raven, 1996.

HEPATITIS, VIRAL: TYPES A, B, C, D, E

HEPATITIS A

Hepatitis A is caused by an RNA virus of the enterovirus family. Mode of transmission of this disease is the fecal-oral route, primarily through ingestion of foods or fluids infected by the virus. The virus is found in the stool of infected patients before the onset of symptoms and during the first few days of illness. The incubation period is estimated to be from 1 to 7 weeks, with an average of 30 days. The course of illness may last from 4 to 8 weeks. The virus is present only briefly in the serum; by the time jaundice appears the patient is likely to be noninfectious.

CLINICAL MANIFESTATIONS

1. Many patients are anicteric (without jaundice) and symptomless.
2. When symptoms appear, they are of a mild, flulike, upper respiratory infection, with low-grade fever.
3. Anorexia is an early symptom and often severe.
4. Later, jaundice and dark urine may be apparent.
5. Indigestion is present in varying degrees.
6. Liver and spleen may be moderately enlarged for a few days after onset.
7. Adults are more likely to be symptomatic than children.

MANAGEMENT

1. Bed rest during the acute stage; encourage nutritious diet.
2. Give small frequent feedings supplemented by IV glucose if necessary during period of anorexia.
3. Promote gradual but progressive ambulation to hasten recovery.

PROGNOSIS

1. Recovery from hepatitis A is usual; rarely progresses to acute liver necrosis and fulminant hepatitis.
2. A person who is immune to hepatitis A may contract other forms of hepatitis.
3. No carrier state exists and no chronic hepatitis is associated with hepatitis A.

PREVENTION

1. Administration of immune globulin to prevent hepatitis A if given within 2 weeks of exposure.
2. Also recommended for those who travel to developing countries and settings with poor or uncertain sanitation conditions.
3. Recommended for household members and sexual contacts of persons with hepatitis A.

✎ PATIENT EDUCATION AND HEALTH MAINTENANCE: CARE IN THE HOME AND COMMUNITY

H

1. Patient is usually managed at home unless symptoms are severe.
2. Assist patient and family to cope with the incapacitation and fatigue that are common problems in hepatitis.
3. Be aware of indications to seek additional health care if the symptoms persist or worsen.
4. Instruct patient and family regarding guidelines about diet, rest, follow up blood work, avoidance of alcohol, sanitation and hygiene measures (handwashing) to prevent spread of disease to other family members.
5. Teach patients and families about reducing risk of contracting hepatitis A: good personal hygiene with careful handwashing, environmental sanitation with safe food and water supply and sewage disposal.

HEPATITIS B

Hepatitis B virus (HBV) is a DNA virus. It is transmitted primarily through blood. The virus has been found in saliva, semen, vaginal secretions, and can be transmitted through mucous membranes and breaks in the skin. It replicates in the liver and remains in the serum for long periods, allowing transmission of the virus. Those at risk include all health care workers, patients in hemodialysis and oncology units, homosexually active and bisexual males, and IV drug users. Incubation period is between 1 and 6 months. Mortality ranges from 1% to 10%.

CLINICAL MANIFESTATIONS

1. Symptoms may be insidious and variable; fever and respiratory symptoms are rare; some have arthralgias and rashes.
2. Loss of appetite, dyspepsia, abdominal pain, general aching, malaise, and weakness.
3. Jaundice may or may not be evident. With jaundice there are light-colored stools and dark urine.
4. Liver may be tender and enlarged; spleen is enlarged and palpable in a small number of patients. Posterior cervical lymph nodes may also be enlarged.

MANAGEMENT

1. Clinical trials with interferon have shown promising results.
2. Bed rest and restriction of activities until hepatic enlargement and elevation of serum bilirubin and liver enzymes have disappeared.
3. Maintain adequate nutrition; restrict proteins when the ability of the liver to metabolize protein is impaired.
4. Administer antacids, belladonna, and antiemetics for dyspepsia and general malaise; avoid all medications if vomiting.
5. Convalescence may be prolonged and recovery may take 3–4 months.
6. Encourage gradual activity after complete clearing of jaundice.
7. Consider psychological implications of the long disease course.
8. Include family in planning patient's care and activities.

PROGNOSIS

Mortality is as high as 10%. Another 10% progress to a carrier state or develop chronic hepatitis. Hepatitis B is the chief cause of cirrhosis and hepatocellular carcinoma worldwide.

CONTROL AND PREVENTION

1. Interrupt the chain of transmission.
2. Protect those people at high risk with active immunization through use of hepatitis B vaccine.
3. Use passive immunization for unprotected people exposed to hepatitis B.

✎ PATIENT EDUCATION AND HEALTH MAINTENANCE: CARE IN THE HOME AND COMMUNITY

1. Educate patient and family in home care and convalescence.
2. Provide adequate rest and nutrition prior to discharge.
3. Inform family/friends about risks of contracting hepatitis B.
4. Arrange for them to receive hepatitis B vaccine or hepatitis B immune globulin (HBIG). Hepatitis B vaccine is given in three doses, the second and third doses 1 and 6 months after the first dose.
5. Both active and passive immunization (HBIG) are recommended when exposed through sexual contact or percutaeous or transmucosal routes.
6. Inform family that follow-up home visits by community health nurse are indicated to assess progress and answer questions.
7. Encourage patient to avoid sexual intercourse or use condoms to prevent exchange of body fluids.
8. Caution against using alcohol.

✪ Gerontologic Considerations

Elderly patients who contract hepatitis B have a serious risk of severe liver cell necrosis or fulminant hepatic failure. The patient is seriously ill and prognosis is poor.

HEPATITIS C

A significant portion of cases of viral hepatitis are neither A, B, nor D; they are classified as hepatitis C. It is the primary form of hepatitis associated with transfusions. The incubation period is variable and may range from 15 to 160 days. The clinical course of hepatitis C is similar to that of hepatitis B; symptoms are usually mild. A chronic carrier state occurs frequently, and significant chronic liver disease often occurs with hepatitis C. There is increased risk of cirrhosis and liver cancer after hepatitis C. Long-term, low-dose interferon therapy has been effective in preliminary trials in some patients with hepatitis C.

HEPATITIS D

Hepatitis D (delta agent) occurs in some cases of hepatitis B. Only individuals with hepatitis B are at risk. The virus requires hepatitis B surface antigen for its replication. It is common in persons who are IV drug users, hemodialysis patients, and recipients of multiple blood transfusions. Sexual contact with those with hepatitis B is a mode of transmission of hepatitis B and D. Incubation varies between 21 and 140 days. The symptoms are similar to those of hepatitis B except that patients are more likely to have fulminant hepatitis and progress to chronic active hepatitis and cirrhosis. Treatment is similar to other forms of hepatitis.

HEPATITIS E

The hepatitis E virus (newest hepatitis virus) is transmitted by the fecal-oral route. Incubation is variable and estimated to range between 15 and 65 days. Onset and symptoms are similar to those of other types of viral hepatitis. The major method of prevention is avoiding contact with the virus through hygiene (handwashing). Effectiveness of immune globulin in protecting against hepatitis E virus is uncertain.

For more information see Chapter 38 in Smeltzer and Bare: *Brunner and Suddarth's Textbook of Medical–Surgical Nursing*, 8th Edition. Philadelphia: Lippincott–Raven, 1996.

HERNIA, HIATAL

H

See Hiatal Hernia

HERNIATION OR RUPTURE OF AN INTERVERTEBRAL DISC

In herniation of the intervertebral disc (ruptured disc), the nucleus of the disc protrudes into the annulus (the fibrous ring around the disc), with subsequent nerve compression. Rupture of the disc is usually preceded by degenerative changes that occur with aging. In most patients, the immediate symptoms of trauma are short lived, and those resulting from injury to the disc do not appear for months or years. A herniated disc with accompanying pain may occur in any portion of the spine.

CLINICAL MANIFESTATIONS

Depend on location, rate of development (acute or chronic), and effect on surrounding structures.

1. Pain.
2. Changes in sensation and reflex action.

DIAGNOSTIC EVALUATION

MRI, CT, myelogram.

MANAGEMENT

Herniation of cervical and lumbar discs: conservative management with bed rest and medication.

Surgical Interventions

The goal of surgical treatment is to relieve pressure on the nerve root to relieve pain and reverse neurologic deficits.

1. Discectomy: removal of herniated or extruded fragments of intervertebral disc.
2. Discectomy with fusion: a bone graft is used to fuse the vertebral spinous process; the objective is to bridge over the defective disc to stabilize the spine and reduce the rate of recurrence.
3. Laminectomy: removal of the lamina to expose the neural elements in the spinal canal; allows the surgeon to inspect the spinal canal, identify and remove pathology, and relieve compression of the cord and roots.
4. Laminotomy: division of the lamina of the vertebra.

For more information see Chapter 60 in Smeltzer and Bare: *Brunner and Suddarth's Textbook of Medical–Surgical Nursing,* 8th Edition. Philadelphia: Lippincott–Raven, 1996.

HHNK SYNDROME

See Hyperglycemic Hyperosmolar Nonketotic Syndrome

HIATAL HERNIA

In a hiatal hernia the opening in the diaphragm through which the esophagus passes becomes enlarged and part of the upper stomach tends to move up into the lower portion of the thorax. There are two types of hernias: axial and paraesophageal.

AXIAL

Axial, or sliding hiatal hernias, occur when the upper stomach and the gastroesophageal junction are displaced upward and slide in and out of the thorax. About 90% of patients with hiatal hernias have sliding hernias.

PARAESOPHAGEAL

The less frequent paraesophageal hernias occur when all or part of the stomach pushes through the diaphragm next to the gastroesophageal junction. Fewer than 10% of patients experience paraesophageal herniation.

H

CLINICAL MANIFESTATIONS

Axial (Sliding) Hernia

1. Heartburn, regurgitation, and dysphagia.
2. At least 50% are asymptomatic.
3. Often implicated in reflux.

Paraesophageal Hernia

1. Sense of fullness after eating or may be asymptomatic.
2. Reflux does not usually occur.
3. Complications of hemorrhage, obstruction, and strangulation can occur.

DIAGNOSIS AND MANAGEMENT

Axial (Sliding) Hernia

1. Diagnosis is confirmed by radiographic studies and fluoroscopy.
2. Medical management includes frequent, small feedings that easily pass through the esophagus.
3. Advise not to recline for 1 hour after eating to prevent reflux or movement of the hernia.
4. Elevate head of the bed to prevent movement of the hernia by gravity.
5. Surgery is indicated in about 15% of patients.

Paraesophageal Hernia

1. Diagnosis is confirmed by x-ray and fluoroscopy.
2. May require emergency surgery.
3. Medical and surgical management are similar to that for gastroesophageal reflux.

For more information see Chapter 34 in Smeltzer and Bare: *Brunner and Suddarth's Textbook of Medical–Surgical Nursing,* 8th Edition. Philadelphia: Lippincott–Raven, 1996.

HIGH BLOOD PRESSURE

See Hypertension

HIV

See Acquired Immunodeficiency Syndrome

HODGKIN'S DISEASE

Hodgkin's disease is a malignant disease of unknown origin that originates in the lymphatic system and involves the lymph nodes. It is more common in men and tends to peak in the early 20s and after age 50. The Reed-Sternberg cell, a gigantic atypical tumor cell, is the pathologic hallmark and essential diagnostic criterion for Hodgkin's disease.

CLINICAL MANIFESTATIONS

1. Painless enlargement of the lymph nodes on one side of the neck. (a) Individual nodes are rubbery and painless. (b) Lymph nodes of other regions (the other side of the neck) also enlarge in the same manner.
2. Mediastinal and retroperitoneal lymph nodes may also enlarge, causing severe pressure symptoms:

(a) dyspnea from pressure against the trachea; (b) dysphagia from pressure against the esophagus; (c) laryngeal paralysis and brachial, lumbar, or sacral neuralgias from pressure on nerves; (d) edema of one or both extremities and effusion into the pleura from pressure on veins; (e) obstructive jaundice from pressure on the bile duct.

3. Later, spleen may become palpable and liver may enlarge.
4. In some patients the first nodes to enlarge are in the axillae or groin; occasionally mediastinal or peritoneal nodes; or enlargement of spleen may be the only sign.
5. Eventually progressive anemia develops.
6. Fever varies with pathologic involvement.
7. Untreated, this is a progressive disease causing weight loss, cachexia, infection, anemia, anasarca, and hypotension.
8. Death is likely in 1 to 3 years without treatment.

DIAGNOSTIC EVALUATION

Depends on identification of characteristic histologic features in an excised lymph node. Once diagnosis is confirmed, assess total extent of tumor involvement and define distribution.

1. Laboratory studies: complete blood studies; liver and renal function studies.
2. Bone marrow biopsy and liver and spleen scans.
3. Chest x-ray and extensive bone scans.

MANAGEMENT

Treatment is determined by the stage of the disease instead of the histologic type. Hodgkin's disease is potentially curable by radiotherapy if it has not extended beyond the lymph node chains, spleen, and oronasopharnyx.

1. Patients who do not have extension of the disease should have the benefit of "curative" radiotherapy.

2. Patients who have any sign of spread beyond treatable areas should receive a combination of chemotherapy and palliative radiotherapy.

STAGING OF HODGKIN'S DISEASE

Staging is determined by the extent and location of node involvement.

1. Stage I: disease limited to a single node and contiguous structures or a single organ or site.
2. Stage II: disease involves more than a single node or group of contiguous nodes, but confined to one side of the diaphragm.
3. Stage III: disease is present above and below the diaphragm and may include solitary involvement of the spleen, one extra lymphatic site, or both.
4. Stage IV: disease has disseminated diffusely to one or more extralymphatic sites with or without associated lymph node involvement.
5. Stages are further subdivided on basis of presence or absence of one or more of these symptoms: fever, night sweats, unexplained weight loss. Without symptoms, staging is designated A, and with symptoms, the designation is B.
6. Patients diagnosed IA or IIA have a 5-year survival rate of 90%.
7. Survival rates decrease progressively with more advanced stages.

NURSING INTERVENTIONS

1. Help patient to cope with undesirable effects of radiation therapy, i.e., esophagitis, anorexia, loss of taste, dry mouth, nausea and vomiting, diarrhea, skin reactions, and lethargy.
2. Serve bland, soft foods at mild temperatures.
3. Provide anesthetic throat lozenges to relieve mouth discomfort that interferes with eating.
4. Teach patient there is an increased risk of dental caries and instruct in proper dental hygiene.

5. Administer antiemetics during peak times of nausea.

6. Teach patient that skin reactions and the appearance of sunburned or tanned skin are common; rubbing the area and applying heat, cold, or lotion should be avoided.

7. Encourage patient to rest and sleep to maintain a reasonable energy level; lethargy accompanies radiation.

8. Give support to help patients tolerate toxic effects of chemotherapy, i.e., bone marrow depression, gastrointestinal disturbances, and alopecia. Provide for anticipatory nausea and vomiting with prompt recognition and treatment. Help patients to prepare for alopecia by encouraging them to purchase a wig prior to the time of hair loss.

9. Encourage patient to report any sign of infection for immediate treatment.

10. Teach that they are extremely vulnerable to infection as a result of radiation and chemotherapy; avoid contact with persons with infection.

11. Use contraception during chemotherapy to prevent cytotoxic effects on the fetus.

12. Encourage patient to keep all follow-up appointments.

13. Inform that there is a high incidence of acute leukemia developing years after treatment with radiation and chemotherapy.

For more information see Chapter 32 in Smeltzer and Bare: *Brunner and Suddarth's Textbook of Medical–Surgical Nursing,* 8th Edition. Philadelphia: Lippincott–Raven, 1996.

HUMAN IMMUNODEFICIENCY VIRUS

See Acquired Immunodeficiency Syndrome

HUNTINGTON'S DISEASE

Huntington's disease (HD) is a chronic, hereditary disease of the nervous system that results in progressive involuntary choreiform (dancelike) movements and dementia. It affects men and women of all races. It is transmitted as an autosomal-dominant genetic disorder. Each child of a parent with HD has a 50% risk of inheriting the illness. A genetic marker for HD has been located. It offers no hope of cure or even specific determination of onset.

CLINICAL MANIFESTATIONS

1. Most prominent clinical features are abnormal involuntary movements (chorea), intellectual decline, and emotional disturbance.
2. Constant writhing, twisting, and uncontrollable movements of the entire body occur as the disease progresses.
3. Facial movements produce ticks and grimaces; speech is affected, becoming slurred to eventually unintelligible.
4. Chewing and swallowing are difficult and aspiration is a danger.
5. Gait becomes disorganized and ambulation eventually impossible; patient is eventually confined to a wheelchair.
6. Bowel and bladder control is lost.
7. Progressive intellectual impairment occurs.
8. Uncontrollable emotional changes occur, but become less acute as the disease progresses. Patient may be nervous, clumsy, irritable, or impatient. During the early stages of illness: uncontrollable fits of anger; profound, often suicidal depression; apathy; or euphoria.
9. Hallucinations, delusions, and paranoid thinking may precede appearance of disjointed movements.

10. Eventually patient succumbs from heart failure, pneumonia, infection, or dies as a result of fall or choking.

MANAGEMENT

1. Medications such as phenylthiazines, butyrophenones, and thioxanthenes that block dopamine receptors improve chorea in many patients.
2. Continually assess and evaluate patient's motor signs.
3. Psychotherapy aimed at allaying anxiety and reducing stress may be beneficial; antidepressants for depression or suicidal ideation.
4. Focus on patient's needs and capabilities.

H

✎ PATIENT EDUCATION AND HEALTH MAINTENANCE: CARE IN THE HOME AND COMMUNITY

1. HD takes emotional, physical, social, and financial tolls on every member of the patient's family.
2. Encourage crucial genetic counseling, access to long-term psychological counseling, marriage counseling, and financial and legal support.
3. Provide information about the Huntington's Disease Foundation of America, which gives information, referrals, education, and support for research.

For more information see Chapter 60 in Smeltzer and Bare: *Brunner and Suddarth's Textbook of Medical–Surgical Nursing,* 8th Edition. Philadelphia: Lippincott–Raven, 1996.

HYPERCORTISOLISM

See Cushing's Syndrome

HYPERGLYCEMIC HYPEROSMOLAR NONKETOTIC SYNDROME

Hyperglycemic hyperosmolar nonketotic (HHNK) syndrome is a situation in which hyperglycemia and hyperosmolarity predominate with alterations of the sensorium (sense of awareness). Ketosis is minimal or absent. The basic biochemical defect is lack of effective insulin. The persistent hyperglycemia causes osmotic diuresis, resulting in water and electrolyte losses. While there is not enough insulin to prevent hyperglycemia, the small amount of insulin present is enough to prevent fat breakdown. This condition occurs most frequently in older people (50–70 years) who have had no previous history of diabetes or only mild Type II diabetes. The acute development of the condition can be traced to some precipitating event, i.e., acute illness (pneumonia, myocardial infarction, stroke), ingestion of medications known to provoke insulin insufficiency (thiazide diuretics, propranolol), or therapeutic procedures (peritoneal dialysis/hemodialysis, hyperalimentation).

CLINICAL MANIFESTATIONS

1. History of days to weeks of polyuria and polydipsia.
2. Hypotension, tachycardia.
3. Profound dehydration (dry mucous membranes, poor skin turgor).
4. Variable neurological signs (alterations of sensorium, seizures, hemiparesis).

MANAGEMENT

The overall treatment of HHNK syndrome is similar to that of diabetic ketoacidosis (DKA): fluids, electrolytes, and insulin.

1. Monitor fluid volume and electrolyte status for prevention of congestive heart failure and cardiac

dysrhythmias (because of increased age of typical patient).

2. Start fluid treatment with 0.9% or 0.45% normal saline depending on sodium level and severity of volume depletion.

3. Central venous or arterial pressure monitoring may be necessary to guide fluid replacement.

4. Add potassium to replacement fluids when urinary output is adequate and is guided by continuous ECG monitoring and laboratory determinations of potassium.

5. Insulin is usually given at a continuous low rate to prevent hyperglycemia.

6. Dextrose is added to replacement fluids when the glucose level decreases to the 250–300 mg/dl range.

7. Other treatment modalities are determined by the underlying illness of the patient and results of continuing clinical and lab evaluation.

8. Treatment is continued until metabolic abnormalities are corrected and neurological symptoms clear (may take 3–5 days for neurological symptoms to resolve).

9. After recovery from HHNK syndrome many patients can control diabetes with diet alone or diet and oral hypoglycemic agents. Insulin may not be needed once the acute hyperglycemic complication is resolved.

For more information see Chapter 39 in Smeltzer and Bare: *Brunner and Suddarth's Textbook of Medical–Surgical Nursing*, 8th Edition. Philadelphia: Lippincott–Raven, 1996.

HYPERPARATHYROIDISM

Hyperparathyroidism is due to overproduction of parathyroid hormone by the parathyroid glands and is characterized by bone calcification and development of renal stones containing calcium. Primary hyperparathyroidism occurs two to four times more often in women than in men and is most frequently seen in patients between 60 and 70 years of age. Secondary hyperparathyroidism with similar manifestations occurs in patients with chronic renal failure and renal rickets.

CLINICAL MANIFESTATIONS

The patient may have no symptoms or may experience signs and symptoms resulting from involvement of several body systems.

1. Apathy, fatigue, muscular weakness, nausea, vomiting, constipation, hypertension, and cardiac dysrhythmias may occur.
2. Psychological manifestations vary from emotional irritability and neuroses to psychoses due to the effect of calcium on the brain and nervous system.
3. Stones in one or both kidneys may occur, causing obstruction, polynephritis, and renal failure.
4. Musculoskeletal symptoms result from demineralization of the bones or bone tumors. Skeletal pain and tenderness in the back and joints; pain on weight bearing; pathologic fractures; deformities; and shortening of body stature.
5. Incidence of peptic ulcer and pancreatitis is increased.

DIAGNOSTIC EVALUATION

1. Persistent increased serum calcium levels and elevated level of parahormone.
2. Ultrasound, MRI, thallium scan, and fine-needle biopsy.

MANAGEMENT

1. Surgical removal of abnormal parathyroid tissue for primary hyperparathyroidism: in the preoperative period encourage patient to have a fluid intake of 2000 ml or more to prevent calculus formation.
2. Avoid thiazide diuretics because they decrease renal excretion of calcium.

3. Mobility is encouraged because bones subjected to normal stress give up less calcium.
4. Oral phosphates are administered to lower serum calcium levels.
5. Limit foods high in calcium and phosphorus.
6. Nursing management of the patient undergoing parathyroidectomy is essentially the same as that for a thyroidectomy patient.
7. Monitor closely to detect symptoms of tetany, an early postoperative complication.
8. Remind patient and family of importance of follow-up to assure normal serum calcium levels.

H

HYPERCALCEMIC CRISIS

Acute hypercalcemic crisis can occur when serum calcium levels exceed 15 mg/dl. This results in neurologic, cardiovascular, and renal symptoms that can be life-threatening.

1. Treatment includes rehydration with large volume of IV fluids, diuretic agents for renal excretion of excess calcium, and phosphate therapy to correct hypophosphatemia and decrease serum calcium levels.
2. Cytotoxic agents, calcitonin, and dialysis may be used in emergency situations to decrease serum calcium quickly.
3. Monitor patients in hypercalcemic crisis very closely for complications, deterioration of condition, and reversal of serum calcium levels.
4. Assess and care for patient to minimize complications and reverse the life-threatening hypercalcemia.

For more information see Chapter 40 in Smeltzer and Bare: *Brunner and Suddarth's Textbook of Medical–Surgical Nursing,* 8th Edition. Philadelphia: Lippincott–Raven, 1996.

HYPERTENSION

Hypertension can be defined as persistent levels of blood pressure in which the systolic pressure is above 140 mmHg and the diastolic pressure is above 90 mmHg. In the elderly population, hypertension is defined as systolic pressure above 160 mmHg and diastolic above 90 mmHg. Hypertension is a major cause of heart failure, stroke, and kidney failure. Hypertension carries the risk of premature morbidity or mortality, which increases as the systolic and diastolic pressure rises.

ESSENTIAL (PRIMARY) HYPERTENSION

1. About 20% of the adult population develops hypertension; more than 90% of these have essential (primary) hypertension, which has no identifiable medical cause.
2. On occasion it appears abruptly and severely and takes a "malignant" course that causes rapid deterioration in condition.
3. Emotional disturbances, obesity, excessive alcohol intake, and overstimulation with coffee, tobacco, and stimulatory drugs play a role.
4. Strongly familial.
5. Affects more women than men, but African-American men are less able to tolerate the disease.

SECONDARY HYPERTENSION

Elevations in blood pressure with specific cause, e.g., arterial disease, renal disease, certain medications, tumors, and pregnancy.

CLINICAL MANIFESTATIONS

1. Physical examination may reveal no abnormality other than high blood pressure.
2. Changes in the retinae with hemorrhages, exudates, narrowed arterioles, and papilledema may be seen.

3. Symptoms usually indicate vascular damage related to organ systems served by involved vessels.
4. Coronary artery disease with angina is the most common sequela.
5. Left ventricular hypertrophy; left heart failure ensues.
6. Pathologic changes in the kidney (nocturia and azotemia).
7. Cerebral vascular involvement (stroke or transient ischemic attack [TIA, i.e., temporary hemiplegia, blackouts, alterations in vision]).

H

DIAGNOSTIC EVALUATION

1. History and physical examination including retinae exam, laboratory studies for organ damage, ECG for left ventricular hypertrophy.
2. Special studies: renograms, intravenous pyelograms, renal arteriograms, split renal function studies, and renin levels.

MANAGEMENT

The objective of any treatment program is to prevent associated morbidity and mortality by achieving and maintaining an arterial blood pressure below 140/90 mmHg, whenever possible.

1. Nonpharmacologic approaches: i.e., weight reduction; restriction of alcohol, sodium, tobacco; exercise and relaxation.
2. Pharmacologic approaches should be initiated when the diastolic blood pressure is persistently over 85–89 mmHg and the systolic is 130–139 mmHg when the individual is at high risk (men, smokers).
3. Select a drug class that has the greatest effectiveness, fewest side effects, and best chance of acceptance by the patient. Promote compliance by avoiding complicated drug schedules.
4. Two classes of drugs are available as first-line therapy: diuretics and beta-blockers.

NURSING PROCESS

Assessment

Assess blood pressure at frequent intervals; know baseline level. Note changes in pressure that would require a change in medication. Include the following in the physical examination:

1. Apical and peripheral pulse rate, rhythm, and character.
2. Symptoms such as nosebleeds, anginal pain, shortness of breath, alterations in vision, vertigo, headaches, or nocturia.

Major Nursing Diagnosis

1. Knowledge deficit regarding the relationship between the treatment regimen and control of the disease process.
2. Potential noncompliance to the self-care program related to negative side effects of prescribed therapy.

Collaborative Problems

1. Retinal hemorrhage.
2. Congestive heart failure.
3. Renal insufficiency.
4. Cerebral vascular accident (CVA).

Planning and Implementation

The major goals include understanding of the disease process and its treatment, and compliance with self-care program.

 PATIENT EDUCATION AND HEALTH MAINTENANCE: CARE IN THE HOME AND COMMUNITY

Lower Blood Pressure to Normal Levels

1. Promote adherence to therapy in a cost-effective manner, i.e., antihypertensive medications, dietary restrictions of sodium and fat, weight control,

lifestyle changes, exercise program, and follow-up health care at regular intervals.
2. Encourage counseling, education and self-help groups for family and patient.

Promote Compliance with the Self-Care Program

1. Encourage active participation of the patient in the program, including self-monitoring of blood pressure and diet for increased compliance.
2. Encourage patient to abstain from alcohol because alcohol may have a synergistic effect with medication.
3. Discourage use of tobacco and nicotine products.
4. Give patient written information regarding expected effects and side effects of medication.
5. Teach patient how to take own blood pressure.

✪ GERONTOLOGIC CONSIDERATIONS

Compliance with the therapeutic program is even more difficult for elderly people because medication therapy must be continuous, it may be complicated, and it may be expensive for a person on a fixed income.

Monotherapy, treatment with a single agent, may be an appropriate option for simplifying the medication regimen and making it less expensive. Make sure that the patient understands the medication regimen and is able to read the instructions.

Be aware of postural hypotensive effects of antihypertensive medications (change position slowly, use supportive devices).

Include the family in the teaching program so they understand the patient's needs, support adherence to the therapeutic program, and know when to seek guidance from health professionals.

Encourage return to the outpatient setting for follow-up care. Assess all body systems to detect evidence of vascular damage to vital organs, i.e., eyes (blurred vision, spots in front of eyes, diminished visual activity), heart, nervous system, and kidney function.

✚ Clinical Alert: Hypertensive Emergency

Exists when an elevated blood pressure must be lowered within 1 hour. Requires prompt treatment in an intensive care setting because of serious organ damage.

Medication regimen (e.g., nitroprusside, labetalol hydrochloride) requires extremely close hemodynamic monitoring.

For more information see Chapter 31 in Smeltzer and Bare: *Brunner and Suddarth's Textbook of Medical–Surgical Nursing,* 8th Edition. Philadelphia: Lippincott–Raven, 1996.

HYPERTHYROIDISM (GRAVES' DISEASE)

Hyperthyroidism constitutes a well-defined disease entity, with Graves' disease the most common cause. An excessive output of thyroid hormones is thought to be due to abnormal stimulation of the thyroid gland by circulating immunoglobulins. Long-acting thyroid stimulator (LATS) is found in significant concentration in the serum of many of these patients. The disorder affects women five times more frequently than men and peaks in incidence in the third and fourth decades. It may appear after an emotional shock, stress, or infection, but the exact significance of these relationships is not understood. Other common causes include thyroiditis and excessive ingestion of thyroid hormone.

CLINICAL MANIFESTATIONS

Present a characteristic group of signs and symptoms (thyrotoxicosis).

1. Nervousness (emotionally hyperexcitable), irritable, apprehensive; cannot sit quietly; suffer from palpitations, and rapid pulse on rest and exertion.
2. Tolerate heat poorly and perspire freely; skin is flushed, and is likely to be warm, soft, and moist.

3. Elderly patients may report dry skin and diffuse pruritus.
4. Fine tremor of the hands may be observed.
5. May exhibit exophthalmos (bulging eyes).
6. Other symptoms include increased appetite and dietary intake, progressive loss of weight, abnormal muscle fatigability, weakness, amenorrhea, and changes in bowel function (constipation or diarrhea).
7. Pulse ranges between 90 and 160 beats per minute; systolic (but not diastolic) blood pressure is elevated.
8. Atrial fibrillation may occur and cardiac decompensation in the form of congestive heart failure, especially in the elderly.
9. Osteoporosis and fracture.
10. The disease may be mild, with remissions and exacerbations, terminating with spontaneous recovery in a few months or years.
11. It may progress relentlessly, causing emaciation, intense nervousness, delirium, disorientation, and eventually heart failure.
12. Symptoms may be caused by excessive administration of thyroid hormone for treatment of hypothyroidism.

DIAGNOSTIC EVALUATION

1. Thyroid gland is enlarged; it is soft and may pulsate; a thrill may be felt and a bruit heard over thyroid arteries.
2. Laboratory tests; increase in serum T_4; increase in ^{131}I uptake

MANAGEMENT

No treatment directed toward the cause is available. Management depends on the etiology of the hyperthyroidism.

1. Pharmacotherapy with antithyroid drugs.
2. Irradiation involving the administration of ^{131}I or ^{125}I for destructive effects on the thyroid gland.

3. Surgery with the removal of most of the thyroid gland.

Pharmacotherapy

1. The objective of pharmacotherapy is to inhibit hormone synthesis or release.
2. The most commonly used medications are propylthiouracil (Propacil, PTU) or methimazole (Tapazole) until patient is euthyroid.
3. Establish maintenance dose, followed by gradual withdrawal of the medication over the next several months.
4. Antithyroid drugs are contraindicated in late pregnancy; risk for goiter and cretinism in the fetus.

Beta-adrenergic Agents

1. May be used to control the sympathetic nervous system effects that occur in hyperthyroidism.
2. Propranolol is used for nervousness, tachycardia, tremor, anxiety, and heat intolerance.

Radioactive Iodine (^{131}I)

1. [131]I is given to destroy the overactive thyroid cells.
2. [131]I is contraindicated in pregnancy and nursing mothers because radioiodine crosses the placenta and is secreted in breast milk.

SURGICAL INTERVENTION

1. Surgical intervention removes about five-sixths of the thyroid tissue.
2. Before surgery the patient is given propylthiouracil until signs of hyperthyroidism have disappeared.
3. Iodine is prescribed to reduce thyroid size and vascularity.
4. Risk of relapse and complications necessitate long-term follow-up of patient undergoing treatment of hyperthyroidism.

NURSING PROCESS

Assessment

1. Health history including family history of hyperthyroidism.
2. Stressors and the patient's ability to cope with stress.
3. Nutritional status and presence of symptoms; note excessive nervousness and changes in vision and appearance of eyes.

Major Nursing Diagnosis

1. Altered nutrition related to exaggerated metabolic rate, excessive appetite, and increased gastrointestinal activity.
2. Ineffective coping related to irritability, hyperexcitability, apprehension, and emotional instability.
3. Disturbance in self-esteem related to changes in appearance, excessive appetite, and weight loss.
4. Altered body temperature.

Collaborative Problems

1. Thyrotoxicosis or thyroid storm.
2. Hypothyroidism.

Planning and Implementation

The patient's goals may be improved nutritional status, improved coping ability, improved self-esteem, maintenance of normal body temperature, and absence of complications.

Interventions

MONITORING AND MANAGING POTENTIAL COMPLICATIONS

1. Monitor closely for signs and symptoms indicative of thyroid storm.
2. Assess cardiac and respiratory function, i.e., vital signs, cardiac output, ECG monitoring, arterial blood gases, pulse oximetry.
3. Administer oxygen to prevent hypoxia.

4. Give intravenous fluids to maintain blood glucose levels and replace lost fluids.
5. Prescribe antithyroid medications to reduce thyroid hormone levels.
6. Prescribe propranolol and digitalis to treat cardiac symptoms.
7. Implement strategies to treat shock if needed.

IMPROVING NUTRITIONAL STATUS

1. Provide several small, well-balanced meals (up to six meals a day) to satisfy patient's increased appetite.
2. Replace food and fluids lost through diarrhea and diaphoresis and control diarrhea that results from increased peristalsis.
3. Reduce diarrhea by avoiding highly seasoned foods and stimulants such as coffee, tea, cola, and alcohol; encourage high-calorie, high-protein foods.
4. Provide quiet atmosphere during mealtime to aid digestion.
5. Record patient's weight and dietary intake daily.

ENHANCING COPING MEASURES

1. Reassure family and friends that symptoms are expected to disappear with treatment.
2. Maintain a calm, unhurried approach and minimize stressful experiences.
3. Keep the environment quiet and uncluttered.
4. Provide information regarding thyroidectomy to alleviate patient anxiety.
5. Assist patient to take medications as prescribed and encourage adherence to the therapeutic regimen.

IMPROVING SELF-ESTEEM

1. Convey to the patient an understanding of concern regarding problems in appearance, appetite, and weight.
2. Provide eye protection if experiencing eye changes secondary to hyperthyroidism; instruct regarding

correct installation of eyedrops or ointment to soothe the eyes and protect the exposed cornea.
3. Arrange for the patient to eat alone, if desired and if embarrassed by the large meals consumed due to increased metabolic rate.

MAINTAINING NORMAL BODY TEMPERATURE

1. Provide a cool, comfortable environment and fresh bedding and gown as needed.
2. Give cool baths and provide cool fluids; monitor body temperature.
3. Explain to patient and family the importance of providing a cool environment.

H

✎ PATIENT EDUCATION AND HEALTH MAINTENANCE: CARE IN THE HOME AND COMMUNITY

1. Instruct how and when to take prescribed medications.
2. Teach patient how the medication regimen fits in with the broader therapeutic plan.
3. Provide an individualized written plan of care for use at home.
4. Teach patient and family members about the desired effects and side effects of medications.
5. Instruct patient and family about which adverse effects should be reported to the physician.
6. Stress long-term follow-up care because of the possibility of hypothyroidism following thyroidectomy or treatment with antithyroid drugs or [131]I.
7. Teach patient about what to expect from a thyroidectomy if this is to be performed.
8. Teach to avoid situations that have the potential of stimulating thyroid storm.
9. Refer to home care for assessment of the home and family environment.
10. Assess patient's and family's understanding of the importance of the therapeutic regimen and compliance with it; recommend follow-up monitoring.

11. Assess for changes indicating return to normal thyroid function; also physical signs of hyper- and hypothyroidism.

✪ GERONTOLOGIC CONSIDERATIONS

The major symptoms of the elderly patient may be depression and apathy, accompanied by significant weight loss. The patient may report cardiovascular symptoms and difficulty climbing stairs or rising from a chair because of muscle weakness.

The elderly may experience a single manifestation such as atrial fibrillation, anorexia, or weight loss. These general symptoms may mask underlying thyroid disease. Spontaneous remission of hyperthyroidism is rare in the elderly. Measurement of T_4 and T_3 uptake is indicated in elderly patients with unexplained physical or mental deterioration.

Use of ^{131}I is generally recommended for treatment of thyrotoxicosis rather than surgery unless an enlarged thyroid gland is pressing on the airway. Thyrotoxicosis must be controlled by antithyroid drugs before ^{131}I is used because radiation may precipitate thyroid storm, which has a high mortality rate in the elderly.

Use of beta-blockers may be indicated to decrease cardiovascular and neurologic signs; use these agents with extreme caution and monitor closely for granulocytopenia.

Modify dosages of other medications because of the altered rate of metabolism in hyperthyroidism.

For more information see Chapter 43 in Smeltzer and Bare: *Brunner and Suddarth's Textbook of Medical–Surgical Nursing*, 8th Edition. Philadelphia: Lippincott–Raven, 1996.

HYPERURICEMIA

See Gout

HYPOFUNCTION, ADRENAL

See Chronic Primary Adrenocorticol Insufficiency

HYPOGLYCEMIA (INSULIN REACTION)

Hypoglycemia (abnormally low blood glucose level) occurs when the blood glucose falls below 50–60 mg/dl. It can be caused by too much insulin or oral hypoglycemic agents, too little food, or excessive physical activity. Hypoglycemia may occur at any time. It often occurs before meals, especially if delayed or if snacks are omitted. Middle-of-the-night hypoglycemia may occur because of peaking evening NPH or Lente insulins, especially in patients who have not eaten a bedtime snack.

H

CLINICAL MANIFESTATIONS

1. The symptoms of hypoglycemia may be grouped into two categories: adrenergic symptoms and central nervous system symptoms.
2. Hypoglycemic symptoms may occur suddenly and unexpectedly and vary from person to person.
3. Patients who have blood glucose in the hyperglycemic range (200s or greater) may feel hypoglycemic.
4. Adrenergic symptoms occur when blood glucose drops to 120 mg/dl or less.
5. Decreased hormonal (adrenergic) response may occur in patients who have diabetes for many years.
6. As the glucose falls, the normal surge of adrenaline does not occur and patient does not feel the usual adrenergic symptoms, i.e., sweating and shakiness.

Mild Hypoglycemia

The sympathetic nervous system is stimulated, producing sweating, tremor, tachycardia, palpitations, nervousness, and hunger.

Moderate Hypoglycemia

1. Produces impaired function of the central nervous system.
2. Inability to concentrate, headache, lightheadedness, confusion, and memory lapses.
3. Numbness of the lips and tongue.
4. Slurred speech, incoordination, emotional changes, irrational behavior, double vision, and drowsiness.

Severe Hypoglycemia

1. Central nervous system function is further impaired.
2. Patient needs the assistance of another for treatment.
3. Disoriented behavior, seizures, difficulty arousing from sleep, or loss of consciousness.

MANAGEMENT

1. Usual recommendation is 10–15 g of a fast-acting sugar orally: (a) 2–4 commercially prepared glucose tablets; (b) 4–6 oz of fruit juice or regular soda; (c) 6–10 Lifesavers or other hard candies; (d) 2–3 teaspoons of sugar or honey.
2. Avoid adding table sugar to juice, even "unsweet-ened" juice, which may cause sharp increase in glucose and patient may experience hyperglycemia later.
3. Repeat treatment if the symptoms persist more than 10–15 minutes.
4. Provide a snack containing protein and starch (milk, or cheese and crackers) after the symptoms resolve.
5. Recommend that diabetic patients always carry a form of simple sugar with them at all times.
6. Discourage from eating high-calorie, high-fat dessert foods to treat hypoglycemia. High-fat content may slow absorption of the glucose.

MANAGEMENT OF SEVERE HYPOGLYCEMIA

1. Glucagon 1 mg subcutaneously or intramuscularly for patients who are unable to swallow, or refuse treatment. May take up to 20 minutes to regain consciousness. Give a simple sugar followed by snack when awake.
2. Instruct patient to notify physician after severe hypoglycemia has occurred.
3. 25–50 ml of 50% dextrose in water ("D-50") administered IV to patients who are unconscious or unable to swallow in hospital situation.

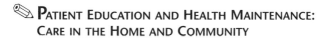

✎ PATIENT EDUCATION AND HEALTH MAINTENANCE: CARE IN THE HOME AND COMMUNITY

1. Prevent hypoglycemia by following a regular pattern for eating, administering insulin, and exercising. Consume between-meal and bedtime snacks to counteract the maximum insulin effect.
2. Routine blood glucose tests are performed so changing insulin requirements may be anticipated and adjusted.
3. Encourage patients taking insulin to wear identification bracelet or tag indicating they have diabetes.
4. Instruct patients and family members on symptoms of hypoglycemia and use of glucagon.
5. Teach family members hypoglycemia can cause irrational and unintentional behavior.
6. Teach patients the importance of performing blood glucose tests on a frequent and regular basis.
7. Teach Type II diabetic patients who take oral hypoglycemic agents that symptoms of hypoglycemia may also develop.

✿ GERONTOLOGIC CONSIDERATIONS

Elderly people frequently live alone and may not recognize symptoms of hypoglycemia. With decreasing renal function, it takes longer for oral hypoglycemic agents to be excreted by the kidneys. Teach patient to avoid skipping meals because of decreased appetite or financial limitations on meal planning.

Decreased visual acuity may lead to errors in insulin administration.

For more information see Chapter 39 in Smeltzer and Bare: *Brunner and Suddarth's Textbook of Medical–Surgical Nursing,* 8th Edition. Philadelphia: Lippincott–Raven, 1996.

HYPOPARATHYROIDISM

The most common cause of hypoparathyroidism is inadequate secretion of parathyroid hormone following interruption of the blood supply or surgical removal of parathyroid gland tissue during thyroidectomy, parathyroidectomy, or radical neck dissection. Atrophy of the parathyroid glands of unknown etiology is a less common cause. Symptoms are due to deficiency of parathormone that results in an elevation of blood phosphate and decrease in blood calcium.

CLINICAL MANIFESTATIONS

Tetany is the chief symptom.

1. Latent tetany: numbness, tingling, and cramps in the extremities; stiffness in the hands and feet.
2. Overt tetany: bronchospasm, laryngospasm, carpopedal spasm, dysphagia, photophobia, cardiac dysrhythmias, and convulsions.
3. Other symptoms: anxiety, irritability, depression, and delirium.

DIAGNOSTIC EVALUATION

1. Latent tetany is suggested by positive Trousseau's sign or positive Chvostek's sign.
2. Diagnosis is difficult because of vague symptoms; laboratory studies show decreased serum calcium,

increased serum phosphate; increased bone density on x-ray; brain calcification on x-ray.

MANAGEMENT

1. Raise the serum calcium level to 9–10 mg/dl.
2. When hypocalcemia and tetany occur following thyroidectomy, give calcium gluconate IV immediately. Sedatives may be administered. Parenteral parathormone may be given; watch for allergic reaction.
3. Reduce neuromuscular irritability by providing environment free of noise, sudden drafts, bright lights, or sudden movement.
4. Provide emergency management with tracheostomy or mechanical ventilation for respiratory distress.

H

Nursing Interventions

1. Anticipate signs of tetany, convulsions, and respiratory difficulty.
2. Keep calcium gluconate at bedside and observe for cardiac problems, i.e., dysrhythmias. If receiving digitalis, then calcium gluconate must be administered slowly and cautiously.
3. Provide continuous cardiac monitoring and careful assessment; calcium and digitalis increase systolic contraction and potentiate each other and the risk for fatal dysrhythmias.
4. Provide diet high in calcium and low in phosphorus for patients with chronic hypoparathyroidism. Restrict milk, milk products, and egg yolk since they contain high levels of phosphorus. Eliminate spinach because it contains oxalate, which forms insoluble calcium substances.
5. Provide oral tablets of calcium salts, i.e., calcium gluconate; aluminum hydroxide gel is given after meals to bind phosphate.
6. Provide vitamin D preparations to enhance calcium absorption from the GI tract.
7. Teach about medications and diet therapy and reason for high calcium and low phosphate intake;

teach patient to contact physician if symptoms occur.

For more information see Chapter 40 in Smeltzer and Bare: *Brunner and Suddarth's Textbook of Medical–Surgical Nursing,* 8th Edition. Philadelphia: Lippincott–Raven, 1996.

HYPOPITUITARISM

Hypopituitarism is pituitary insufficiency from destruction of the anterior lobe of the pituitary gland. Panhypopituitarism (Simmond's disease) is total absence of all pituitary secretions and is rare. Postpartum pituitary necrosis (Sheehan's syndrome) is another uncommon cause of failure of the anterior pituitary. It is more likely to occur in women with severe blood loss, hypovolemia, and hypotension at the time of delivery. Hypopituitarism is also a complication of radiation therapy to the head and neck. Total destruction of the pituitary gland by trauma, tumor, or vascular lesion removes all stimuli that are normally received by the thyroid, gonads, and adrenal glands. The result is extreme weight loss, emaciation, atrophy of all endocrine glands and organs, hair loss, impotence, amenorrhea, hypometabolism, and hypoglycemia. Coma and death will occur without replacement of missing hormones.

For more information see Chapter 40 in Smeltzer and Bare: *Brunner and Suddarth's Textbook of Medical–Surgical Nursing,* 8th Edition. Philadelphia: Lippincott–Raven, 1996.

HYPOPROLIFERATIVE ANEMIA

See Anemia, Aplastic

HYPOTHYROIDISM AND MYXEDEMA

Hypothyroidism is a condition of thyroid hypofunction followed by thyroid failure. It results from suboptimal levels of thyroid hormone. Types of hypothyroidism include primary, which refers to dysfunction of the thyroid gland itself (95% of patients have this type); central, due to failure of the pituitary gland, hypothalamus, or both; secondary or pituitary, which is due entirely to a pituitary disorder; hypothalamic or tertiary, due to a disorder of the hypothalamus resulting in inadequate secretion of TSH from decreased stimulation by TRH. Causes include autoimmune thyroiditis (Hashimoto's thyroiditis, most common type in adults); therapy for hyperthyroidism (radioiodine, surgery, or antithyroid drugs); medications (lithium and iodine compounds); radiation therapy for head and neck cancer; infiltrative diseases of the thyroid (amyloidosis and scleroderma); iodine deficiency and iodine excess. When thyroid deficiency is present at birth, the condition is known as cretinism. Myxedema refers to the accumulation of mucopolysaccharides in subcutaneous and other interstitial tissue. The term *myxedema* is used only to describe the extreme symptoms of severe hypothyroidism.

CLINICAL MANIFESTATIONS

1. General early symptoms are nonspecific.
2. Extreme fatigue.
3. Hair loss, brittle nails, dry skin, and numbness and tingling of the fingers.
4. Husky voice and hoarseness.
5. Mental disturbances; menorrhagia or amenorrhea; loss of libido.
6. In severe hypothyroidism, temperature and pulse rate become subnormal; weight gain without corresponding increase of food intake.
7. Patient often complains of being cold in a warm environment.

8. Emotional responses become subdued as the condition progresses; mental processes are dulled and the patient appears apathetic.

9. Speech is slow; tongue enlarges; hands and feet increase in size; constipation; and deafness may occur.

10. Hypothyroidism affects women five times more frequently than men and there is an associated tendency toward atherosclerosis with all consequences.

11. Advanced hypothyroidism: personality changes, pleural effusion, pericardial effusion, and respiratory muscle weakness.

12. Myxedema: skin becomes thickened, hair thins and falls out; face becomes expressionless and masklike.

13. A patient with advanced myxedema is hypothermic, abnormally sensitive to sedatives, opiates, and anesthetic agents; these drugs are given with extreme caution.

MANAGEMENT

The primary objective is to restore a normal metabolic state by replacing thyroid hormone.

1. Synthetic levothyroxine (Synthroid or Levothroid) is the preferred preparation.

2. Additional treatment consists of maintaining vital functions; monitoring arterial blood gases, and administering fluids cautiously because of danger of water intoxication.

3. Avoid external heat application because it increases oxygen requirements and may lead to vascular collapse.

4. Concentrated glucose may be given if hypoglycemia is evident.

5. If myxedema coma is present, thyroid hormone is given intravenously until consciousness is restored.

Interaction of Thyroid Hormones with Other Drugs

1. Thyroid hormones increase blood glucose levels, which may necessitate adjustment in doses of insulin or oral hypoglycemic agents.
2. The effects of thyroid hormone may be increased by phenytoin and tricyclic antidepressants.
3. Thyroid hormone may increase the pharmacologic effect of digitalis, glycosides, anticoagulants, and indomethacin, requiring careful observation and assessment for side effects of these drugs.
4. Severe untreated hypothyroidism increases susceptibility to all hypnotic and sedative drugs.

H

Nursing Interventions

MODIFYING ACTIVITIES

1. Support the patient by assisting with care and hygiene while encouraging to participate in activities within tolerance to prevent complications of immobility (major role of nurse).
2. Monitor vital signs and cognitive level closely during diagnostic work-up and initiation of treatment to detect (1) deterioration of physical and mental status, (2) symptoms indicating that an increased metabolic rate exceeds the ability of the cardiovascular and pulmonary systems to respond, and (3) continued limitations and complications of myxedema.
3. Administer medications cautiously.

REGULATING TEMPERATURE

1. Provide extra clothing and blankets for chilling and extreme intolerance to cold.
2. Avoid heating pads; patient could be burned because of delayed responses and decreased mental status.

PROVIDING EMOTIONAL SUPPORT

1. Assist patient and family in dealing with emotional reactions to changes in appearance and body image.
2. Inform that symptoms subside if hypothyroidism is treated successfully.
3. Provide assistance and counseling to deal with the emotional concerns and reactions that result.

✎ PATIENT EDUCATION AND HEALTH MAINTENANCE: CARE IN THE HOME AND COMMUNITY

1. Provide follow-up, teaching, and health care prior to hospital discharge.
2. Provide dietary instruction to promote weight loss once medication has been initiated and to promote return of normal bowel pattern.
3. Inform and instruct family member about treatment goals, medication schedules, and side effects to be reported.
4. Give encouragement and assistance in the daily administration of medications.
5. Reinforce knowledge that continued thyroid hormone replacement is necessary.
6. Arrange a weekly visit from the home care nurse to assess the physical and cognitive status, and ability to cope with recent changes.
7. Document and report subtle signs and symptoms that indicate inadequate thyroxine hormone.

✪ GERONTOLOGIC CONSIDERATIONS

The higher prevalence of hypothyroidism in the elderly may be related to alterations in immune function with age. Depression, apathy, or decreased mobility or activity may be the major initial symptom.

The effects of analgesics, sedatives, and anesthetic agents are prolonged in all patients with hypothyroidism, so they should be administered with caution. Thyroid hormone replacement must be started with low doses and gradually increased to prevent serious cardiovascular and neurological side effects, i.e., angina.

Myxedema and myxedema coma generally occur exclusively in patients over 50.

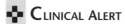 Cʟɪɴɪᴄᴀʟ Aʟᴇʀᴛ

Patients with unrecognized hypothyroidism undergoing surgery are at increased risk for intraoperative hypotension, postoperative congestive heart failure, and altered mental status. Myocardial ischemia or infarction may occur in response to therapy in patients with severe, longstanding hypothyroidism, or myxedema coma. Nurses must be alert for signs of angina, especially during early phase of treatment.

Discontinue administration of thyroid hormone immediately if symptoms occur.

For more information see Chapter 40 in Smeltzer and Bare: *Brunner and Suddarth's Textbook of Medical–Surgical Nursing,* 8th Edition. Philadelphia: Lippincott–Raven, 1996.

HYPOVOLEMIC SHOCK

See Shock, Hypovolemic

ICP

See Increased Intracranial Pressure

IDDM

See Diabetes Mellitus

IDIOPATHIC THROMBOCYTOPENIA PURPURA

Idiopathic thrombocytopenia purpura (ITP) is a disease of all ages, but is more common in children and young women. Although the precise cause remains unknown, viral infection sometimes precedes the disease in children. Antiplatelet antibodies are produced; platelet life span is markedly shortened. Usually the diagnosis is made from decreased platelet count, survival time, and increased bleeding time.

CLINICAL MANIFESTATIONS

1. Petechiae, mucosal bleeding, and heavy menses in women.
2. Platelet count is generally below 20,000 mm^3.

MANAGEMENT

1. Corticosteroids are the treatment of choice.
2. Splenectomy.
3. Immunosuppressive drugs are given to patients who do not respond to splenectomy.

4. Instruct to avoid all drugs that interfere with platelet function.

For more information see Chapter 32 in Smeltzer and Bare: *Brunner and Suddarth's Textbook of Medical–Surgical Nursing,* 8th Edition. Philadelphia: Lippincott–Raven, 1996.

IMPETIGO

Impetigo is a superficial infection of the skin caused by staphylococci, streptococci, or multiple bacteria. Exposed areas of the body, face, hands, neck, and extremities are most frequently involved. Impetigo is contagious and may spread to other parts of the patient's skin or to other members of the family who touch the patient, or use towels or combs that are soiled with the exudate of the lesion. Impetigo is particularly common among children living in poor hygienic conditions. In adults, ill health, poor hygiene, and malnutrition may predispose to impetigo. Bullous impetigo, a superficial infection of the skin caused by *Staphylococcus aureus* is characterized by the formation of bullae from original vesicles. The bullae rupture, leaving a raw, red area.

CLINICAL MANIFESTATIONS

1. Lesions begin as small, red macules that become discrete thin-walled vesicles that rupture and become covered with a honey-yellow crust.
2. These crusts, when removed, reveal smooth, red, moist surfaces on which new crusts develop.
3. If the scalp is involved, the hair is matted, distinguishing the condition from ringworm.

MANAGEMENT

Systemic Antibiotic Therapy

1. Usual treatment for impetigo.
2. Reduces contagious spread and prevents possible aftermath of glomerular nephritis.

3. Nonbullous impetigo: benzathine penicillin, or oral penicillin.
4. Bullous impetigo: penicillinase-resistant penicillin.

Topical Antibacterial Therapy

1. Apply to lesions several times daily for 1 week.
2. Soak or wash lesions with soap solution to remove bacterial growth and give the topical antibiotic opportunity to reach the infected site.
3. Wear gloves when giving care to these patients.
4. Antiseptic solutions (povidone-iodine) may be used to cleanse the skin and reduce bacterial content and prevent spread.

✎ PATIENT EDUCATION AND HEALTH MAINTENANCE: CARE IN THE HOME AND COMMUNITY

1. Instruct patient and family to bathe at least once daily with bactericidal soap.
2. Encourage cleanliness and good hygienic practices to prevent spread of lesion from one skin area to another and one person to another. Provide each person with separate towel and washcloth. Keep infected child away from other children.

For more information see Chapter 54 in Smeltzer and Bare: *Brunner and Suddarth's Textbook of Medical–Surgical Nursing,* 8th Edition. Philadelphia: Lippincott–Raven, 1996.

INCREASED INTRACRANIAL PRESSURE

Increased intracranial pressure (ICP) is the result of the amount of brain tissue, intracranial blood volume, and cerebrospinal fluid (CSF) within the skull at any one time. The volume and pressure of these three components are usually in a state of equilibrium. Because there is limited space for expansion within the skull, an increase of any of these components causes a change in the volume of the other, by either displacing or shifting CSF, increasing the absorption of CSF, or decreasing cerebral blood volume. The normal ICP varies depending on the position of the patient and is considered to be less than or equal to 15 mmHg. Although elevated ICP is most commonly associated with head injury, an elevated pressure may be seen secondary to brain tumors, subarachnoid hemorrhage, and toxic and viral encephalopathies. Increased ICP from any cause affects cerebral perfusion and produces distortion and shifts of brain tissue.

CLINICAL MANIFESTATIONS

1. When ICP increases to where the brain's ability to adjust has reached its limits, neural function is impaired. Manifested by changes in level of consciousness and abnormal respiratory and vasomotor responses.
2. Level of responsiveness/consciousness is the most important indicator of the patient's condition.
3. Lethargy is the earliest sign of increasing ICP. Slowing of speech and delay in response to verbal suggestions are early indicators.
4. Sudden change in condition, such as becoming restless (without apparent cause), appearing confused, or displaying increasing drowsiness, has neurologic significance.
5. As pressure increases, patient may react only to loud auditory or painful stimuli. Indicates serious impairment of brain circulation and immediate surgical intervention may be required. Abnormal motor responses in the form of decortication, decerebration, or flaccidity may occur.
6. If stupor deepens, patient responds to deep, painful stimuli by moaning but may not withdraw.
7. As condition worsens, extremities become flaccid and reflexes are absent. Jaw sags, tongue becomes flaccid, airway obstruction and inadequate respiratory exchange may occur.

8. When coma is profound, pupils dilate and fix, respirations are impaired, and a fatal outcome is usually inevitable.

MANAGEMENT

1. Increased ICP constitutes a true emergency and must be treated promptly. The immediate management for relief of ICP is based on decreasing cerebral edema, lowering the volume of CSF, and decreasing blood volume.
2. Administer osmotic diuretics and corticosteroids, restrict fluids, drain CSF, hyperventilate the patient, control fever, and reduce cellular metabolic demands.
3. If patient is not responsive to conventional treatment, reduction of cellular metabolic demands may be accomplished through administration of high doses of barbiturates or administration of pharmacologic paralyzing agents, i.e., pancuronium (Pavulon). Requires care in a critical care unit.

NURSING PROCESS

Assessment

Use the Glasgow Coma Scale to assess three types of behavior: verbal response, motor response, and eye opening.

SUBTLE CHANGES

Restlessness, headache, forced breathing, purposeless movements, and mental cloudiness may be early indications of rising ICP.

CHANGES IN VITAL SIGNS

1. Alterations in vital signs may be a late sign of increased ICP.
2. As ICP increases, pulse rate and respiratory rate decrease and blood pressure and temperature rise.

3. Observe for arterial hypertension, bradycardia, and respiratory irregularity, i.e., Cheyne-Stokes breathing and ataxic breathing.
4. Observe for widened pulse pressure—a serious development.
5. Immediate surgical intervention is indicated if the major circulation begins to fall as a result of brain compression.

HEADACHE

Headache is constant, increasing in intensity, and aggravated by movement or straining.

PUPILLARY CHANGES

1. Inspect pupils for size, configuration, and reaction to light.
2. Evaluate gaze as to whether it is conjugate (paired; working together) or dysconjugate.
3. Assess ability of eyes to abduct or adduct.
4. Inspect retina and optic nerve for hemorrhage and papilledema.

VOMITING

Assess for recurrent or projectile vomiting, which indicates increased pressure.

ICP MONITORING

ICP monitoring is an essential part of management.

MAJOR NURSING DIAGNOSIS

1. Altered cerebral tissue perfusion related to the effects of ICP.
2. Ineffective breathing patterns related to neurologic dysfunction (brain stem compression, structural displacement).

3. Ineffective airway clearance related to accumulation of secretions secondary to depression of level of responsiveness.
4. Risk for fluid volume deficit related to dehydration procedures.
5. Altered urine and bowel elimination related to effects of medication, indwelling urethral catheter, and diminished fluid/food intake.
6. Risk for infection related to ICP monitoring system (intraventricular catheter).

Collaborative Problems

1. Brain stem herniation.
2. Diabetes insipidus.
3. Syndrome of inappropriate antidiuretic hormone (SIADH).

Planning and Implementation

The goals may include achievement of cerebral tissue perfusion through reduction of ICP, normalization of respiration, achievement of airway clearance, restoration of fluid balance, normal urine and bowel elimination, absence of infection, and absence of complications.

Interventions

ACHIEVING CEREBRAL TISSUE PERFUSION

1. Monitor for bradycardia and a rising blood pressure (Cushing's reflex).
2. Avoid raising jugular venous pressure and ICP by keeping patient's head in a neutral (midline) position and maintain slight elevation of the head to aid in venous drainage.
3. Avoid extreme rotation and flexion of the neck because compression or distortion of the jugular veins increases the ICP.
4. Avoid extreme hip flexion because this position causes an increase in intra-abdominal and intrathoracic pressures, which produce a rise in ICP.

5. Avoid the Valsalva maneuver or even moving in bed; provide stool softeners and high-fiber diet if patient is able to eat.
6. Avoid isometric muscle contractions.
7. Avoid suctioning longer than 15 seconds; hyperventilate using sigh mode on ventilator with 100% oxygen prior to suctioning.
8. Maintain a calm atmosphere and reduce environmental stimuli.
9. Avoid enemas and cathartics.
10. During nursing care ICP should not rise above 25 mmHg and should return to baseline levels within 5 minutes.

ATTAINING NORMAL RESPIRATORY PATTERN

1. Monitor constantly for respiratory irregularities.
2. Collaborate with respiratory therapist in monitoring arterial carbon dioxide pressure ($PaCO_2$), which is usually maintained between 25 and 30 mmHg when hyperventilation therapy is used.
3. Maintain continuous neurologic observation record.

ACHIEVING AIRWAY CLEARANCE

1. Maintain patency of the airway; oxygenate patient before and after suctioning.
2. Auscultate lung fields for presence of adventitious sounds.
3. Elevate head of bed to aid in clearing secretions and improve venous drainage of the brain.

ATTAINING FLUID BALANCE

1. Assess patient's skin turgor, mucous membranes, serum and urine osmolality for signs of dehydration.
2. Monitor vital signs to assess fluid volume status.
3. Give oral hygiene for mouth dryness.

ATTAINING NORMAL URINE AND BOWEL ELIMINATION

1. Insert indwelling catheter to assess renal and fluid status.

2. Assess lower abdomen for bowel distention and bowel sounds.
3. Test stools for blood if patient is on high doses of corticosteroids (GI bleeding is a complication).
4. Caution to avoid straining during a bowel movement because the Valsalva maneuver increases ICP.

PREVENTING INFECTION

1. Strictly adhere to the written protocols for managing ICP monitoring systems in the health care facility.
2. Keep dressings over ventricular catheters dry because wet dressings are conducive to bacterial growth.
3. Use aseptic technique at all times when managing the ventricular drainage system.
4. Check carefully for any loose connections that cause leaking and contamination of the ventricular system and contamination of CSF, as well as inaccurate ICP readings.
5. Monitor for signs and symptoms of meningitis: fever, chills, nuchal (neck) rigidity, and increasing or persistent headache.

MONITORING AND MANAGING POTENTIAL COMPLICATIONS

1. ICP elevation: monitor ICP closely for continuous elevation or significant increase over baseline; assess vital signs at time of ICP increase.
2. Impending brain herniation: increase in blood pressure, decrease in pulse, and change in pupillary response.
3. Patients not on paralyzing agents may change from decerebrate to decorticate posturing to a flaccid or rag doll appearance; requires rapid intervention of mannitol or drainage of CSF. Monitor urine output closely.
4. Diabetes insipidus requires volume and electrolyte replacement and administration of vasopressin; monitor serum electrolytes for replacement.

5. SIADH requires fluid restriction and serum electrolyte monitoring.

For more information see Chapter 59 in Smeltzer and Bare: *Brunner and Suddarth's Textbook of Medical–Surgical Nursing*, 8th Edition. Philadelphia: Lippincott–Raven, 1996.

INFECTIVE ENDOCARDITIS

See Endocarditis, Infective

INFLAMMATION OF THE MYOCARDIUM

See Myocarditis

INFLAMMATION OF THE PERICARDIUM

See Pericarditis

INFLAMMATION OF THE PERITONEUM

See Peritonitis

INFLAMMATION OF THE PROSTATE

See Prostatitis

INFLAMMATION OF THE STOMACH

See Gastritis

INFLAMMATION OF THE THYROID

See Thyroiditis

INFLUENZA

Influenza is an acute viral disease that occurs in epidemic proportions every 2–3 years with a highly variable degree of severity. The virus is easily spread from host to host. Previous infection with influenza does not guarantee protection from future exposure. Epidemics are sudden and have high attack rates. Peak activity for influenza outbreaks is 6–8 weeks in winter months. Transmission is most likely to occur in the first 3 days of illness.

CLINICAL MANIFESTATIONS

1. Chills, fever, headache, muscle aches, anorexia, cough, and upper respiratory symptoms.
2. Recovery starts about the fourth day; cough and some degree of debilitation may persist.
3. Complications: viral pneumonia or superimposed bacterial pneumonia. Those at risk for progression of the disease include the elderly, those with immunosuppression, diabetes, chronic renal failure, or chronic pulmonary disease.

MANAGEMENT

The goals of management are to relieve symptoms, treat complications, and prevent transmission to others.

1. Cough is controlled with an expectorant-antitussive combination.
2. Acetaminophen for headache and myalgias.
3. Encourage rest at home for greater comfort and reduction of transmission.
4. Avoid giving aspirin to children because of its association with Reye's syndrome.
5. Amantadine hydrochloride and rimantadine hydrochloride have been effective against influenza A.

PREVENTION

1. Annual influenza vaccinations are recommended for those at high risk for complications of influenza: those over 65 years of age; residents of extended care facilities; those with chronic pulmonary or cardiovascular diseases, diabetes, immunosuppression, or renal dysfunction; children who require long-term aspirin therapy, which puts them at increased risk of developing Reye's syndrome; and health care personnel who have extensive contact with high-risk patients.
2. Restrict visitation of those who may have febrile illness and screen elective admissions to decrease influenza transmission.

✪ GERONTOLOGIC CONSIDERATIONS

Adverse effects of amantadine occur mainly in the elderly: central nervous system toxicity, confusion, dizziness, slurred speech, headache, sleep disturbances, and visual hallucinations.

For more information see Chapter 65 in Smeltzer and Bare: *Brunner and Suddarth's Textbook of Medical–Surgical Nursing,* 8th Edition. Philadelphia: Lippincott–Raven, 1996.

INTERSTITIAL CYSTITIS

Interstitial cystitis (chronic inflammation of the bladder) is not caused by bacteria and does not respond to antibiotics. It occurs mostly in women (ages 40–50). The cause is unknown. There is some suggestion of an inflammatory or autoimmune basis. Suggested causes include penetration of urinary irritants into the urothelium or suburothelial tissues due to a defect in the barrier between the urine and bladder wall mucosa. Interstitial cystitis is a progressive disease if not treated; early diagnosis may improve the response to treatment. It is a physical disorder with psychological consequences.

CLINICAL MANIFESTATIONS

1. Severe irritable voiding symptoms and markedly diminished bladder capacity: urinary frequency, nocturia, urgency, suprapubic pressure, and pain with bladder filling. Pain may occur in abdomen or perineum or radiate to the groin.
2. Urine contains both red and white blood cells even though uninfected and cytology is benign.
3. Increased number of mast cells in urine.
4. Presence of Hunner's ulcers (superficial erosions of the bladder wall) is considered diagnostic; however, these do not occur in all women.

DIAGNOSTIC EVALUATION

Elimination of other causes; history, micturition chart or diary, abnormal x-ray findings of a characteristic small bladder.

MANAGEMENT

1. Goals include use of tricyclic antidepressants that may decrease excitability of smooth muscle in the bladder.
2. Destruction of ulcers with laser photo irradiation.
3. Bladder instillation (i.e., silver nitrate, dimethyl sulfoxide, chlorpactin).
4. Bladder removal and urinary diversion.
5. TENS (transcutaneous electrical nerve stimulation) to relieve symptoms.

NURSING PROCESS

Interventions

1. Convey to patient the belief that symptoms exist and appreciate their severity and effects on lifestyle.
2. Provide explanations about diagnostic tests and treatment modalities.
3. Assess the effectiveness of the patient's ability to cope.

4. Provide psychologic support.

For more information see Chapter 43 in Smeltzer and Bare: *Brunner and Suddarth's Textbook of Medical-Surgical Nursing,* 8th Edition. Philadelphia: Lippincott-Raven, 1996.

INTRACRANIAL ANEURYSM

See Aneurysm, Intracranial

IRON DEFICIENCY ANEMIA

See Anemia, Iron Deficiency

ITP

See Idiopathic Thrombocytopenia Purpura

JOINT DISEASE, DEGENERATIVE

See Osteoarthritis

KAPOSI'S SARCOMA

Kaposi's sarcoma (KS) is the most common HIV-related malignancy involving the endothelial layer of blood and lymphatic vessels. KS characteristically presented as lower-extremity skin lesions in elderly men of eastern European ancestry, when first noted (classic KS). The endemic form found in children and young men in equatorial Africa is more virulent than the classic form. Acquired KS occurs when individuals are treated with immunosuppressive agents. Epidemic KS is most often seen in male homosexuals and bisexuals.

CLINICAL MANIFESTATIONS

Cutaneous lesions anywhere on the body; brownish pink to deep purple color. AIDS-related KS is a more variable and aggressive disease course.

1. Lesions may be flat or raised and surrounded by ecchymosis and edema; rapid development with extensive disfigurement.
2. Location and size of lesions can lead to venous stasis, lymphedema, and pain.
3. Common sites of visceral involvement include the lymph nodes, gastrointestinal tract, and lungs.
4. Internal organ involvement leads to organ failure, hemorrhage, infection, and death.

DIAGNOSIS AND PROGNOSIS

1. Diagnosis confirmed by biopsy of suspected lesions.
2. Prognosis depends on extent of tumor, presence of constitutional symptoms, and the CD4+ count.
3. Death occurs from tumor progression; more often from other complications of HIV disease.

For more information see Chapter 50 in Smeltzer and Bare: *Brunner and Suddarth's Textbook of Medical–Surgical Nursing*, 8th Edition. Philadelphia: Lippincott–Raven, 1996.

KETOACIDOSIS, DIABETIC

See Diabetic Ketoacidosis

KIDNEY CANCER

See Cancer of the Kidneys

KIDNEY DISEASE

See Glomerulonephritis

LARGE BOWEL OBSTRUCTION

See Bowel Obstruction, Large

LARYNGEAL CANCER

See Cancer of the Larynx

LEUKEMIA

The common feature of the leukemias is an unregulated proliferation or accumulation of white cells in the bone marrow, replacing normal marrow elements. There is also proliferation in the liver, spleen, and lymph nodes, and invasion of nonhematologic organs. The leukemias are often classified as either lymphocytic or myelocytic and according to the maturity of the malignant cells. Cause is unknown. There is some evidence that genetic influence and viral pathogenesis may be involved. Bone marrow damage due to radiation exposure or chemicals (benzine) can cause leukemia.

For more information see Chapter 32 in Smeltzer and Bare: *Brunner and Suddarth's Textbook of Medical–Surgical Nursing*, 8th Edition. Philadelphia: Lippincott–Raven, 1996.

LEUKEMIA, LYMPHOCYTIC, ACUTE

Acute lymphocytic leukemia (ALL) is believed to be a malignant proliferation of lymphoblasts. It is most common in young children; males are affected more than females, with a peak incidence at 4 years of age. After age 15, ALL is uncommon. Therapy for this childhood leukemia has improved to the extent that approximately 60% of children survive at least 5 years.

CLINICAL MANIFESTATIONS

Skeletal

1. Immature lymphocytes proliferate in marrow and peripheral tissue and crowd development of normal cells.
2. Normal hematopoiesis inhibited and leukopenia, anemia, and thrombocytopenia develop.

Circulatory System

1. Erythrocyte and platelet counts low.
2. Leukocyte counts low or high but always include immature cells.

Malignancy

Manifestations of leukemic cell infiltration into other organs more common with ALL than other forms of leukemia.

MANAGEMENT

Major form of treatment is chemotherapy.
1. Combinations of vincristine, prednisone, daunorubicin, and asparaginase used for initial therapy.
2. Combinations of mercaptopurine, methotrexate, vincristine, and prednisone for maintenance.
3. Irradiation of the cerebrospinal region and intrathecal injection of chemotherapeutic drugs help prevent central nervous system recurrence.

For more information see Chapter 32 in Smeltzer and Bare: *Brunner and Suddarth's Textbook of Medical–Surgical Nursing*, 8th Edition. Philadelphia: Lippincott–Raven, 1996.

LEUKEMIA, LYMPHOCYTIC, CHRONIC

Chronic lymphocytic leukemia (CLL) tends to be a mild disorder that primarily affects persons between 50 and 70 years of age. Western countries report this as the most common leukemia. It is diagnosed during physical examination or treatment for another disease.

CLINICAL MANIFESTATIONS

1. Many are asymptomatic.
2. Possible manifestations are those of anemia, infection, or enlargement of lymph nodes and abdominal organs.
3. Erythrocyte and platelet counts may be normal or decreased.
4. Lymphocytosis is always present.

MANAGEMENT AND PROGNOSIS

1. If mild, CLL may require no treatment. When symptoms are severe, chemotherapy with steroids and chlorambucil (Leukeran) is often used.
2. Patients who do not respond to ordinary therapy may achieve remission by, e.g., fludarabine monophosphate or pentostatin.
3. Intravenous immunoglobulin (IVIG) is an effective prophylactic treatment for selected patients.
4. The average survival is 7 years.

COMPLICATIONS

1. Bleeding and infection are the major causes of death.
2. Renal stone formation, anemia, and gastrointestinal problems.
3. Bleeding correlates with level of thrombocytopenia: presents with petechiae, ecchymoses, and major hemorrhages when platelet count below 20,000 mm^3. Fever or infection increases bleeding.

NURSING PROCESS FOR A PATIENT WITH LEUKEMIA

Assessment

1. Identify range of signs and symptoms reported by patient in nursing history and physical examination.
2. Clinical picture will vary with the type of leukemia involved, i.e., weakness and fatigue, bleeding tendencies, petechiae and ecchymosis, pain, headache, vomiting, fever, and infection.
3. Blood studies may show alterations of white blood cells, anemia, and thrombocytopenia.

Major Nursing Diagnosis

1. Pain related to leukocytic infiltration of systemic tissues.
2. Altered nutrition, less than body requirements, related to gastrointestinal proliferative changes and toxic effects of chemotherapeutic agents.
3. Fatigue and activity intolerance related to anemia.
4. Grieving related to anticipatory loss and altered role functioning.
5. Impaired skin integrity, alopecia related to toxic effects of chemotherapy.
6. Disturbance in body image related to change in appearance, function, and roles.

Collaborative Problems

1. Infection.
2. Bleeding.

Planning and Implementation

Major goals may include ability to cope with the diagnosis and prognosis, tolerance of activity, attainment or maintenance of comfort, attainment or maintenance of adequate nutrition, promotion of positive body image, and absence of complications.

Interventions

COPING WITH THE DIAGNOSIS AND PROGNOSIS

1. Contribute to patient comfort by explaining procedures, anticipating side effects of medication, and encouraging to participate in the therapeutic regimen.
2. Be a sympathetic listener and help patients and family mobilize defenses to cope with emotional and physical stresses.

PREVENTING BLEEDING

1. Assess for thrombocytopenia, granulocytopenia, and anemia.
2. Report any increase in petechiae, melena, hematuria, or nosebleeds.
3. Avoid trauma and injections; use small-gauge needles when analgesics are administered parenterally and apply pressure after injections to avoid bleeding.
4. Use acetaminophen instead of aspirin for analgesia.
5. Give prescribed hormonal therapy to prevent menses.
6. Treat hemorrhage with bed rest and transfusions of red blood cells and platelets.

PREVENTING INFECTION (A MAJOR CAUSE OF DEATH)

1. Assess temperature elevation, flushed appearance, chills, tachycardia; appearance of white patches in the mouth.
2. Observe for redness, swelling, heat, or pain in eyes, ears, throat, skin, joints, abdomen, rectal and perineal areas.
3. Assess for cough and changes in character or color of sputum.
4. Give frequent oral hygiene.
5. Wear sterile gloves to start infusions.
6. Provide daily IV site care; observe for signs of infection.

7. Ensure normal elimination; avoid rectal thermometers, enemas, and rectal trauma; avoid vaginal tampons.
8. Avoid catheterization unless essential. Practice scrupulous asepsis if catheterization necessary.

IMPROVING ACTIVITY TOLERANCE

1. Assist in choosing activity priorities.
2. Offer alternate rest and activity periods if patient weak and easily fatigued.
3. Assess for dyspnea, tachycardia, and other evidence of inadequate oxygen supply to vital organs.

PROMOTING COMFORT

1. Prevent undue pain in the abdomen, lymph node areas, bones, and joints with careful positioning of patient.
2. Avoid sudden movements and promote comfort with soft supports such as pillows.
3. Administer acetaminophen rather than aspirin for analgesia.
4. Give high fluid intake to prevent crystallization of uric acid and subsequent painful stone formation.

ATTAINING/MAINTAINING ADEQUATE NUTRITION

1. Supply good nutrition by careful timing of chemotherapeutic drug administration; prophylactic use of antiemetics; and encouragement of foods and fluids that are the least irritating.
2. Give frequent oral hygiene to prevent oral lesions and promote appetite.
3. Maintain nutrition with small, frequent feedings of foods and fluids that are high in protein and vitamins, and palatable.

PROMOTING POSITIVE BODY IMAGE

1. Prepare patient for the occurrence of alopecia and help to express and resolve feelings.

2. Help patient adjust to body image problems by encouraging involvement and support of family or support system.

✎ Patient Education and Health Maintenance: Care in the Home and Community

1. Ensure that patients and their families have a clear understanding of disease and prognosis.
2. Respect patient's choices about treatment, including measures to prolong life, when they no longer respond to therapy. Provide for advanced directives and living wills to give patient control during terminal phase.
3. Support families and coordinate home care services to alleviate anxiety about managing patient's care in the home.
4. Teach family members about home care while patient is still in hospital.
5. Provide respite for caregivers and patient with hospice volunteers.
6. Give patient and caregivers assistance to cope with changes in their roles and responsibilities, i.e., anticipatory grieving.
7. Provide information concerning hospital-based hospice programs for patients to receive palliative care in the hospital when care at home is no longer possible.

✪ Gerontologic Considerations

Aging is accompanied by a gradual decline of physiologic processes, among which is a reduction in the immune function, resulting in increased susceptibility to infections.

Older patients often delay reporting symptoms because of lack of knowledge, financial resources, or support systems. The complications of leukemia can be devastating to the already decreased reserves of the elderly.

Comprehensive nursing care is critical in assisting the older patient to tolerate the side effects and treatment of the disease as well as cope with the psychological and financial aspects.

✚ CLINICAL ALERT

The usual manifestations of infection are altered in patients with leukemia. Corticosteroid therapy may blunt the normal febrile and inflammatory responses to infection.

For more information see Chapter 32 in Smeltzer and Bare: *Brunner and Suddarth's Textbook of Medical–Surgical Nursing*, 8th Edition. Philadelphia: Lippincott–Raven, 1996.

LEUKEMIA, MYELOGENOUS, ACUTE

Acute myelogenous leukemia (AML) affects the hematopoietic stem cell that differentiates into all myeloid cells: monocytes, granulocytes (basophils, neutrophils, eosinophils), erythrocytes, and platelets. All age groups are affected; incidence rises with age. It is the most common nonlymphocytic leukemia.

CLINICAL MANIFESTATIONS

1. Most signs and symptoms evolve from insufficient production of normal blood cells. (a) Vulnerability to infection results from granulocytopenia. (b) Weakness and fatigue are due to anemia. (c) Bleeding tendencies are a result of thrombocytopenia.

2. Proliferation of leukemic cells within organs leads to a variety of additional symptoms: (a) pain from enlarged liver or spleen; (b) lymphadenopathy; (c) headache or vomiting secondary to meningeal leukemia; (d) bone pain from expansion of marrow.

3. Onset insidious with symptoms occurring over 1–6 months.

4. Peripheral blood shows decreased erythrocyte and platelet counts.
5. Leukocyte count low, normal, or high, percentage of normal cells usually decreased.

DIAGNOSTIC EVALUATION

1. Bone marrow specimen (excess of immature blast cells).
2. Auer rods present in the cytoplasm.

MANAGEMENT

Chemotherapy is the major form of therapy and in some instances results in remissions lasting a year or longer.

Chemotherapy

1. Daunorubicin hydrochloride (Cerubidine).
2. Cytarabine (Cytosar-U).
3. Mercaptopurine (Purinephol).

Supportive Care

1. Administration of blood products.
2. Prompt treatment of infections.

Bone Marrow Transplantation

1. Used when a tissue match of a close relative can be obtained.
2. Transplant follows destruction of leukemic marrow by chemotherapy.

PROGNOSIS

Survival of treated patients averages only 1 year, with death usually a result of infection or hemorrhage. Untreated patients survive only about 2–5 months.

For more information see Chapter 32 in Smeltzer and Bare: *Brunner and Suddarth's Textbook of Medical–Surgical Nursing,* 8th Edition. Philadelphia: Lippincott–Raven, 1996.

LEUKEMIA, MYELOGENOUS, CHRONIC

Chronic myelogenous leukemia (CML) is believed to be a malignancy of myeloid stem cells. More normal cells are present than in the acute form, however, and the disease is milder. A genetic abnormality termed the Philadelphia chromosome is found in 90–95% of patients. Uncommon before age 20, the incidence of CML rises with age.

CLINICAL MANIFESTATIONS

Clinical picture is similar to that of AML, but signs and symptoms are less severe. Many patients are without symptoms for years.

1. Onset insidious.
2. Leukocytosis always present, sometimes at extraordinary levels.
3. Splenomegaly is common.

MANAGEMENT

1. Therapies of choice are busulfan (Myleran) and hydroxyurea, chlorambucil (Leukeran) alone or with steroids.
2. Bone marrow transplantation increases survival significantly.
3. Other drug choices: alpha-interferon and fludarabine (Fludara).

PROGNOSIS

Overall, patients live for 3–4 years. Death usually results from infection or hemorrhage.

NURSING PROCESS

Similar to that of chronic lymphocytic leukemia.

For more information see Chapter 32 in Smeltzer and Bare: *Brunner and Suddarth's Textbook of Medical–Surgical Nursing*, 8th Edition. Philadelphia: Lippincott–Raven, 1996.

LIVER

See Hepatic Coma; Hepatic Failure, Fulminant;
Hepatitis, Viral

LIVER CANCER

See Cancer of the Liver

LOU GEHRIG'S DISEASE

See Amyotrophic Lateral Sclerosis

L

LOWER BACK PAIN

See Back Pain, Low

LUNG ABSCESS

A lung abscess is a localized necrotic lesion of the lung parenchyma containing purulent materials; the lesion collapses and forms a cavity. Most lung abscesses occur because of aspiration of nasopharyngeal or oropharyngeal material.

Abscesses also may occur secondary to mechanical or functional obstruction of the bronchi. At-risk patients include those with impaired cough reflexes, loss of glottal closures, or swallowing difficulties, which may cause aspiration of foreign material. Other at-risk patients include those with altered states of consciousness, esophageal disease, and those fed by nasogastric tube.

The posterior segment of the upper right lobe is the most common site. The aerobic organism most frequently associated with lung abscess is *Staphylococcus aureus.*

CLINICAL MANIFESTATIONS

1. Vary from a mild productive cough to acute illness.
2. Fever and a productive cough of foul-smelling sputum, often bloody.
3. Pleurisy, or dull chest pain, dyspnea, weakness, anorexia, and weight loss are common.

DIAGNOSTIC EVALUATION

Chest x-ray, sputum culture, and fiberoptic bronchoscopy.

MANAGEMENT

Findings of history, physical examination, chest x-ray, and sputum culture will indicate type of organism and treatment.

1. Intravenous (IV) antimicrobial therapy: clindamycin (Cleocin) is the medication of choice, followed by penicillin with metronidazole (Flagyl). Large intravenous doses are required because antibiotic must penetrate necrotic tissue and abscess fluid.
2. High-protein, high-calorie diet.
3. Signs of improvement, i.e., normal temperature, lowering of white blood cell count, improvement of chest x-ray, reduction in size of cavity, antibiotic administered orally instead of IV.
4. Antibiotic therapy may be from 6 to 16 weeks.
5. Surgical intervention is rare. Pulmonary resection (lobectomy) performed when there is massive hemoptysis, a malignancy, or no response to medical management.
6. Prevention (reduce risk of lung abscess): give appropriate antibiotic therapy before dental procedures; maintain adequate dental and oral hygiene. Give appropriate antimicrobial therapy for pneumonia.

Nursing Interventions

1. Administer antibiotic and intravenous therapy as prescribed and monitor for any adverse effects.

2. Initiate chest physiotherapy as prescribed to drain abscess.
3. Teach patient deep breathing and coughing exercises.
4. Encourage diet high in protein and calories.
5. Provide emotional support; abscess may take a long time to resolve.

Patient Education and Health Maintenance: Care in the Home and Community

1. Teach patient or caregiver how to change dressings to prevent skin excoriation and offensive odor.
2. Perform deep breathing and coughing exercises every 2 hours during the day.
3. Teach postural drainage and percussion techniques to caregiver.
4. Provide counseling for attaining and maintaining an optimal state of nutrition.
5. Emphasize importance of completing antibiotic regimen, rest, and appropriate activity levels to prevent relapse.
6. Arrange home visits by an IV therapy nurse to administer IV antibiotic therapy.

For more information see Chapter 24 in Smeltzer and Bare: *Brunner and Suddarth's Textbook of Medical–Surgical Nursing,* 8th Edition. Philadelphia: Lippincott–Raven, 1996.

LUNG CANCER

See Cancer of the Lung

LYMPHATIC CANCER

See Hodgkin's Disease

L

LYMPHEDEMA AND ELEPHANTIASIS

Lymphedemas are classified as primary (congenital mal-formations), or secondary (acquired obstruction). A swelling of tissues in the extremities occurs due to increased lymph that results from an obstruction of the lymphatics. It is especially marked when the extremity is in a dependent position. The most common type is congenital lymphedema (lymphedema praecox), caused by hypoplasia of the lymphatic system of the lower extremity. It is usually seen in women, and appears first between the ages of 15 and 25 years. The obstruction may be in both the lymph nodes and the lymphatic vessels. At times it is seen in the arm after a radical mastectomy, and in the leg in association with varicose veins or a chronic phlebitis. Lymphatic obstruction caused by a parasite (filaria) is seen frequently in the tropics. When chronic swelling is present, there may be frequent bouts of infection (high fever and chills) and increased residual edema after inflammation has resolved. This leads to chronic fibrosis, thickening of the subcutaneous tissues, and hypertrophy of the skin. This condition, in which chronic swelling of the extremity recedes only slightly with elevation, is referred to as elephantiasis.

MANAGEMENT

The goal of medical therapy is to reduce and control the edema and prevent infection.

Rest, Activity, and Comfort

1. Strict bed rest with leg elevation to aid in mobilizing fluids.
2. Active and passive exercises to assist in movement of lymphatic fluid into bloodstream.
3. External compression devices.
4. Custom-fitted elastic stockings, when patient is ambulatory.

LYMPHEDEMA AND ELEPHANTIASIS

Pharmacologic Treatment

1. Furosemide (Lasix) initially to prevent fluid overload.
2. Diuretics, palliatively for lymphedema.
3. Antibiotic therapy, if lymphangitis or cellulitis is present.

Surgical Treatment Performed If

1. Edema is severe and uncontrolled by medical therapy.
2. Mobility is severely compromised.
3. There is persistent infection.

Postoperative Management

1. Skin grafts and flaps cared for the same as when therapies are used for other conditions.
2. Prophylactic antibiotics prescribed for 5–7 days.
3. Elevate affected extremity and observe for complications constantly.
4. Complications may include flap necrosis, hematoma or abscess under the flap, and cellulitis.

For more information see Chapter 31 in Smeltzer and Bare: *Brunner and Suddarth's Textbook of Medical–Surgical Nursing,* 8th Edition. Philadelphia: Lippincott–Raven, 1996.

MALIGNANT MELANOMA

A malignant melanoma is a malignant neoplasm in which atypical melanocytes (pigment cells) are present in both the epidermis and the dermis (and sometimes the subcutaneous cells). It is the most lethal of all skin cancers. It can occur in one of several forms: superficial spreading melanoma, lentigo-maligna melanoma, nodular melanoma, and acral-lentiginous melanoma. Most melanomas derive from cutaneous epidermal melanocytes; some appear in preexisting nevi (moles) in the skin or develop in the uveal tract of the eye. Melanomas frequently appear simultaneously with cancer of other organs. Incidence and mortality rate are increasing, probably related to increased recreational sun exposure.

CAUSES AND PERSONS AT RISK

Etiology is unknown; ultraviolet rays are strongly suspected.

1. Fair complexions, blue eyes, red or blond hair, and freckles.
2. Persons of Celtic or Scandinavian origin.
3. Persons who burn and do not tan.
4. Older Americans retiring to southwestern United States.
5. Family history of melanoma, have giant congenital nevi, or significant history of severe sunburn.
6. Persons with dysplastic nevus syndrome.

CLINICAL MANIFESTATIONS

Superficial spreading melanoma

1. Most common form, usually affects the middle-aged, occurs most frequently on trunk and lower extremities.
2. Lesions tend to be circular with irregular outer portions.
3. Margins of lesion may be flat or elevated and palpable.
4. May appear in combination of colors, with hues of tan, brown, and black mixed with gray, bluish-black, or white.

Nodular Melanoma

1. Second most common type, spherical, blueberry-like nodule with relatively smooth surface and uniform blue-black color.
2. May have other shadings of red, gray, or purple.
3. May appear as irregularly shaped plaques.
4. May be described as a blood blister that fails to resolve.
5. Invades directly into adjacent dermis (vertical growth); poor prognosis.

M

Lentigo-Maligna Melanomas

1. Slowly evolving pigmented lesions.
2. Occur on exposed skin areas; head and neck in elderly people.
3. First appear as tan, flat lesions; in time undergo changes in size and color.

Acral-Lentiginous Melanoma

1. Occurs in areas not excessively exposed to sunlight.
2. Found on the palms of the hands, soles, in nail beds, and mucous membranes in dark-skinned persons.
3. Appear as irregular pigmented macules that develop nodules.
4. Become invasive early.

DIAGNOSTIC EVALUATION

Excisional biopsy specimen.

PROGNOSIS

1. Prognosis is related to the depth of dermal invasion and the thickness of lesion.
2. Malignant melanoma can spread through both bloodstream and lymphatic routes and can metastasize to the bones, liver, lungs, spleen, central nervous system, and lymph nodes.

MANAGEMENT

The therapeutic approach to malignant melanoma depends on the level of invasion and the depth of the lesion.

Surgery

1. Treatment of choice for small superficial lesions.
2. Deeper lesions require wide local excision and skin graft.
3. A regional lymph node dissection may be performed to rule out metastasis.

NURSING PROCESS

Assessment

Assessment is based on history and symptoms.
1. Question specifically about pruritus, tenderness, and pain, which are not features of a benign nevus.
2. Question about changes in preexisting moles or development of new pigmented lesions.
3. Assess persons at risk carefully.

Assess Skin

1. Use a magnifying lens to examine for irregularity and changes in the mole.
2. Signs that suggest malignant changes: variegated color, irregular border, irregular surface.

3. Pay attention to common sites of melanoma occurrence.
4. Measure diameter of mole; melanomas are often larger than 6 mm.

Major Nursing Diagnosis

1. Pain related to surgical incision and grafting.
2. Anxiety and depression related to possible life-threatening consequences of melanoma and disfigurement.
3. Knowledge deficit about early signs of melanoma.

Collaborative Problems

Metastasis.

Planning and Implementation

The major goals may include relief of pain and discomfort, reduction of anxiety, and absence of complications.

M

Interventions

RELIEVING PAIN AND DISCOMFORT

Anticipate need for and administer appropriate analgesic.

REDUCING ANXIETY

1. Give support and allow patient to express feelings.
2. Convey understanding of anger and depression.
3. Answer questions and clarify information during the diagnostic work-up and staging of the tumor.
4. Point out patient resources, past effective coping mechanisms, and support systems to help cope with diagnosis and treatment.

Monitoring and managing potential complications: Metastasis

1. Present treatment is largely unsuccessful and cure is generally not possible.
2. Surgical intervention may be performed to debulk the tumor or to remove part of the organ involved.

3. More extensive surgery is for relief of symptoms, not for cure.
4. Chemotherapy may be effective in controlling the metastasis.
5. Provide time for patient to express fears and concerns about the future; arrange for hospice/palliative care services.

 ## PATIENT EDUCATION AND HEALTH MAINTENANCE: CARE IN THE HOME AND COMMUNITY

Teach Patients to:

1. Recognize the early signs of melanoma.
2. Examine the skin and scalp monthly in an orderly manner.
3. Use a full-length mirror and a small hand mirror to aid in examination.
4. Learn where moles and birthmarks are located.
5. Inspect all moles and other pigmented lesions; report to physician/clinic immediately moles that change colors, enlarge, become raised or thicker, itch, or bleed.
6. Inform person who has had a malignant melanoma to have lifelong follow-up; higher risk of developing a second one.
7. Avoid exposure to sunlight.

For more information see Chapter 54 in Smeltzer and Bare: *Brunner and Suddarth's Textbook of Medical–Surgical Nursing,* 8th Edition. Philadelphia: Lippincott–Raven, 1996.

MASTOIDITIS

Mastoiditis is an inflammation of the mastoid resulting from an infection of the middle ear; if it is untreated, osteomyelitis may occur.

CLINICAL MANIFESTATIONS

1. Pain and tenderness behind the ear.
2. Discharge from the middle ear.
3. Swelling of the mastoid.

MANAGEMENT

1. Usually general symptoms are successfully treated with antibiotics; occasionally myringotomy is required.
2. If recurrent or persistent tenderness, fever, headache, and discharge from the ear, mastoidectomy may be necessary.

NURSING PROCESS: MASTOID SURGERY

Assessment

1. During health history, data collected about duration and intensity, causation, previous treatments, other health problems, current medications, and drug allergies.
2. Physical assessment to include observation for erythema, edema, otorrhea, lesions, and odor of discharge.
3. Review results of audiogram.

Major Nursing Diagnosis

1. Acute pain related to mastoid surgery.
2. Risk for infection related to mastoidectomy, placement of grafts, prostheses, and/or electrodes; surgical trauma to surrounding tissues and structures.
3. Knowledge deficit about mastoid disease, surgical procedure, and postoperative care and expectations.

Planning and Implementation

The major goals for mastoidectomy include reduction of anxiety; freedom from discomfort; prevention of infection; stabilization or improvement of hearing; absence of injury or vertigo; absence of, or adjustment to, altered

sensory perception; return of skin integrity; and knowledge regarding disease process, surgical procedure, and
postoperative care.

Interventions

REDUCING ANXIETY

1. Reinforce information the otologic surgeon has
   discussed.
2. Encourage patient to discuss any anxiety or
   concerns.

RELIEVING PAIN

1. Give prescribed analgesic for the first 24 hours
   postoperatively and then only as needed.
2. Instruct patient in use of and side effects of
   medication.

PREVENTING INFECTION

1. Give prescribed prophylactic antibiotics; instruct to
   prevent water from entering the ear for 2 weeks.
2. Keep postauricular incision dry for 2 weeks.
3. Observe for and report signs of infection.

IMPROVING COMMUNICATION

1. Initiate measures to improve communication, i.e.,
   reduce environmental noise, face patient when
   speaking, and speak clearly.
2. Instruct family members that patient will have temporarily reduced hearing from surgery, i.e., edema,
   packing, fluid in middle ear.

IMPROVING KNOWLEDGE

Discuss postoperative expectations, information about
the surgery, and operating room environment.

For more information see Chapter 57 in Smeltzer and
Bare: *Brunner and Suddarth's Textbook of Medical–Surgical
Nursing,* 8th Edition. Philadelphia: Lippincott–Raven, 1996.

MD

See Muscular Dystrophy

MEGALOBLASTIC ANEMIA

See Anemia, Megaloblastic

MENIERE'S DISEASE

Ménière's disease is an inner ear fluid balance problem. The etiology is unknown. Some attribute the impairment of the microvasculature of the inner ear to abnormally high levels of metabolites (glucose, insulin, triglycerides, and cholesterol) in the blood. It is more common in adults, with the average age of onset in the 40s. There is no cure for this disease.

M

CLINICAL MANIFESTATIONS

1. Quadrad of symptoms: episodic incapacitating vertigo, tinnitus, and fluctuating sensorineural hearing loss, feeling of pressure or fullness in the ear.
2. At the onset, only one or two symptoms are manifested.
3. Vertigo lasting from minutes to hours; nausea and vomiting.
4. Attacks occur with increasing frequency.
5. Diaphoresis, persistent feeling of disequilibrium; may last for days.
6. Usually only one ear is involved.

DIAGNOSTIC EVALUATION

1. Disease not diagnosed until quadrad of symptoms is present.
2. There is no absolute diagnostic test for this disease.

MANAGEMENT

The goals of treatment may include recommendations for changes in lifestyle and habits or surgical treatment. The treatment is designed to eliminate vertigo or stop the progression of, or stabilize, the disease. Treatment approaches include rehabilitative, dietary strategies, medical, and surgical treatment.

Medications

1. Use to suppress the vestibular system, i.e., tranquilizers and antihistamines.
2. Diuretics to lower pressure in the endolymphatic system.
3. Antiemetics.
4. Ototoxic medications, i.e., streptomycin, gentamicin by systemic injections or infusion into the middle and inner ear to eliminate vertigo; procedure has significant risk of hearing loss.

Dietary Management

1. Low sodium (2000 mg per day).
2. Alcohol, nicotine, and caffeine are avoided.

Surgical Management

1. Endolymphatic sac decompression or shunt.
2. Labyrinthectomy (destruction of the inner ear).
3. Vestibular nerve section (8th cranial nerve).

NURSING PROCESS FOR THE PATIENT WITH VERTIGO

Major Nursing Diagnosis

1. Risk for injury related to altered mobility because of gait disturbance and vertigo.
2. Impaired adjustment related to disability requiring change in lifestyle due to unpredictability of vertigo.
3. Risk for fluid volume deficit related to increased fluid output, altered intake, and medications.

4. Anxiety related to threat of, or change in, health status and disability effects of vertigo.
5. Self-care deficit: feeding, bathing/hygiene, dressing/grooming, toileting, related to labyrinth dysfunction and episodes of vertigo.

Planning and Implementation

Patient goals include remaining free of any injuries associated with imbalance and/or falls; adjusting to or modifying lifestyle to decrease disability and exert maximum control and independence; maintaining a normal fluid–electrolyte balance; experiencing less or no anxiety; ability to care for self; and freedom from complications.

Interventions

PREVENTING INJURY

1. Assess for vertigo.
2. Encourage to lie down; side rails up on bed.
3. Place pillow on each side of head to restrict movement.
4. Assist patient in identifying aura that suggests an attack.
5. Recommend patient keep eyes open and stare straight ahead when lying down and experiencing vertigo.
6. Administer or teach administration of antivertiginous medication and/or vestibular sedation; instruct in side effects.

ADJUSTING TO DISABILITY

1. Encourage to identify personal strengths and roles.
2. Provide information about vertigo and what to expect.
3. Include family and significant others in rehabilitative process.

MAINTAINING FLUID VOLUME

1. Assess intake and output; monitor laboratory values.
2. Assess indicators of dehydration.

3. Encourage oral fluids as tolerated; avoid caffeine (a vestibular stimulant).
4. Teach administration of antiemetics and antidiarrheal medications.

RELIEVING ANXIETY

1. Assess level of anxiety; help identify successful coping skills.
2. Encourage to discuss anxieties and explore concerns about vertigo attacks.
3. Teach stress management; provide comfort measures.

CARING FOR SELF

1. Administer antiemetic and other prescribed medications to relieve nausea and vomiting.
2. Encourage patient to care for bodily needs when free of vertigo.
3. Review diet with patient and caregivers.

Monitoring and Managing Complications

1. Assist patient in preparing for diagnostic tests.
2. Prepare patient for surgery if indicated.
3. Observe for potential complications.
4. Assist unsteady patient as required; expect vertigo and nausea after labyrinthectomy.
5. Arrange for psychosocial and family support as necessary.
6. Provide patient and family with the appropriate hearing aid service information.

For more information see Chapter 57 in Smeltzer and Bare: *Brunner and Suddarth's Textbook of Medical–Surgical Nursing,* 8th Edition. Philadelphia: Lippincott–Raven, 1996.

MENINGITIS

Meningitis is an inflammation of the meninges (membranes surrounding the brain and spinal cord) and is caused by a viral, bacterial, or fungal organism. Types of meningitis include aseptic, septic, and tuberculosis. Aseptic refers to viral meningitis or meningeal irritation, e.g., encephalitis. Septic refers to a bacterial cause, e.g., influenza bacillus. Tuberculosis meningitis is caused by the tubercle bacillus. Meningeal infections generally originate in one of two ways: either through the bloodstream from other infections (cellulitis) or by direct extension (after a traumatic injury to the facial bones). In a small number of cases the cause is iatrogenic or secondary to invasive procedures (lumbar puncture) or devices (ICP monitoring devices).

BACTERIAL MENINGITIS

Bacterial meningitis is the most significant form. The common bacteria are *Neisseria meningitidis* (meningococcal meningitis), *Streptococcus pneumoniae* (in adults), and *Haemophilus influenzae* (in children and young adults). These three organisms account for about 75% of the cases. Mode of transmission is direct contact, including droplets and discharges from nose and throat of carriers or infected persons. Bacterial meningitis starts as an infection of the oropharynx and is followed by septicemia, which extends to the meninges of the brain and upper region of the spinal cord.

CLINICAL MANIFESTATIONS

1. Symptoms result from infection and increased intracranial pressure (ICP).
2. Headache and fever are frequently initial symptoms.
3. Changes in level of consciousness are associated with bacterial type.
4. Disorientation and memory impairment are common early in the illness.
5. Lethargy, unresponsiveness, and coma may develop as illness progresses.

Signs of Meningeal Irritation

1. Nuchal rigidity (stiff neck) is an early sign.
2. Positive Kernig's sign: when lying with thigh flexed on abdomen, cannot completely extend leg.
3. Positive Brudzinski's sign: when neck is flexed, flexion of the knees and hips is produced; when passive flexion of lower extremity of one side is made, similar movement is seen for opposite extremity.
4. Photophobia.

Seizures and Increased ICP

1. Seizures secondary to focal areas of cortical irritability.
2. Signs of increasing ICP: widened pulse pressure and bradycardia, respiratory irregularity, headache, vomiting, and depressed levels of consciousness.

Rash (Neisseria meningitidis)

Ranges from petechial rash with purpuric lesions to large areas of ecchymosis.

Meningococcal meningitis

Ten percent present with a fulminating infection, with signs of overwhelming septicemia.
1. Abrupt onset of high fever.
2. Extensive purpuric lesions (over face and extremities).
3. Shock, and signs of disseminated intravascular coagulopathy (DIC).
4. Death may occur within a few hours of onset of infection.

DIAGNOSTIC EVALUATION

Infecting organisms usually identified through culture of cerebrospinal fluid and blood.

MANAGEMENT

1. Antimicrobial therapy: penicillin, ampicillin, or chloramphenicol, or cephalosporins.
2. Treat dehydration or shock with fluid volume expanders.
3. Control seizures with diazepam or phenytoin.
4. Treat cerebral edema with an osmotic diuretic (mannitol).

Nursing Interventions

1. Prognosis depends on supportive care given.
2. Monitor vital signs constantly, determine arterial blood gases, insert cuffed endotracheal tube (or tracheostomy), and place on mechanical ventilation as prescribed.
3. Give oxygen to maintain arterial partial pressure of oxygen (PO_2).
4. Monitor central venous pressure (CVP) for incipient shock, which precedes cardiac or respiratory failure.
5. Note generalized vasoconstriction, circumoral cyanosis, and cold extremities.
6. Reduce high fever to decrease load on heart and brain oxygen demands.
7. Rapid intravenous fluid replacement may be prescribed, but care is taken not to overhydrate patient because of risk of cerebral edema.
8. If inappropriate antidiuretic hormone (ADH) secretion is suspected, monitor closely for body weight, serum electrolytes, urine volume, specific gravity, and osmolality.
9. Ongoing assessment required for clinical status, attention to skin and oral hygiene, promotion of comfort, and protection during seizures and while comatose.
10. Advise respiratory isolation for 24 hours after start of antibiotic therapy.

M

PREVENTION

1. Persons having close contact with patient should be considered candidates for antimicrobial prophylaxis (Rifampin).
2. Observe and examine immediately close contacts if fever or other signs and symptoms of meningitis develop.
3. GA meningococcal vaccination may be of benefit for some travelers visiting countries that are experiencing epidemic meningococcal disease.
4. Vaccination should be considered as an adjunct to antibiotic chemoprophylaxis for anyone living with a patient who has meningococcal disease.
5. Polysaccharide vaccine (*Haemophilus b* polysaccharide vaccine) against invasive *Haemophilus influenzae* type b is used routinely in pediatrics for prevention of meningitis.

MENINGITIS IN AIDS

Aseptic cryptococcal and tuberculosis meningitis have been reported in patients with AIDS. Acute and chronic forms of aseptic meningitis may occur with AIDS; both are accompanied by headache; signs of meningeal irritation generally occur with the acute form. Aseptic meningitis with AIDS may be accompanied by cranial nerve palsies.

Cryptococcal Meningitis

1. Most common fungal infection of central nervous system in patients with AIDS.
2. May experience headache, nausea, vomiting, seizures, confusion, and lethargy.
3. Some develop few if any symptoms because of blunted inflammatory response occurring in the immunocompromised patient.
4. Cryptococcal meningitis treatment is intravenous administration of amphotericin B, may be used with or without 5-flucytosine.

5. Maintenance therapy with amphotericin B to prevent relapse.

MENINGITIS IN LYME DISEASE

1. Lyme disease is a multisystem inflammatory process caused by the tick-transmitted spirochete *Borrelia burgdorferi.*
2. Neurologic abnormalities (seen in later stages) include meningitis, chronic lymphocytic meningitis, and encephalitis.

For more information see Chapter 60 in Smeltzer and Bare: *Brunner and Suddarth's Textbook of Medical–Surgical Nursing,* 8th Edition. Philadelphia: Lippincott–Raven, 1996.

METASTATIC BONE CANCER

See Bone Tumors

M

MI

See Myocardial Infarction

MIGRAINE

See Headache

MITRAL INSUFFICIENCY (REGURGITATION)

Mitral insufficiency results when the margins of the mitral valve are unable to close during systole. The chordae tendinae become shortened, preventing closure of the leaflets. At each beat the left ventricle forces some blood back into the left atrium, causing dilation and hypertrophy. This backward flow of blood from the ventricle causes the lungs to eventually become congested.

CLINICAL MANIFESTATIONS

1. Palpitation of the heart, shortness of breath on exertion, and cough due to chronic passive pulmonary congestion.
2. Irregular pulse as a result of either extra systoles or atrial fibrillation may persist indefinitely.

MANAGEMENT

Management is the same as that for congestive heart failure. Surgical intervention consists of mitral valve replacement.

For more information see Chapter 29 in Smeltzer and Bare: *Brunner and Suddarth's Textbook of Medical–Surgical Nursing,* 8th Edition. Philadelphia: Lippincott–Raven, 1996.

MITRAL REGURGITATION

See Mitral Insufficiency

MITRAL STENOSIS

Mitral stenosis is the progressive thickening and contracture of the mitral valve cusps, which causes narrowing of the orifice and progressive obstruction to blood flow. Normally, the mitral valve opening is as wide as three fingers. In cases of marked stenosis, the opening narrows to the width of a lead pencil.

CLINICAL MANIFESTATIONS

1. Progressive fatigue (result of low cardiac output), hemoptysis and dyspnea (due to pulmonary venous hypertension), cough, and repeated respiratory infections.

2. Weak and often irregular pulse (because of atrial fibrillation).

DIAGNOSTIC EVALUATION

1. Electrocardiography (EKG).
2. Echocardiography.
3. Cardiac catheterization with angiography.

MANAGEMENT

1. Antibiotic therapy to prevent recurrence of infections.
2. Cardiotonics and diuretics for treatment of congestive heart failure.
3. Surgical intervention (valvotomy or replacement of the mitral valve).
4. Percutaneous transluminal valvuloplasty for palliation of symptoms.

For more information see Chapter 29 in Smeltzer and Bare: *Brunner and Suddarth's Textbook of Medical–Surgical Nursing*, 8th Edition. Philadelphia: Lippincott–Raven, 1996.

M

MITRAL VALVE PROLAPSE SYNDROME

The mitral valve prolapse syndrome is a dysfunction of the mitral valve leaflets that prevents the mitral valve from closing completely and results in valvular regurgitation. It occurs more frequently in women.

CLINICAL MANIFESTATIONS

The syndrome may produce no symptoms or may progress rapidly and result in sudden death.

Symptoms Identified During Physical Examination

1. A mitral click is identified.
2. Presence of a click indicates early valvular incompetence.

3. The mitral click may deteriorate into a murmur over time as the valve leaflets become more dysfunctional.
4. As the murmur progresses there may be signs and symptoms of heart failure.

MANAGEMENT

Medical management is directed at controlling symptoms.

1. Antidysrhythmic agents.
2. In advanced stages, mitral valve replacement may be necessary.
3. Educate patients about the need for prophylactic antibiotic therapy before invasive procedures, e.g., dental work.
4. Consult physician about risk factors and need for antibiotics.

For more information see Chapter 29 in Smeltzer and Bare: *Brunner and Suddarth's Textbook of Medical–Surgical Nursing,* 8th Edition. Philadelphia: Lippincott–Raven, 1996.

MOUTH CANCER

See Cancer of the Oral Cavity

MS

See Multiple Sclerosis

MULTIPLE MYELOMA

Multiple myeloma is a malignant disease of plasma cells that infiltrates bone, lymph nodes, liver, spleen, and kidneys. It is not classified as a lymphoma. The malignant cell is the plasma cell, the neoplastic proliferation taking place mainly in the bone marrow. Median survival is 2–5 years, with death resulting from infection or renal failure.

CLINICAL MANIFESTATIONS

1. Normochromic, normocytic anemia, back pain, and sometimes leukopenia or thrombocytopenia due to bone marrow infiltration by malignant plasma cells.
2. Constant bone pain that may be incapacitating.
3. Hypercalcemia and bone fractures are common especially in the vertebrae or ribs.

DIAGNOSTIC EVALUATION

1. Aspiration or biopsy of the bone marrow.
2. Bence Jones proteins (fragments of abnormal globulins) are excreted in urine.

MANAGEMENT

1. Melphalan (Alkeran), cyclophosphamide, and steroids to decrease tumor mass and relieve bone pain.
2. Radiation for relieving bone pain.
3. Good hydration to prevent renal damage resulting from Bence Jones proteins in the renal tubules, hypercalcemia, and hyperuricemia.
4. Assess patients for signs and symptoms of renal insufficiency.
5. Narcotic analgesics and local radiation for severe pain.
6. Keep patients as active as possible to prevent pathologic fractures.
7. Observe for bacterial infections (pneumonia).
8. Avoid fasting regimens for diagnostic tests because dehydrating procedures can precipitate acute renal failure.

M

❂ GERONTOLOGIC CONSIDERATIONS

Incidence of multiple myeloma increases with age, rarely occurring before age 40. Closely investigate any back pain, which is often presented as a complaint.

For more information see Chapter 32 in Smeltzer and Bare: *Brunner and Suddarth's Textbook of Medical–Surgical Nursing,* 8th Edition. Philadelphia: Lippincott–Raven, 1996.

MULTIPLE SCLEROSIS

Multiple sclerosis (MS) is a chronic, degenerative, progressive disease of the central nervous system characterized by small patches of demyelination in the brain and spinal cord. Demyelinization refers to the destruction of myelin and results in impaired transmission of nerve impulses. The cause of MS is not known but a defective immune response probably plays a major role. MS is more common in people living in northern temperate climate zones. It is one of the most disabling neurologic diseases of young adults (20–40 years), affecting twice as many women as men.

COURSE TYPES

1. Relapsing-remitting course with complete recovery between relapses.
2. Chronic progressive course from the onset with a progressive decline in function.
3. Benign course with a normal life span; symptoms so mild that patients do not seek health care and treatment.

CLINICAL MANIFESTATIONS

Signs and symptoms are varied and multiple, reflecting the location of the lesion or combination of lesions.

1. Primary symptoms are fatigue, weakness, numbness, difficulty in coordination, and loss of balance.
2. Visual disturbances: blurring of vision, patchy blindness (scotoma), or total blindness may occur.
3. Spastic weakness of the extremities and loss of abdominal reflexes.
4. Sensory dysfunction.

5. Cognitive and psychosocial problems.
6. Emotional lability and euphoria.
7. Ataxia and tremor.
8. Bladder, bowel, and sexual problems.

Secondary Manifestations Related to Complications

1. Urinary tract infections, constipation.
2. Pressure ulcers, contracture deformities, dependent pedal edema.
3. Pneumonia.
4. Reactive depressions.
5. Emotional, social, marital, economic, and vocational problems.

Exacerbations and Remissions

1. Relapses may be associated with periods of emotional and physical stress.
2. There is evidence that remyelinization occurs in some patients.

DIAGNOSTIC EVALUATION

1. Magnetic resonance imaging (MRI) (primary diagnostic tool) to visualize small plaques, evaluate course and effect of treatment.
2. Electrophoresis study of the cerebrospinal fluid (CSF). Abnormal IG antibody appears in the CSF; up to 95% of patients.

MANAGEMENT

No cure exists for MS. An individualized treatment program is indicated to relieve symptoms and provide support.

Pharmacotherapy

1. Pharmacologic agents modulate the immune response and reduce the rate at which the disease progresses, frequency, and severity of exacerbations (azathioprine, interferon, cyclophosphamide).

2. Corticosteroids and ACTH are used as anti-inflammatory agents and may improve nerve conduction.
3. Baclofen is treatment of choice for spasticity.
4. Beta interferon (Betaseron) is used for relapsing-remitting MS.

Radiation

May be used for immunosuppression.

Bowel and Bladder Management

1. Medications and intermittent self-catheterization.
2. Assess urinary tract infections; give ascorbic acid to acidify urine; prescribe antibiotics when appropriate.

NURSING PROCESS

Assessment

1. Assess actual and potential problems associated with the disease: neurologic problems, secondary complications, and impact of the disease on patient and family.
2. Assess patient's function when well rested and when fatigued; look for weakness, spasticity, visual impairment, and incontinence.
3. Assess sexual history for specific areas of concern.

Major Nursing Diagnosis

1. Impaired physical mobility related to weakness, muscle paresis, spasticity.
2. Risk for injury related to sensory and visual impairment.
3. Altered urinary and bowel elimination related to spinal cord dysfunction.
4. Altered thought processes (loss of memory, dementia, euphoria) related to cerebral dysfunction.
5. Ineffective coping.
6. Impaired home maintenance management related to physical, psychological, and social limits imposed by MS.

7. Potential for sexual dysfunction related to spinal cord involvement or psychological reactions to condition.

Planning and Implementation

The major goals may include promotion of physical mobility, avoidance of injury, achievement of bladder and bowel continence, improvement of cognitive function, development of coping strengths, improved self-care, and adaptation to sexual dysfunction.

Interventions

PROMOTING PHYSICAL MOBILITY

1. Encourage progressive resistive exercises to strengthen weak muscles.
2. Encourage patient to work up to the point just short of fatigue.
3. Advise to take frequent short rest periods, preferably lying down, to prevent extreme fatigue.
4. Encourage walking exercises to improve gait.
5. Provide warm packs to spastic muscles.
6. Encourage daily exercises for muscle stretching to minimize joint contractures.
7. Encourage swimming, stationary bicycling, and progressive weight-bearing to relieve spasticity in legs.
8. Avoid hurrying the patient in any activity because hurrying increases spasticity.
9. Prevent complications of immobility by assessment and maintenance of skin integrity, and coughing and deep breathing exercises.

PREVENTING INJURY

1. Teach patient to walk with feet wide apart to increase walking stability if motor dysfunction causes incoordination.
2. Teach patient to watch the feet while walking if there is a loss of position sense.

M

3. Provide a wheelchair if gait remains insufficient after gait training (walker, cane, braces, crutches, parallel bars, and physical therapy).
4. Assess skin for pressure ulcers when patient is confined to wheelchair.

PROMOTING BLADDER AND BOWEL CONTROL

1. Keep bedpan or urinal readily available because the need to void must be heeded immediately.
2. Set up a voiding schedule, with gradual lengthening of time intervals.
3. Instruct to drink a measured amount of fluid every 2 hours and then attempt to void 30 minutes after drinking.
4. Encourage to take prescribed medications for bladder spasticity.
5. Encourage intermittent self-catheterization, if necessary.
6. Provide adequate fluids, dietary fiber, and a bowel-training program for bowel problems including constipation, fecal impaction, and incontinence.

IMPROVING SENSORY AND COGNITIVE FUNCTION

1. Provide an eye patch or eyeglass occluder to block visual impulses of one eye when diplopia (double vision) occurs.
2. Advise patient about free talking book services from the library.
3. Refer patient and family to a speech-language pathologist when mechanisms of speech are involved.
4. Provide compassion and emotional support to patients and family to adapt with new self-image and cope with life disruption.
5. Keep a structured environment; use lists and other memory aids to help patient maintain a daily routine.

STRENGTHENING COPING MECHANISMS

1. Alleviate stress and make referrals for counseling and support to minimize adverse effects of dealing with chronic illness.
2. Provide information on the illness to patient and family.
3. Help patient define problems and develop alternatives for management.

IMPROVING SELF-CARE

1. Suggest modifications that allow independence in self-care activities at home (raised toilet seat, bathing helps, telephone modifications, long-handled comb, tongs, modified clothing).
2. Avoid physical and emotional stress when possible.
3. Maintain moderate environmental temperature; heat increases fatigue and muscle weakness; extreme cold may increase spasticity.

M

ADAPTING TO SEXUAL DYSFUNCTION

Suggest a sexual counselor to assist patient and partner with sexual dysfunction, i.e., erectile and ejaculatory disorders in males; orgasmic dysfunction and adductor spasms of the thigh muscles in females; bladder and bowel incontinence; urinary tract infections.

PATIENT EDUCATION AND HEALTH MAINTENANCE: CARE IN THE HOME AND COMMUNITY

1. Encourage to contact the local chapter of the National Multiple Sclerosis Society for services, publications, and contact with other MS patients
2. Assist patient and family to deal with new disabilities and changes as disease progresses.
3. Teach and reinforce new self-care techniques.
4. Assess changes in patient's health status and coping strategies.

For more information see Chapter 60 in Smeltzer and Bare: *Brunner and Suddarth's Textbook of Medical–Surgical Nursing,* 8th Edition. Philadelphia: Lippincott–Raven, 1996.

MUSCULAR DYSTROPHIES

Muscular dystrophies are a group of chronic muscle disorders characterized by a progressive weakening and wasting of the skeletal or voluntary muscles. Most are inherited. The pathologic features include degeneration and loss of muscle fibers, variation in muscle fiber size, phagocytosis and regeneration, and replacement of muscle tissue by connective tissue. Types of symptoms are affected by patterns of inheritance, muscles involved, age of onset, and rate of progression.

CLINICAL MANIFESTATIONS

1. Muscle wasting and weakness.
2. Abnormal elevation in serum creatinine phosphokinase (CPK).
3. Myopathic electromyography (EMG) pattern.
4. Myopathic findings on muscle biopsy.

MANAGEMENT

Treatment focuses on supportive care and prevention of complications. Supportive management is intended to keep the patient active and functioning as normally as possible, and to minimize functional deterioration.

1. A therapeutic exercise program is individualized. Prevent muscle tightness, contractures, and disuse atrophy. Use night splints and stretching exercises to delay joint contractures.
2. Fit patient with orthotic jacket to improve sitting stability and reduce trunk deformity from spinal deformity. Spinal fusion may be performed to maintain spinal stability.

3. Treat vigorously all upper respiratory infections and fractures from falls to minimize immobilization and to prevent joint contractures.
4. Advise genetic counseling because of the genetic nature of this disease.

Other Difficulties

Should be treated symptomatically.

1. Dental and speech problems.
2. Gastrointestinal tract problem resulting in gastric dilation, rectal prolapse, and fecal impaction.
3. Cardiomyopathy (common complication in all forms of muscular dystrophy).

NURSING INTERVENTIONS

The goals of the patient and the nurse are to maintain function at optimal levels and enhance the quality of life.

M

1. Attend to patient's physical requirements and emotional and developmental needs.
2. Involve patient and family in decision making.

✎ PATIENT EDUCATION AND HEALTH MAINTENANCE: CARE IN THE HOME AND COMMUNITY

1. Encourage use of self help devices to achieve a greater degree of independence.
2. Encourage range-of-motion exercises to prevent disabling contractures.
3. In teaching family to monitor patient for respiratory problems, give specific information regarding appropriate respiratory support, i.e., negative-pressure devices, positive-pressure ventilators.
4. Assist family in adjusting home environment to maximize functional independence; patient may require manual or electric wheelchair, gait aids, seating systems, bathroom equipment, lifts, ramps, and additional ADL aids.

5. Assess for signs of depression, prolonged anger, bargaining, or denial and help patient to cope and adapt to chronic disease.
6. Provide a hopeful, supportive, and nurturing environment.

For more information see Chapter 60 in Smeltzer and Bare: *Brunner and Suddarth's Textbook of Medical–Surgical Nursing,* 8th Edition. Philadelphia: Lippincott–Raven, 1996.

MYASTHENIA GRAVIS

Myasthenia gravis is a disorder affecting the neuromuscular transmission of the voluntary muscles of the body. Excessive weakness and fatigability occur. It affects women between the ages of 15 and 35 years and men over 40. It is considered an autoimmune disease in which antibodies directed against acetylcholine receptor (AChR) impair neuromuscular transmission.

CLINICAL MANIFESTATIONS

Extreme muscular weakness and easy fatigability; worse after effort and relieved by rest.

Varied Symptoms According to Muscles Affected

1. Diplopia and ptosis are early symptoms.
2. Sleepy, masklike expression because facial muscles are affected.
3. Dysphonia (voice impairment).
4. Problems with chewing and swallowing present danger of choking and aspiration.
5. Complaints of weakness of arm and hand muscles; less commonly in leg muscles.
6. Progressive weakness of the diaphragm and intercostal muscles may produce respiratory distress or myasthenic crisis.

DIAGNOSTIC EVALUATION

1. Presumptive diagnosis based on history and physical examination.
2. Injection of edrophonium (Tensilon) is used to confirm diagnosis.
3. Improvement in muscle strength represents a positive test and usually confirms diagnosis.

MANAGEMENT

Management is directed at improving function through the administration of anticholinesterase medications and reducing and removing circulating antibodies.

Anticholinesterase Medications

1. Pyridostigmine bromide (Mestinon), ambenonium chloride (Mytelase), neostigmine bromide (Prostigmin).
2. Given to increase response of the muscles to nerve impulses and improve strength; results expected within 1 hour after administration.

Immunosuppressive Therapy

1. Directed toward reducing production of antireceptor antibody or removing it directly by plasma exchange.
2. Corticosteroids suppress the immune response, decreasing the amount of blocking antibody.
3. Plasma exchange (plasmapheresis) produces a temporary reduction in the titer of circulating antibodies.
4. Thymectomy (surgical removal of the thymus) causes substantial remission, especially in patients with tumor or hyperplasia of the thymus gland.

MYASTHENIC CRISIS VS. CHOLINERGIC CRISIS

Myasthenic Crisis

1. Sudden onset of muscular weakness that is usually the result of undermedication or no cholinergic medication at all.

M

2. May result from progression of the disease, emotional upset, systemic infections, drugs, surgery, or trauma.
3. Manifested by sudden onset of acute respiratory distress and inability to swallow or speak.

Cholinergic Crisis

1. Caused by overmedication with cholinergic or anticholinesterase drugs.
2. In addition to muscle weakness and respiratory depression of myasthenic crisis, these patients experience GI symptoms (nausea, vomiting, diarrhea), sweating, increased salivation, and bradycardia.

NURSING PROCESS

Assessment

1. Assess health history and focus on the patient and family's knowledge about the disease and the drug treatment program.
2. Assess patient's functional capability and support system to determine discharge needs for services.
3. Patients with myasthenia gravis are usually managed on an outpatient basis unless hospitalization is required for managing symptoms or complications.

Major Nursing Diagnosis

1. Ineffective breathing pattern related to respiratory muscle weakness.
2. Impaired physical mobility due to voluntary muscle weakness.
3. Risk for aspiration related to weakness of bulbar muscles.

Collaborative Problems

1. Myasthenic crisis.
2. Cholinergic crisis.

Planning and Implementation

The major goals may include improved respiratory function, increased physical mobility, avoidance of aspiration, and absence of potential complications (myasthenic and cholinergic crisis).

Interventions

IMPROVING RESPIRATORY FUNCTION

1. Assess respiratory status frequently to detect pulmonary problems before changes in arterial blood gas levels appear.
2. Provide chest physical therapy, including postural drainage to mobilize secretions; suction to remove secretions.
3. Acknowledge patient's fears and give assurance.

INCREASING PHYSICAL MOBILITY

1. Teach patient facts about anticholinergic drugs: action, timing, dosage, symptoms of overdose, and toxic effects.
2. Emphasize taking medication on time to improve strength and endurance.
3. Encourage patient to keep a diary to determine fluctuation of symptoms.
4. Teach patient factors that may increase weakness and precipitate myasthenic crisis: emotional upset, infections (respiratory), vigorous physical activity, exposure to heat and cold.
5. Advise to wear an identification bracelet, such as Medic Alert.

IMPROVING COMMUNICATION

Teach patients with weakened speech muscles techniques for improving communication, e.g., blink eyes, wiggle fingers or toes.

M

PROVIDING EYE CARE

Help cope with impaired vision; taping eyes open for short intervals, instilling artificial tears to prevent corneal damage, using a patch over one eye for double vision, and wearing sunglasses diminish the effects of bright light that increase eye problems.

PREVENTING ASPIRATION

1. Assess for drooling, regurgitation through the nose, and choking while attempting to swallow.
2. Provide standby suction.
3. Encourage rest before meals; place in an upright position to facilitate swallowing.
4. Provide soft foods that are easily swallowed.
5. Schedule meals to coincide with the peak effects of anticholinesterase.
6. Assist with gastrostomy feedings if necessary.

MONITORING AND MANAGING POTENTIAL COMPLICATIONS: MYASTHENIC AND CHOLINERGIC CRISIS

1. Respiratory distress combined with various signs of dysphagia (difficulty swallowing), dysarthria (difficulty speaking), eyelid ptosis, diplopia, and prominent muscle weakness are symptoms of crisis of either type.
2. Provide immediate adequate ventilatory assistance.
3. Suction patient as needed.
4. Monitor arterial blood gases, serum electrolytes, intake and output, and daily weights.
5. Assist with endotracheal intubation and mechanical ventilation; place patient in ICU for constant monitoring.
6. Assist with administration of IV edrophonium (Tensilon) to differentiate type of crisis; improves patient in myasthenic crisis; temporarily worsens patient in cholinergic crisis.
7. Assist with nasogastric tube feedings if patient is unable to swallow.

8. Avoid sedatives and tranquilizing drugs. They aggravate hypoxia and hypercapnia and can cause respiratory and cardiac depression.

✎ Patient Education and Health Maintenance: Care in the Home and Community

1. Teach patient to consult with physician before taking any new medications. Many prescription and nonprescription medications aggravate myasthenia gravis.
2. Avoid novocaine and advise the patient's dentist.

✚ Clinical Alert

A nursing priority is to give the prescribed anticholinesterase drug according to an exact time schedule to control patient symptoms; delay in drug administration may result in inability to swallow.

For more information see Chapter 60 in Smeltzer and Bare: *Brunner and Suddarth's Textbook of Medical–Surgical Nursing,* 8th Edition. Philadelphia: Lippincott–Raven, 1996.

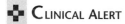

MYOCARDIAL INFARCTION

Myocardial infarction (MI) refers to the process by which myocardial tissue is destroyed in regions of the heart that are deprived of an adequate blood supply because of reduced coronary blood flow. The cause is either a critical narrowing of a coronary artery due to atherosclerosis or complete occlusion of an artery due to embolus or thrombus. Decreased coronary blood flow may also result from shock and hemorrhage. In each case, there is an imbalance between myocardial oxygen supply and demand.

CLINICAL MANIFESTATIONS

1. Chest pain that occurs suddenly and continues unabated, usually over the lower sternal region and upper abdomen, is the primary presenting symptom.
2. Pain may increase steadily in severity until it becomes almost unbearable.
3. It is a heavy, viselike pain that may radiate to the shoulders and down the arms (usually left).
4. It begins spontaneously (not after effort or emotional upset), persists for hours or days, and is not relieved by rest or nitroglycerin (NTG).
5. Pain may radiate to the jaw and neck.
6. Pain is often accompanied by shortness of breath, pallor, cold, clammy diaphoresis, dizziness or light-headedness, and nausea and vomiting.
7. Patients with diabetes mellitus may not experience severe pain because the neuropathy that accompanies diabetes can interfere with neuroreceptors (dulling the pain experience).

DIAGNOSTIC EVALUATION

1. Patient history.
2. Electrocardiogram.
3. Serial serum enzymes and isoenzymes.
4 Echocardiogram

MEDICAL MANAGEMENT

The goal of medical management is to minimize myocardial damage by relieving pain, providing rest, and preventing complications such as lethal dysrhythmias and cardiogenic shock.

1. Oxygen administration initiated at the onset of chest pain.
2. Analgesics (morphine sulfate).

Pharmacotherapy

1. Vasodilators to increase oxygen supply (NTG).
2. Anticoagulants (heparin).

3. Thrombolytics (streptokinase, tissue-type plasminogen activator [t-PA], anistreplase) are only effective if administered within 6 hours of the onset of chest pain, before transmural tissue necrosis occurs.
4. Coronary artery bypass is the viable alternative for revascularization of the myocardium in persons for whom clot lysis is ineffective or contraindicated.

NURSING PROCESS

Assessment

Establish a baseline management to get information on present status of patient so deviations may be noted immediately. Include history of chest pain, dyspnea, palpitations, faintness, or sweating.

COMPLETE PHYSICAL ASSESSMENT

Critical to detect complications and should include the following:

M

1. Level of consciousness.
2. Chest pain (most important clinical finding).
3. Heart rate and rhythm; dysrhythmias may indicate not enough oxygen to the myocardium.
4. Heart sounds; S_3 can be an early sign of impending left ventricular failure.
5. Blood pressure: measured to determine response to pain and treatment; note pulse pressure, which may be narrowed after an MI, suggesting ineffective ventricular contraction.
6. Peripheral pulses: assess rate, rhythm, and volume.
7. Skin color and temperature.
8. Lungs: auscultate lung fields at frequent intervals for signs of ventricular failure (crackles in lung bases).
9. Gastrointestinal function: assess bowel motility; mesenteric artery thrombosis is a potentially fatal complication.
10. Fluid volume status: observe urinary output; check for edema; note early sign of cardiogenic shock is hypotension with oliguria.

Major Nursing Diagnosis

1. Chest pain related to reduced coronary blood flow.
2. Potential ineffective breathing patterns related to fluid overload.
3. Potential altered tissue perfusion related to decreased cardiac output.
4. Anxiety related to fear of death.
5. Potential noncompliance with self-care program related to denial of diagnosis of MI.

Collaborative Problems

1. Dysrhythmias.
2. Acute pulmonary edema.
3. Congestive heart failure.
4. Thromboembolism.

Planning and Implementation

The major goals include relief of chest pain, absence of respiratory difficulties, maintenance or attainment of adequate tissue perfusion, reduction of anxiety, and adherence to self-care program.

Interventions

RELIEVING CHEST PAIN

1. Administer vasodilator (NTG) and anticoagulant (heparin) medications to preserve heart muscle.
2. Provide thrombolytic therapy if patient clinically qualifies.
3. Administer analgesic agents (morphine sulfate).
4. Administer oxygen in tandem with analgesia to assure maximum relief of pain (inhalation of oxygen reduces pain associated with low levels of circulating oxygen).
5. Assess vital signs as long as patient is experiencing pain.
6. Provide physical rest with back elevated or in cardiac chair to decrease chest discomfort and dyspnea.

IMPROVING RESPIRATORY FUNCTION

1. Assess respiratory function to detect early signs of complications.
2. Pay attention to fluid volume status to prevent overloading the heart and the lungs.
3. Encourage patient to breathe deeply and change position to prevent pooling of fluid in lung bases.

PROMOTING ADEQUATE TISSUE PERFUSION

1. Keep patient on bed or chair rest to reduce cardiac workload.
2. Check skin temperature and peripheral pulses frequently to determine adequate tissue perfusion.
3. Administer oxygen to enrich supply of circulating oxygen.

REDUCING ANXIETY

1. Develop a trusting and caring relationship with patients.
2. Provide frequent and private opportunities to share concerns and fears.
3. Provide an atmosphere of acceptance to help know their feelings are both realistic and normal.

MONITORING AND MANAGING COMPLICATIONS

Monitor closely for cardinal signs and symptoms that signal onset of complications.

CARDIAC REHABILITATION

Goals of rehabilitation for the patient with an MI are to extend and improve quality of life.

Immediate Objectives

Return the patient as rapidly as possible to a normal or near-normal lifestyle.

1. Encourage physical activity and physical conditioning.
2. Educate both patient and family.
3. Initiate psychosocial and vocational counseling when necessary.

Four Phases of Cardiac Rehabilitation

1. Phase 1 begins while the patient is still in the coronary care unit.
2. Phase 2 occurs during the remainder of hospitalization.
3. Phase 3 begins with the patient's discharge to home and continues through convalescence.
4. Phase 4 focuses on long-term conditioning and maintaining cardiovascular stability.

✎ PATIENT EDUCATION AND HEALTH MAINTENANCE: CARE IN THE HOME AND COMMUNITY

Educate about the disease process and work with patients in development of plans to meet their specific needs to enhance compliance.

✪ GERONTOLOGIC CONSIDERATIONS

The elderly patient may not experience the typical vise-like pain associated with MI because of diminished responses of neurotransmitters that occur in the aging process. Often the pain is atypical such as jaw pain or fainting.

Arteriosclerosis that accompanies aging may compromise tissue perfusion. The elderly may have a well-established collateral circulation of the myocardium and are often spared the lethal complications associated with MI.

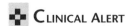 **C**LINICAL **A**LERT

The resolution of pain is the prmary clinical indicator that myocardial oxygen demand and supply are in equilibrium.

For more information see Chapter 28 in Smeltzer and Bare: *Brunner and Suddarth's Textbook of Medical–Surgical Nursing,* 8th Edition. Philadelphia: Lippincott–Raven, 1996.

MYOCARDITIS

Acute myocarditis is an inflammatory process involving the myocardium. When the muscle fibers of the heart are damaged, life is threatened. Myocarditis usually results from an infectious process, e.g., viral, bacterial, mycotic, parasitic, protozoal, or spirochetal. It may be produced from hypersensitivity states such as rheumatic fever. Other risk factors are immunosuppressive therapy or infective endocarditis. Myocarditis can cause heart dilation, mural thrombi, and degeneration of the muscle fibers.

M

CLINICAL MANIFESTATIONS

1. Depend on type of infection, degree of myocardial damage, and capacity of the myocardium to recover.
2. Symptoms may be mild or absent; fatigue and dyspnea, palpitations, occasional discomfort in the chest and upper abdomen.
3. Cardiac enlargement, faint heart sounds, gallop rhythm, and systolic murmur may be found on clinical examination.
4. Pericardial friction rub may be heard if associated with pericarditis.

5. Pulsus alternans may be present.
6. Fever and tachycardia are frequently seen and symptoms of congestive heart failure may develop.

DIAGNOSTIC EVALUATION

Confirmed by endomyocardial biopsy.

MANAGEMENT

1. Treat the specific underlying cause.
2. Bed rest to decrease cardiac workload and prevent complications.
3. Continuous cardiac monitoring if dysrhythmia occurs.
4. Medications to slow the heart rate and augment myocardial contractility (digitalis) when there is evidence of congestive heart failure.
5. Because patients with myocarditis are sensitive to digitalis, they should be monitored for digitalis toxicity (dysrhythmia, anorexia, nausea, vomiting, bradycardia, headache, malaise).
6. Use elastic stockings and passive and active exercises to prevent thrombosis.

PREVENTION

1. Appropriate immunizations and early treatment to decrease the incidence of myocarditis.
2. Increase physical activity slowly and instruct to report any symptoms that occur with increased activity, i.e., rapid heart rate.
3. Avoid competitive sports and alcohol.

For more information see Chapter 29 in Smeltzer and Bare: *Brunner and Suddarth's Textbook of Medical–Surgical Nursing,* 8th Edition. Philadelphia: Lippincott–Raven, 1996.

MYXEDEMA

See Hypothyroidism and Myxedema

NEPHROTIC SYNDROME

Nephrotic syndrome is a clinical disorder characterized by proteinuria, hypoalbuminemia, edema, and hypercholesterolemia. It is seen in any condition that seriously damages the glomerular capillary membrane. Generally a disorder of childhood, it does occur in adults, including the elderly. Causes include chronic glomerular nephritis, diabetes mellitus with intercapillary glomerulosclerosis, amyloidosis of the kidney, systemic lupus erythematosus, and renal vein thrombosis.

CLINICAL MANIFESTATIONS

1. Major manifestation is edema (usually soft, pitting, and periorbital, in dependent areas [sacrum, ankles, and hands], and ascites).
2. Malaise, headache, irritability, and fatigue.

DIAGNOSTIC EVALUATION

1. Microscopic hematuria, urinary casts.
2. Needle biopsy of the kidney for histologic examination to confirm diagnosis.

Collaborative Problems

1. Infection due to deficient immune response.
2. Thromboembolism (renal vein).
3. Pulmonary emboli.
4. Accelerated atherosclerosis.

MANAGEMENT

The objective of management is to preserve renal function.

1. Bed rest for a few days to promote diuresis and reduce edema.

2. High-protein diet to replenish urinary losses.
3. Low-sodium diet for severe edema.
4. Diuretics for severe edema.
5. Adrenocorticosteroids to reduce proteinuria.
6. Antineoplastic agents (Cytoxan) or immunosuppressive agents (Imuran, Leukeran, or cyclosporine) may be used.

Nursing Interventions

1. In the early stages, nursing management is similar to that of the patient with acute glomerulonephritis.
2. As the disease worsens, management is similar to that of the patient with chronic renal failure.
3. Instruct patient receiving steroids or cyclosporine regarding medication and signs and symptoms that must be reported to the physician.
4. Instruct patient in selecting a high-protein diet while restricting cholesterol and fat intake.

For more information see Chapter 43 in Smeltzer and Bare: *Brunner and Suddarth's Textbook of Medical–Surgical Nursing,* 8th Edition. Philadelphia: Lippincott–Raven, 1996.

NIDDM

See Diabetes Mellitus

NONCARDIOGENIC PULMONARY EDEMA

See Adult Respiratory Distress Syndrome

NOSEBLEEDS

See Epistaxis

OA

See Osteoarthritis

OBSTRUCTION, LARGE BOWEL

See Bowel Obstruction, Large

OBSTRUCTION, SMALL BOWEL

See Bowel Obstruction, Small

OPEN PNEUMOTHORAX

See Pneumothorax

ORAL CANCER

See Cancer of the Oral Cavity

OSTEOARTHRITIS

Osteoarthritis (OA), also known as degenerative joint disease or osteoarthrosis, is the most common and frequently disabling of the joint disorders. OA is characterized by a progressive loss of joint cartilage. Besides age, risk factors for OA include female gender; genetic predisposition; obesity; mechanical joint stress; joint trauma; previous bone and joint disorders; inflammatory joint diseases; and endocrine and metabolic diseases. OA has been classified as primary (idiopathic) and secondary (related to risk factors). Obese women have been shown to have an incidence of OA of the knee nearly four times that of women of average weight. OA peaks between the fifth and sixth decades.

CLINICAL MANIFESTATIONS

1. Pain, stiffness, and functional impairment are primary clinical manifestations.
2. Stiffness is most common in the morning after awakening and usually lasts less than 30 minutes.
3. Functional impairment is due to pain on movement and limited joint motion when structural changes develop.
4. Osteoarthritis occurs most often in weight-bearing joints (hips, knees, cervical, and lumbar spine); finger joints are also involved.
5. Bony nodes may be present (painless unless inflamed).

DIAGNOSTIC EVALUATION

X-ray shows narrowing of joint space and osteophytes (spurs) at the joint margins and on the subchondral bone. These two findings together are sensitive and specific.

MANAGEMENT

The goals of management focus on treating symptoms because there is no treatment available that stops the degenerative joint disease process.

Preventive Measures

1. Weight reduction.
2. Reducing injuries.
3. Perinatal screening for congenital hip disease.
4. Ergonomic approaches to job stress modification.

Pharmacotherapy

1. Acetaminophen; NSAIDs if joint symptoms persist.
2. Intra-articular injections of corticosteroids for acute joint inflammation.

Conservative Measures

1. Heat, weight reduction, joint rest, and avoidance of joint overuse.
2. Orthotic devices to support inflamed joints (splints, braces).
3. Isometric and postural exercises.
4. Occupational and physical therapy.

Surgical Approaches

When pain is intractable and function is lost.

1. Tidal irrigation, arthroscopic debridement, drilling of osteochrondal defects, or abrasion arthroplasty.
2. Joint arthroplasy (replacement).

NURSING PROCESS

The nursing care of the patient with OA is generally the same as the basic care plan for the patient with rheumatic disease.

✪ GERONTOLOGIC CONSIDERATIONS

Many older people expect and accept the immobility and self-care problems related to the rheumatic diseases and do not seek help. Careful diagnosis and appropriate treatment can improve the quality of life for older persons with OA.

OA is a more prevalent rheumatic disease with advancing age. It is the most prevalent activity-limiting condition among older persons and accounts for more total disability than many more serious diseases, e.g., stroke or cancer.

It is difficult to differentiate problems associated with aging from those caused by a rheumatic disease.

Special techniques for promoting patient safety and self-management need to be employed because of poor hearing, diminished vision, forgetfulness, and depression, contributing to noncompliance. The cumulative effect of medications is accentuated because of the physiologic changes of aging.

The elderly person has developed a lifelong pattern of dealing with stress. Those positive coping skills can help the elderly maintain a positive attitude and self-esteem when faced with a rheumatic disease, especially with the support of a skillful nurse.

For more information see Chapter 52 in Smeltzer and Bare: *Brunner and Suddarth's Textbook of Medical–Surgical Nursing,* 8th Edition. Philadelphia: Lippincott–Raven, 1996.

OSTEOMALACIA

Osteomalacia is a metabolic bone disease characterized by inadequate mineralization of bone. (Rickets, a similar condition, afflicts children.) It is thought that the primary defect is a deficiency in activated vitamin D (calcitrol), which causes an imbalance of calcium and phosphate and faulty bone mineralization. In adults, the condition is chronic and skeletal deformities are not as severe as in children. Risk factors include dietary deficiencies, malabsorption, gastrectomy, chronic renal failure, prolonged anticonvulsant therapy, and insufficient vitamin D.

CLINICAL MANIFESTATIONS

1. Bone pain and tenderness.
2. Muscle weakness from calcium deficiency.
3. Waddling or limping gait.
4. Legs become bowed in the more advanced disease.
5. Pathologic fractures.
6. Softened vertebra become compressed, shortening the patient's trunk and deforming the thorax (kyphosis).

7. The sacrum is forced down and forward, compressing the pelvis laterally; pelvic distortion often necessitates cesarean section.
8. Weakness and unsteadiness present risk of falls and fractures.

DIAGNOSTIC EVALUATION

1. X-ray.
2. Laboratory studies show low serum calcium and phosphorus levels; moderately elevated alkaline phosphatase level; urine calcium and creatinine excretion is low.

MANAGEMENT

1. Correct underlying cause when possible, e.g., diet, vitamin D and calcium supplements, sunlight.
2. Long-term monitoring to ensure stabilization or reversal.
3. Treat orthopedic deformities with braces or surgery.

NURSING PROCESS

O

Assessment

1. Assess for generalized bone pain in the low back and extremities, with associated tenderness.
2. Assess for fracture.
3. Obtain information concerning coexisting diseases (malabsorption syndrome) and dietary habits.
4. Note skeletal deformities on physical exam and any muscle weakness.

Major Nursing Diagnosis

1. Knowledge deficit about the disease process and the treatment regimen.
2. Pain related to bone tenderness and possible fracture.
3. Self-concept disturbance related to bowing legs, waddling gait, spinal deformities.

Planning and Implementation

The major goals may include knowledge of the disease process and treatment regimen, relief of pain, and improved self-concept.

Interventions

UNDERSTANDING THE DISEASE PROCESS AND TREATMENT REGIMEN

1. Educate patient on the cause of osteomalacia and approaches to controlling it.
2. Instruct about dietary sources of calcium and vitamin D.
3. Review safe use of vitamin D supplements.
4. Inform patient that high doses of vitamin D are toxic and enhance risk of hypercalcemia.
5. Note importance of monitoring serum calcium levels.
6. Encourage outdoor activities to expose skin to sunshine.

RELIEVING PAIN

1. Assist patient in reducing discomfort by physical, psychological, and pharmaceutical measures.
2. Change positions often to decrease discomfort from immobility.
3. Administer prescribed analgesics as needed.

IMPROVING SELF-CONCEPT

1. Establish a trusting relationship and encourage patient to discuss any changes in body image and methods for coping.
2. Encourage to recognize and use existing strengths.
3. Include patient in plan of care to promote self-control and improve feelings of self-worth.

✿ GERONTOLOGIC CONSIDERATIONS

Promote adequate intake of calcium and vitamin D and a nutritious diet in disadvantaged elderly persons.

Encourage to spend time in the sun.

Reduce incidence of fractures with prevention, identification, and management of osteomalacia. When osteomalacia is combined with osteoporosis, the incidence of fracture increases.

For more information see Chapter 63 in Smeltzer and Bare: *Brunner and Suddarth's Textbook of Medical–Surgical Nursing,* 8th Edition. Philadelphia: Lippincott–Raven, 1996.

OSTEOMYELITIS

Osteomyelitis is an infection of the bone. It is more difficult to cure than a soft-tissue infection because of limited blood supply, inflammatory tissue response, increased tissue pressure, and involucrum formation. It may become a chronic problem that affects quality of life or loss of an extremity. The infection may be due to hematogenous (blood-borne) spread from other foci of infection. *Staphylococcus aureus* causes 70–80% of bone infection. Other pathogenic organisms frequently found include *Proteus, Pseudomonas,* and *Escherichia coli.* Patients at risk include poorly nourished, elderly, obese, or diabetic patients. In addition, patients who have had long-term corticosteroid therapy, joint surgery, concurrent sepsis, lengthy orthopedic surgery, prolonged wound drainage, and wound dehiscence are susceptible. The condition may be prevented by prompt treatment and management of focal and soft-tissue infections.

CLINICAL MANIFESTATIONS

Hematogenous Infection

1. Onset is sudden, occurring with clinical manifestations of septicemia.
2. Chills, high fever, rapid pulse, and general malaise.
3. The extremity becomes painful, swollen, and tender.
4. Patient may describe a constant pulsating pain that intensifies with movement (due to the pressure of collecting pus).

Adjacent Infection or Direct Contamination

1. There are no symptoms of septicemia.
2. Area is swollen, warm, painful, and tender to touch.

Chronic Osteomyelitis

Continually draining sinus or recurrent periods of pain, inflammation, swelling, and drainage.

DIAGNOSTIC EVALUATION

1. Early x-rays show only soft-tissue swelling.
2. In about 2 weeks, irregular decalcification, periosteal elevation, and new bone formation is evident.
3. Blood studies and blood cultures.
4. Chronic osteomyelitis: x-ray shows large, irregular cavities, a raised periosteum, sequestrae, or dense bone formations.

MANAGEMENT

The initial goal is to control and arrest the infective process.

1. Immobilize affected area; provide warm saline soaks for 20 minutes several times a day.
2. Blood cultures; abscess fluid smears performed to identify organisms and select the antibiotic.
3. Intravenous antibiotic therapy around-the-clock.
4. Administer antibiotic orally when infection appears to be controlled; continue for 3 months.
5. Surgical debridement of bone if no response to antibiotic therapy; maintain adjunctive antibiotic therapy.

NURSING PROCESS

Assessment

1. Assess for risk factors (e.g., older age, diabetes, long-term steroid therapy) and for previous injury, infection, or orthopedic surgery.

2. Observe for guarded movement of infected area and generalized weakness due to systemic infection.
3. Observe for swelling of affected area, purulent drainage, and elevated temperature.
4. Note that patients with chronic osteomyelitis may have minimal temperature elevations, occurring in the afternoon or evening.

Major Nursing Diagnosis

1. Pain related to inflammation and swelling.
2. Impaired physical mobility associated with pain, immobilization devices, and weight-bearing limitations.
3. Risk for extension of infection: bone abscess formation.
4. Knowledge deficit about the treatment regimen.

Planning and Implementation

The goals may include relief of pain, improved physical mobility within therapeutic limitations, control and eradication of infection, and knowledge of treatment regimen.

Interventions

RELIEVING PAIN

1. Immobilize affected part with splint to decrease pain and muscle spasm.
2. Provide range of motion to joints above and below affected part.
3. Handle wounds gently to avoid pain.
4. Elevate affected part to reduce swelling and discomfort.
5. Administer prescribed analgesics and other techniques for reducing pain perception.

IMPROVING PHYSICAL MOBILITY

1. Teach the rationale for activity restrictions (bone is weakened by the infective process).
2. Encourage activities of daily living within the physical limitations.

CONTROLLING INFECTIOUS PROCESS

1. Monitor the patient's response to antibiotic therapy and observe the IV sites for evidence of phlebitis or infiltration.
2. Ensure adequate circulation (wound suction, elevation of area, avoidance of pressure on grafted area); maintain needed immobility; comply with weight-bearing restriction if surgery performed.
3. Monitor general health and nutrition of patient.
4. Provide a balanced diet high in protein, vitamin C, and vitamin D to ensure positive nitrogen balance and promote healing.

✎ PATIENT EDUCATION AND HEALTH MAINTENANCE: CARE IN THE HOME AND COMMUNITY

1. Teach patient and family rationale for wound care and IV antibiotic therapy at home.
2. Teach patient and family antibiotic protocols, aseptic dressing changes, and warm compress techniques.
3. Instruct patient to observe and report elevated temperature, drainage, odor, and increased inflammation that may indicate development of new infection.

For more information see Chapter 63 in Smeltzer and Bare: *Brunner and Suddarth's Textbook of Medical–Surgical Nursing,* 8th Edition. Philadelphia: Lippincott–Raven, 1996.

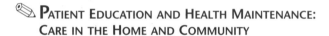

OSTEOPOROSIS

Osteoporosis is a disorder in which there is a reduction of total bone mass. The rate of bone resorption is greater than the rate of bone formation. The bones become progressively porous, brittle, fragile, and fracture easily. Multiple compression fractures of the vertebrae result in skeletal deformity (kyphosis). With the development of kyphoses ("dowager's hump") there is associated loss of height in some postmenopausal women. Risk factors include postmenopausal women; small-framed, nonobese white women of European ancestry; nutrition, lifestyle choices (e.g., smoking, caffeine, and alcohol consumption); and lack of physical activity. Age-related bone loss begins soon after peak bone mass is achieved (about age 35). Withdrawal of estrogens at menopause or oophorectomy causes accelerated bone resorption, which continues during menopausal years. Endogenous and exogenous catabolic agents may contribute to osteoporosis: excessive corticosteroids, Cushing's syndrome, hyperthyroidism, and hyperparathyroidism. Further causes include coexisting medical conditions: malabsorption syndromes, lactose intolerance, renal failure, liver failure, and endocrine disorders. Contributing medications may include isoniazid, heparin, tetracycline, aluminum-containing antacids, furosemide, anticonvulsants, and thyroid supplements. Immobility contributes to the development of osteoporosis.

DIAGNOSTIC EVALUATION

1. Osteoporosis is identified on routine x-ray when there has been 25–40% demineralization.
2. Single-photon absorptiometry to monitor bone mass in wrist.
3. Dual-photon absorptiometry, dual-energy x-ray absorptiometry (DEXA), and CT scan provide information on spine and hip bone mass.

MANAGEMENT

1. Give adequate balanced diet rich in calcium and vitamin D.
2. May increase calcium intake in the middle years or prescribe a calcium preparation.
3. Hormone replacement therapy (HRT) to retard bone loss.
4. Other medications include calcitonin, sodium fluoride, and etidronate sodium.

NURSING PROCESS FOR THE PATIENT WITH A SPONTANEOUS VERTEBRAL FRACTURE RELATED TO OSTEOPOROSIS

Assessment

1. To identify patient's risk for and recognition of problems associated with osteoporosis, interview patient regarding family history, previous fractures, dietary habits, exercise patterns, onset of menopause, and use of steroids.
2. Observe for fracture, kyphosis of the thoracic, or shortened stature upon physical examination.

Major Nursing Diagnosis

1. Knowledge deficit about the osteoporotic process and treatment regimen.
2. Pain related to fracture and muscle spasm.
3. Constipation related to immobility or development of ileus.
4. Risk for injury: fracture related to osteoporotic bone.

Planning and Implementation

The major goals may include knowledge about osteoporosis and the treatment regimen, relief of pain, improved bowel elimination, and absence of additional fracture.

Interventions

UNDERSTANDING OSTEOPOROSIS AND THE TREATMENT REGIMEN

1. Focus patient teaching on factors influencing the development of osteoporosis, interventions to slow the process, and measures to relieve symptoms.
2. Inform patient about adequate dietary or supplemental calcium, regular weight-bearing exercise, and modification of lifestyle, i.e., reduced use of caffeine, cigarettes, and alcohol.
3. Emphasize exercise and physical activity to develop high-density bones.

4. Inform patient about foods high in calcium, i.e., skim or whole milk, swiss cheese, canned salmon with bones.
5. Encourage taking calcium preparations (calcium carbonate).
6. Inform patients that at menopause, HRT may be prescribed.
7. Inform patient that estrogen therapy has been associated with a slightly increased incidence of breast and endometrial cancer; patient must examine her breasts monthly and have regular pelvic examinations.
8. Inform elderly patients to continue to take sufficient calcium, vitamin D, sunshine, and exercise to minimize the process.

RELIEVING PAIN

1. Teach relief of back pain through bed rest and use of a firm, nonsagging mattress.
2. Instruct patient to move the trunk as a unit and avoid twisting; encourage good posture and good body mechanics.
3. Apply lumbosacral corset for temporary support when out of bed.
4. Administer oral narcotic analgesic at onset of back pain; change to nonnarcotic analgesics after a few days.

IMPROVING BOWEL ELIMINATION

1. Encourage a high-fiber diet, increased fluids, and use of prescribed stool softeners.
2. Monitor patient's intake, bowel sounds, and bowel activity; ileus may develop if the vertebral collapse involves T10–L2 vertebra.

PREVENTING INJURY

1. Promote physical activity to strengthen muscles, prevent disuse atrophy, and retard progressive bone demineralization.
2. Encourage isometric exercises to strengthen trunk muscles.

3. Encourage walking, good body mechanics, and good posture.
4. Avoid sudden bending, jarring, and strenuous lifting.
5. Encourage outdoor activity in the sunshine to enhance body's ability to produce vitamin D.

✪ Gerontologic Considerations

The prevalence of osteoporosis in women over 75 is 90%. With the aging of the population, the incidence of fractures, pain, and disability associated with osteoporosis is rising.

Identify and eliminate harmful environmental hazards that may cause the elderly patient to fall; include the patient and family in planning for continued care and preventive management regimens.

Assess home environment for potential hazards, e.g., scatter rugs, pets under foot, cluttered rooms. Create a safe well-lighted environment including grab-bars in the bathroom and properly fitting footwear.

For more information see Chapter 63 in Smeltzer and Bare: *Brunner and Suddarth's Textbook of Medical–Surgical Nursing*, 8th Edition. Philadelphia: Lippincott–Raven, 1996.

OTITIS MEDIA, ACUTE

Acute otitis media is an acute infection of the middle ear. The primary cause is the entrance of pathogenic bacteria into the normally sterile middle ear when there is eustachian tube dysfunction, i.e., obstruction caused by upper respiratory infections, inflammation of surrounding structure (sinusitis), or by allergic reactions (allergic rhinitis). Causative organisms are *Streptococcus pneumoniae, Haemophilus influenzae,* and *Moraxella catarrhalis.* Mode of entry of the bacteria is the eustachian tube from contaminated secretions in the nasopharynx.

CLINICAL MANIFESTATIONS

1. Vary with the severity of the infection and may be either very mild and transient or severe.
2. The condition is usually unilateral in adults.
3. Pain in and about the ear (otalgia) may be intense and relieved only after spontaneous perforation of the eardrum or after myringotomy.
5. Fever, hearing loss, and tinnitus.
6. Tympanic membrane is erythematous and often bulging or perforated.

MANAGEMENT

1. The outcome is dependent on (1) the efficiency of antibiotic therapy, (2) the virulence of the bacteria, and (3) the physical status of the patient.
2. With early and appropriate wide-spectrum antibiotic therapy, otitis media may clear with no serious sequelae. Teach patient to take prescribed doses of antibiotic and all of the prescribed medication.
3. If the condition becomes subacute (3 weeks to 3 months) with purulent discharge, it is rare that it is accompanied by permanent hearing loss.
4. Perforation of the tympanic may persist and develop into chronic otitis media.
5. Secondary complications involve the mastoid, meningitis, or brain abscess (rare but can occur).

Myringotomy (Tympanotomy)

1. An incision is made into the tympanic membrane to relieve pressure and to drain serous or purulent fluid from the middle ear.
2. If mild cases of otitis media are treated effectively, a myringotomy may not be necessary.

For more information see Chapter 57 in Smeltzer and Bare: *Brunner and Suddarth's Textbook of Medical–Surgical Nursing,* 8th Edition. Philadelphia: Lippincott–Raven, 1996.

OTITIS MEDIA, CHRONIC

Chronic otitis media results from repeated episodes of acute otitis media, causing perforation of the eardrum. Chronic infections of the middle ear cause damage to the tympanic membrane, destroy the ossicles, and almost always involve the mastoid.

CLINICAL MANIFESTATIONS

1. Symptoms may be minimal with varying degrees of hearing loss and presence of a persistent or intermittent foul-smelling discharge.
2. Pain may or may not be present.
3. When accompanying acute mastoiditis is present, postauricular area is tender to touch; erythema and edema may be present.
4. Cholesteatoma (cyst filled with degenerated skin and sebaceous material) may be present as a white mass behind the tympanic membrane.
5. If left untreated, cholesteatoma will continue to grow and cause facial nerve paralysis, sensorineural hearing loss, and/or balance disturbance, and brain abscess.

MANAGEMENT

1. Careful cleansing of the ear and instillation of antibiotic drops.
2. Tympanoplasty procedures may be required to prevent further damage to hearing and more serious complications.
3. Mastoidectomy to remove the cholesteatoma.
4. Ossiculoplasty to reconstruct the middle ear bones to restore hearing.

For more information see Chapter 57 in Smeltzer and Bare: *Brunner and Suddarth's Textbook of Medical–Surgical Nursing,* 8th Edition. Philadelphia: Lippincott–Raven, 1996.

OVARIAN CANCER

See Cancer of the Ovaries

O

PANCREATIC CANCER

See Cancer of the Pancreas

PANCREATITIS, ACUTE

Pancreatitis (inflammation of the pancreas) is a serious disorder that can range in severity from a relatively mild self-limiting disorder to a rapidly fatal disease that does not respond to any treatment.

Acute pancreatitis is an autodigestion of this organ by the enzymes it produces, principally trypsin. Common causes of acute episodes are biliary tract disease and long-term alcohol use; 5% of patients with gallstones develop pancreatitis. Other less common forms include bacterial or viral infection, with pancreatitis a complication. There are many disease processes and conditions that have been associated with an increased incidence of pancreatitis: surgery on or near the pancreas, medications, as well as hypercalcemia and hyperlipidemia. Ten percent to 30% of the cases are idiopathic and there is a small incidence of hereditary pancreatitis. Mortality is high because of shock, anoxia, hypotension, or fluid and electrolyte imbalances. Complete recovery may occur or the condition may become chronic.

CLASSIFICATION

Interstitial or Edematous Pancreatitis

1. The patient is acutely ill and at risk of developing shock, fluid and electrolyte disturbances, and sepsis.

Acute Hemorrhagic Pancreatitis (a more advanced form of acute interstitial pancreatitis)

1. Enzymatic digestion of the gland is more wide-spread and complete.
2. Tissue becomes necrotic and the damage extends to the vasculature.
3. Late complications are pancreatic cysts or abscesses.

CLINICAL MANIFESTATIONS

Severe abdominal pain is the major symptom.
1. Pain occurs in the midepigastrium.
2. Frequently acute in onset (24–48 hours after a heavy meal or alcohol ingestion).
3. May be more severe after meals and unrelieved by antacids.
4. May be accompanied by abdominal distention, poorly defined palpable abdominal mass, and decreased peristalsis.

Patient Appears Acutely Ill

1. Abdominal guarding; rigid or boardlike abdomen.
2. Abdomen may be soft in the absence of peritonitis.
3. Ecchymosis in the flank or around the umbilicus may indicate severe hemorrhagic pancreatitis.
4. Nausea and vomiting, fever, jaundice, mental confusion, agitation.

Hypotension Related to Hypovolemia and Shock

1. Acute renal failure is common.
2. May develop tachycardia, cyanosis, and cold, clammy skin.

Respiratory Distress and Hypoxia May Occur

1. Dyspnea.
2. Tachypnea.
3. Abnormal blood gas values.
4. Diffuse pulmonary infiltrates.

Myocardial Depression, Hypocalcemia,
Hyperglycemia, and Disseminated Intravascular
Coagulation (DIC) May Occur

DIAGNOSTIC EVALUATION

1. Based on history of abdominal pain, known risk factors, and selected diagnostic findings.
2. Serum amylase and serum lipase levels are most indicative.

MANAGEMENT

Acute Phase

During the acute phase, management is symptomatic and directed toward preventing or treating complications.

1. Oral intake is withheld to inhibit pancreatic stimulation and secretion of pancreatic enzymes.
2. Total parenteral nutrition (TPN) is administered to the debilitated patient.
3. Nasogastric (NG) suction to relieve nausea and vomiting, decrease painful abdominal distention, and paralytic ileus; and to remove hydrochloric acid so it does not stimulate the pancreas.
4. Cimetidine (Tagamet) is given to decrease hydrochloric acid secretion.
5. Adequate pain medication is administered; avoid morphine and morphine derivatives (causes spasm of the sphincter of Oddi).
6. Adequate correction of fluid, blood loss, and low albumin levels is necessary.
7. Administer antibiotics if infection is present.
8. Insulin is necessary if significant hyperglycemia occurs.
9. Provide aggressive respiratory care for pulmonary infiltrates, effusion, and atelectasis.

10. Biliary drainage results in decreased pain and increased weight gain.
11. Surgical intervention is required for diagnosis, drainage, resection, or debridement.

Postacute Management

1. Antacids are given when the acute episode begins to resolve.
2. Oral feedings low in fat and protein are initiated gradually.
3. Caffeine and alcohol are eliminated.
4. Medications, i.e., thiazide diuretics, glucocorticoids, or oral contraceptives are discontinued.

NURSING PROCESS

Assessment

1. Assess presence and character of pain, its relationship to eating and to alcohol consumption; note effect of patient's efforts to obtain pain relief.
2. Assess nutritional fluid status and history of gallbladder attacks and alcohol use.
3. Elicit history of gastrointestinal problems, i.e., fatty stools, diarrhea, nausea, and vomiting.
4. Assess respiratory status including rate, pattern, and breath sounds.
5. Assess abdomen for pain, tenderness, guarding, and bowel sounds; note boardlike or soft abdomen.

Major Nursing Diagnosis

1. Severe pain related to inflammation, edema, distention of the pancreas, and peritoneal irritation.
2. Altered nutritional status related to reduced food intake and increased metabolic demands.
3. Ineffective breathing pattern related to severe pain, pulmonary infiltrates, early fusion, and atelectasis.

P

Collaborative Problems

1. Fluid and electrolyte disturbances.
2. Necrosis of the pancreas.
3. Shock and multiple organ failure.

Planning and Implementation

The major goals include relief of pain and discomfort, improved fluid and nutritional status, improved respiratory function, and absence of complications.

Interventions

RELIEVING PAIN AND DISCOMFORT

1. Administer meperidine (Demerol) as ordered (drug of choice).
2. Avoid morphine sulfate because it causes spasm of the sphincter of Oddi.
3. Withhold oral fluids to decrease formation and secretion of secretin.
4. Maintain on IV fluids to restore and maintain fluid balance.
5. Use NG suction to remove gastric secretions and relieve abdominal distention; give frequent oral hygiene.
6. Maintain on bed rest to decrease metabolic rate and reduce secretion of pancreatic enzymes; report increased pain (may be pancreatic hemorrhage or inadequate analgesic dosage).
7. Provide adequate explanations about treatment; patient may have clouded sensorium from pain, fluid imbalances, and hypoxemia.

IMPROVING NUTRITIONAL STATUS

1. Monitor laboratory test results, daily weights, anthropometric measures.
2. Assess nutritional status; note increased body temperature, restlessness, increased physical activity, and fluid lost through diarrhea.
3. Medications: NPO during an attack.

4. TPN may be prescribed; monitor physiologic response by serum glucose levels every 4–6 hours.
5. Introduce oral feedings gradually as symptoms subside.
6. Avoid heavy meals and alcoholic beverages; meals should be high in carbohydrates and low in fat and proteins.

IMPROVING BREATHING PATTERN

1. Maintain in semi-Fowler's position to decrease pressure on diaphragm.
2. Change position frequently to prevent atelectasis and pooling of respiratory secretions.
3. Administer anticholinergic medications to decrease gastric and pancreatic secretions, and dry respiratory tract secretions.
4. Assess respiratory status frequently and teach patient techniques of coughing and deep breathing.

MONITORING AND MANAGING COMPLICATIONS: FLUID AND ELECTROLYTE DISTURBANCES

1. Assess fluid and electrolyte status by noting skin turgor and moistness of mucous membranes.
2. Weigh daily; measure all fluid intake and output.
3. Assess for factors that may affect fluid and electrolyte status, e.g., fever, fluid loss through diarrhea, vomiting, NG suction, or wound drainage.
4. Observe for ascites and measure abdominal girth.
5. Administer IV fluids, blood, and albumin to maintain volume and prevent or treat shock.
6. Report decreased blood pressure and reduced urine output.

MONITORING AND MANAGING COMPLICATIONS: PANCREATIC NECROSIS

1. Patient is transferred to intensive care unit for close monitoring.
2. Administer fluids, medications, and blood products.

P

3. Assist with supportive management, i.e., ventilator.
4. Attend to the patient's physical and psychological care.

MONITORING AND MANAGING COMPLICATIONS: SHOCK AND MULTIPLE ORGAN FAILURE

1. Monitor closely for early signs of neurologic, cardiovascular, renal, and respiratory dysfunction.
2. Prepare for rapid changes in patient status; respond quickly.
3. Inform family of status and progress of patient; allow time with patient.

✎ PATIENT EDUCATION AND HEALTH MAINTENANCE: CARE IN THE HOME AND COMMUNITY

1. Provide patient and family with facts and explanations of the acute phase of illness; provide necessary repetition and reinforcement.
2. Reinforce the need for a low-fat diet, avoidance of heavy meals, and avoidance of alcohol.
3. Provide information about resources and support groups particularly if alcohol is the cause of acute pancreatitis.
4. Permit patient and family to discuss their questions and concerns and provide education and emotional support.

✪ GERONTOLOGIC CONSIDERATIONS

The mortality from acute pancreatitis increases with advancing age. Patterns of complications change with age, i.e., the incidence of multiple organ failure increases with age.

Close observation of major organ function (lungs and kidneys) is indicated and aggressive treatment is necessary to reduce mortality in the elderly.

For more information see Chapter 40 in Smeltzer and Bare: *Brunner and Suddarth's Textbook of Medical–Surgical Nursing,* 8th Edition. Philadelphia: Lippincott–Raven, 1996.

PANCREATITIS, CHRONIC

Chronic pancreatitis is an inflammatory disorder characterized by a progressive anatomic and functional destruction of the pancreas. Cells are replaced by fibrous tissue; the end result is mechanical obstruction of the pancreatic and common bile ducts and duodenum. Also, inflammation and destruction of the secreting cells of the pancreas occurs. Alcohol consumption in Western societies and malnutrition worldwide are the major causes. Among alcoholics, the incidence of pancreatitis is 50 times the rate in the nondrinking population. Chronic consumption of alcohol produces hypersecretion of protein in pancreatic secretions. The result is protein plugs and calculi within the pancreatic ducts. Alcohol has a direct toxic effect on the cells of the pancreas. Incidence of chronic pancreatitis is increased in adult men.

CLINICAL MANIFESTATIONS

P

1. Recurring attacks of severe upper abdominal and back pain, accompanied by vomiting; narcotics may not provide relief.
2. There may be continuous severe pain or dull, nagging, constant pain.
3. Risk of addiction to opiates is high because of the severe pain.
4. Weight loss is a major problem.
5. Altered digestion of foods (proteins and fats) results in frequent, frothy, and foul-smelling stools with a high fat content (steatorrhea).
6. As disease progresses calcification of the gland may occur and calcium stones may form within the ducts.

DIAGNOSTIC EVALUATION

Endoscopic retrograde cholangiopancreatography (ERCP) is the most useful study.

MANAGEMENT

1. Treatment is directed toward prevention and management of acute attacks.
2. Relieve pain and discomfort with analgesics.
3. Emphasize importance of avoiding alcohol and other foods that produce abdominal pain and discomfort.
4. Stress that no other treatment will relieve pain if patient continues to consume alcohol.
5. Treat diabetes mellitus resulting from dysfunction of pancreatic islet cells with diet, insulin, or oral hypoglycemic agents.
6. Stress to patient and family members the hazard of severe hypoglycemia related to alcohol use.
7. Provide pancreatic enzyme replacement therapy for malabsorption and steatorrhea.
8. Surgery is done to relieve abdominal pain and discomfort, restore drainage of pancreatic secretions, and reduce frequency of attacks.
9. Morbidity and mortality following surgical procedures is high because of the poor physical condition prior to surgery and concomitant occurrence of cirrhosis.

For more information see Chapter 40 in Smeltzer and Bare: *Brunner and Suddarth's Textbook of Medical–Surgical Nursing,* 8th Edition. Philadelphia: Lippincott–Raven, 1996.

PARALYSIS AGITANS

See Parkinson's Disease

PARALYSIS, FACIAL

See Bell's Palsy

PARKINSON'S DISEASE

Parkinson's disease is a progressive neurologic disorder affecting the brain centers that are responsible for control and regulation of movement. Dopamine is depleted in the substantia nigra and the corpus striatum because of a degeneration process. It results in the characteristic symptoms of bradykinesia (slowness of movement), tremor, and muscle stiffness or rigidity. Regional cerebral blood flow is reduced and there is a high prevalence of dementia. Biochemical and pathologic data suggest that demented patients with Parkinson's may have coexistent Alzheimer's disease. The cause of the disease is mostly unknown. The disease is most prevalent among persons in their 60s and is the second most common neurologic disorder of the elderly.

CLINICAL MANIFESTATIONS

Chief Manifestations

1. Impaired movement.
2. Muscular rigidity.
3. Resting tremors.
4. Muscle weakness.
5. Loss of postural reflexes.

Early Signs

1. Stiffening of the extremities.
2. Waxy rigidity in performance of all movements.
3. Difficulty in initiating, maintaining, and performing motor activities.
4. Experiences some delay in carrying out normal activity.

Later Signs

1. Tremor, frequently begins in one hand and arm, then the other, and later in the head.

P

2. Characteristic tremor is a slow, turning motion of the forearm and hand, and a pill rolling motion of the thumb against the fingers.
3. Tremor is present while at rest and increases with concentration and anxiety.

Other Characteristics Affecting the Face, Stature, and Gait

1. Loss of normal arm swing.
2. Rigid extremities become weaker.
3. Masklike facial expression.
4. Loss of postural reflexes: patient stands with head bent forward and walks with propulsive gait.
5. Depression and psychiatric manifestations (personality changes, psychosis, dementia, and confusion) may occur.

DIAGNOSTIC EVALUATION

Evidence of tremor, rigidity, and bradykinesia.

MANAGEMENT

The goal of treatment is to enhance dopamine transmission.

Pharmacotherapy

1. Levodopa therapy most effective agent to relieve symptoms.
2. Dopamine-agonist-ergot derivatives are useful when added to levodopa to smooth out clinical fluctuations.
3. Antihistamine drugs for allaying tremors.
4. Anticholinergic therapy for controlling the tremor and rigidity.
5. Amantadine hydrochloride, an antiviral agent, is used to reduce rigidity, tremor, and bradykinesia.
6. MAO inhibitors to inhibit dopamine breakdown.
7. Antidepressant drugs.

Surgical Intervention

1. Surgery to destroy a part of the thalamus (stereotaxic thalamotomy) to relieve certain types of excessive muscle contraction.
2. Transplantation of neural cells from fetal tissue of human or animal source to reestablish normal dopamine release.

NURSING PROCESS

Assessment

1. Observe changes in function throughout the day and responses to medication.
2. Observe how patient moves about, walks, and drinks.

Major Nursing Diagnosis

1. Impaired physical mobility related to muscle rigidity and weakness.
2. Self-care deficits (eating, drinking, dressing, hygiene) related to tremor and motor disturbance.
3. Constipation related to medication and reduced activity.
4. Altered nutrition, less than body requirements, related to tremor, slowness in eating, difficulty in chewing and swallowing.
5. Impaired verbal communication related to decreased speech volume, slowness of speech, inability to move facial muscles.
6. Ineffective coping related to depression and dysfunction due to disease progression.

Collaborative Problems

1. Pneumonia.
2. Urinary tract infection.

Planning and Implementation

Goals may include improvement of mobility, attainment of independence in activities of daily living, achievement

P

of adequate bowel elimination, attainment and maintenance of satisfactory nutritional status, achievement of
communication, development of positive coping mechanisms, and absence of complications.

Interventions

IMPROVING MOBILITY

1. Progressive program of daily exercise to increase
   muscle strength, improve coordination and dexterity,
   reduce muscular rigidity, and prevent contractures.
2. Exercises for joint mobility, e.g., stationary bike,
   walking.
3. Teach to walk erect, watch horizon, and use a wide-
   based gait.
4. Postural exercises counter the tendency of the head
   and neck to be drawn forward and down.
5. Warm baths and massage to help relax muscles.

ENHANCING SELF-CARE ACTIVITIES

1. Teach activities of daily living.
2. Modify environment to compensate for functional
   disabilities.

IMPROVING BOWEL FUNCTION

1. Establish a regular bowel routine.
2. Increase fluid intake; eat foods with moderate fiber
   content.
3. Provide raised toilet seat to facilitate toilet activities.

IMPROVING NUTRITION

1. Facilitate swallowing and prevent aspiration by having patient sit in upright position during meal time.
2. Provide semisolid diet with thick liquids that are
   easier to swallow.
3. Remind patient to hold head upright and make conscious effort to swallow to control buildup of saliva.
4. Monitor weight on a weekly basis.

IMPROVING COMMUNICATION

1. Remind patient to face the listener.
2. Exaggerate pronunciation of words.
3. Speak in short sentences.
4. Take a few deep breaths before speaking.

SUPPORTING COPING ABILITIES

1. Maintain faithful adherence to an exercise and walking program.
2. Provide continuous encouragement and reassurance.
3. Assist and encourage to set achievable goals.
4. Encourage to carry out daily tasks to retain independence.

MONITORING AND MANAGING POTENTIAL COMPLICATIONS

1. Pneumonia: implement preventive measures for aspiration.
2. Urinary tract infection: encourage high fluid intake and regular pattern of voiding.

✎ PATIENT EDUCATION AND HEALTH MAINTENANCE: CARE IN THE HOME AND COMMUNITY

P

1. Explain the nature and management of the disease to offset anxieties and fears.
2. Recognize that the family is under stress from living with a disabled member.
3. Include caregiver in planning and counsel to learn stress-reduction techniques.
4. Provide family with information about treatment and care to prevent complications.
5. Encourage caregiver to obtain periodic relief from responsibilities and to have a yearly health assessment.
6. Give family members permission to express feelings of frustration, anger, and guilt.

For more information see Chapter 60 in Smeltzer and Bare: *Brunner and Suddarth's Textbook of Medical–Surgical Nursing,* 8th Edition. Philadelphia: Lippincott–Raven, 1996.

PE

See Pulmonary Edema, Acute

PELVIC INFECTION (PELVIC INFLAMMATORY DISEASE)

Pelvic infection is an inflammatory condition of the pelvic cavity that may involve the fallopian tubes, ovaries, pelvic peritoneum, or pelvic vascular system. Infection may be acute, subacute, recurrent, chronic, and may be localized or widespread. It is usually bacterial but may be caused by virus, fungus, or parasite. Pathogenic organisms usually enter the body through the vagina and pass through the cervical canal into the uterus. One of the most frequent causes of salpingitis is a chlamydia infection, possibly accompanied by gonorrhea. Chlamydial infection involves the cervix and extends upward, infecting the fallopian tubes or the uterus.

CLINICAL MANIFESTATIONS

1. Vaginal discharge, lower abdominal pelvic pain, and tenderness after menses; pain increases during voiding or defecating.
2. Systemic symptoms include fever, general malaise, anorexia, nausea, headache, and possibly vomiting.
3. Intense tenderness noted on pelvic examination.

MANAGEMENT

1. Broad-spectrum antibiotic therapy.
2. Mild to moderate infections are usually treated on an outpatient basis.

3. If acutely ill, patient may require hospitalization.
4. Once hospitalized: bed rest, IV fluids, IV antibiotic therapy are prescribed; nasogastric intubation and suction if ileus present; monitor vital signs.
5. Treatment of sexual partners is necessary to prevent reinfection.

Complications

1. Pelvic or generalized peritonitis, abscess formation, strictures, and obstruction of fallopian tubes.
2. Adhesions that eventually require removal of the uterus, tubes, and ovaries.
3. Bacteremia with septic shock and thrombophlebitis with possible embolization.

Nursing Interventions

1. Support patient nutritionally and administer antibiotic therapy as prescribed.
2. Note vital signs, nature and amount of vaginal discharge.
3. Prevent transmission of infection to others by impeccable use of universal precaution and hospital guidelines for disposing of contaminated articles (i.e., pad).

P

If Hospitalized

1. Maintain on bed rest.
2. Place in semi-Fowler's position to facilitate dependent drainage.
3. Apply heating pad to the abdomen for comfort.
4. Give warm douches as prescribed to improve local circulation.

✎ PATIENT EDUCATION AND HEALTH MAINTENANCE: CARE IN THE HOME AND COMMUNITY

Teach patients how to control and avoid PID, specifically:

1. Inform that intrauterine devices (IUDs) may increase risk for infection.

2. Use proper perineal care, wiping from front to back.
3. Avoid douching, which can reduce natural flora.
4. Consult with health care provider if unusual vaginal discharge or odor is noted.
5. Maintain optimal health with proper nutrition, exercise, weight control, and safer sex practices, i.e., using condoms, avoiding multiple sexual partners.
6. Have a gynecological exam at least once a year.
7. Evaluate any pelvic pain and/or abnormal discharge, particularly after sexual exposure, childbirth, or pelvic surgery.
8. Before and during intercourse, a partner should wear a condom if there is any chance of transmitting infection.
9. All patients who have had PID need information about signs and symptoms of ectopic pregnancy (pain, abnormal bleeding, faintness, dizziness, and shoulder pain).

For more information see Chapter 45 in Smeltzer and Bare: *Brunner and Suddarth's Textbook of Medical–Surgical Nursing,* 8th Edition. Philadelphia: Lippincott–Raven, 1996.

PEMPHIGUS VULGARIS

Pemphigus vulgaris is a serious disease of the skin characterized by appearance of bullae (blisters) on apparently normal skin and mucous membranes (mouth, vagina). Evidence indicates that pemphigus is an autoimmune disease involving IgG, an immunoglobulin. A blister forms from the antigen–antibody reaction. Genetic factors may also play a role, with the highest incidence in those of Jewish descent. It occurs with equal frequency in men and women in middle to old age.

CLINICAL MANIFESTATIONS

1. Most present with oral lesions appearing as irregularly shaped erosions that are painful, bleed easily, and heal slowly.

2. Skin bullae enlarge, rupture, and leave large painful eroded areas with crusting and oozing.
3. A characteristic offensive odor emanates from the bullae.
4. Blistering or sloughing of uninvolved skin occurs when minimal pressure is applied (Nikolsky's sign).
5. Eroded skin heals slowly and eventually huge areas of the body are involved.
6. Bacterial superinfection is common.

DIAGNOSTIC EVALUATION

Confirmed by histologic and immunofluorescent examination of skin biopsies, which show circulating pemphigus antibodies.

MANAGEMENT

Goals of therapy are to bring the disease under control as rapidly as possible, prevent loss of serum and development of secondary infection, and promote re-epithelialization of the skin.

1. Primary treatment: systemic, oral corticosteroids.
2. Adjunct therapy: immunosuppressive agents, e.g., azathioprine (Imuran), cyclophosphamide (Cytoxin).
3. Cure is not possible; control can be achieved.

NURSING PROCESS

Assessment

1. Monitor disease activity by examining skin for appearance of new blisters.
2. Assess for signs and symptoms of infection.

Major Nursing Diagnosis

1. Pain of oral cavity and skin related to blistering and erosions.
2. Impaired skin integrity related to ruptured bullae and denuded areas of the skin.

P

3. Anxiety and ineffective coping related to appearance of the skin and no hope of a cure.

Collaborative Problems

1. Infection and sepsis related to loss of protective barrier of skin and mucous membranes.
2. Fluid volume deficit and electrolyte imbalance related to loss of tissue fluids.

Planning and Implementation

The major goals may include relief of discomfort from lesions, skin healing, anxiety, improved coping capacity, and absence of complications.

Interventions

RELIEVING ORAL DISCOMFORT

1. Provide meticulous oral hygiene for cleanliness and regeneration of epithelium.
2. Provide frequent prescribed mouthwashes to rinse mouth of debris.
3. Avoid commercial mouthwashes.
4. Keep lips moist with lanolin, petrolatum, or lip balm.
5. Humidify environmental air.

ENHANCING SKIN INTEGRITY

1. Provide cool, wet dressings or baths (protective and soothing).
2. Premedicate with analgesics before skin care is initiated.
3. Dry patient's skin carefully and dust with nonirritating powder.
4. Avoid use of tape, which may produce more blisters.
5. Keep patient warm to avoid hypothermia.
6. Nursing management is similar to that of patients with extensive burns.

REDUCING ANXIETY

1. Demonstrate a warm and caring attitude; allow patient to express anxieties, discomfort, and feelings of hopelessness.
2. Educate patient and family regarding the disease.
3. Refer to psychologic counseling as needed.

MONITORING AND MANAGING POTENTIAL COMPLICATIONS: INFECTION AND SEPSIS

1. Keep skin clean to eliminate debris, dead skin, and prevent infection.
2. Inspect oral cavity for secondary infections and *Candida albicans* from high-dose steroid therapy.
3. Investigate all "trivial" complaints or minimal changes because corticosteroids mask typical symptoms of infection.
4. Monitor for chills; secretions and excretions are monitored for changes suggestive of infection.
5. Administer antimicrobials as prescribed and note response to treatment.
6. Employ effective handwashing techniques for health care personnel; use universal precautions.

ACHIEVING FLUID AND ELECTROLYTE BALANCE

P

1. Administer saline infusion for sodium chloride depletion.
2. Administer blood component therapy to maintain blood volume and hemoglobin and plasma protein concentrations if necessary.
3. Encourage adequate oral intake.
4. Monitor serum albumin and protein levels.
5. Provide cool, nonirritating fluids (grape or apple juice) for hydration; provide small, frequent feedings of high-protein, high-calorie foods.
6. Provide total parenteral nutrition if unable to eat.

PATIENT EDUCATION AND HEALTH MAINTENANCE: CARE IN THE HOME AND COMMUNITY

1. Disease is characterized by recurrent relapses that require continuing therapy.
2. Regular monitoring for side effects of cortisone is necessary.
3. Encourage patient to report for health-care follow-up regularly.

For more information see Chapter 54 in Smeltzer and Bare: *Brunner and Suddarth's Textbook of Medical–Surgical Nursing,* 8th Edition. Philadelphia: Lippincott–Raven, 1996.

PEPTIC ULCER

A peptic ulcer is an excavation formed in the mucosal wall of the stomach, pylorus, duodenum, or esophagus. It is frequently referred to as a gastric, duodenal, or esophageal ulcer, depending on its location. It is caused by the erosion of a circumscribed area of mucous membrane. Peptic ulcers are more likely to be in the duodenum than in the stomach. They tend to occur singly but there may be several present at one time. Chronic gastric ulcers usually occur in the lesser curvature of the stomach, near the pylorus. It is known that peptic ulcers only occur in the areas of the gastrointestinal tract that are exposed to hydrochloric acid and pepsin. More men than women are affected, but after menopause the incidence among women is almost equal to that in men. Other predisposing factors include family history of peptic ulcer, chronic use of nonsteroidal anti-inflammatory drugs (NSAIDs), alcohol ingestion, and excessive smoking. It has also been associated with bacterial infection such as *Helicobacter pylori.*

CLINICAL MANIFESTATIONS

Symptoms of duodenal ulcer (most common peptic ulcer) may last days, weeks, or months and may even disappear only to reappear without cause. Many persons have symptomless ulcers.

Pain

1. Dull, gnawing pain; burning sensation in the mide-pigastrium or in the back.
2. Pain relieved by eating or taking alkali; once the stomach has emptied or the alkali wears off, pain returns.
3. Sharply localized tenderness elicited by gentle pressure on the epigastrium or slightly right of the midline.

Pyrosis (Heartburn)

Burning sensation in the esophagus and stomach; sour eructation.

Vomiting

1. Rare in uncomplicated duodenal ulcer.
2. May or may not be preceded by nausea; usually follows a bout of severe pain; relieved by ejection of the acid gastric contents.

Constipation and Bleeding

1. As a result of diet and medications.
2. Some patients who bleed from acute ulcers have no previous digestive complaints, but develop symptoms later.

DIAGNOSTIC EVALUATION

Endoscopy, stool specimens for occult blood, gastric secretory studies, and biopsy and histology with culture to determine presence of *H. pylori* (there is also a breath test for *H. pylori*).

P

MANAGEMENT

The goal is to manage gastric acidity.

Stress Reduction and Rest

1. Help patient identify situations that are stressful or exhausting, e.g., rushed lifestyle and irregular schedules.
2. Patient may benefit from suggestions regarding regular rest periods during the day, during acute phase of the disease.
3. Biofeedback, hypnosis, or behavioral modification.

Smoking

1. Acidity of the duodenum is higher with smoking.
2. Cigarette smoking significantly inhibits ulcer repair.
3. Strongly encourage to stop smoking; support groups are helpful.

Diet

1. Encourage patients to eat whatever agrees with them; little evidence to support the theory that bland diets are beneficial.
2. Minimize oversecretion and hypermotility of the GI tract by avoiding extremes of temperature and over-stimulation by meat extracts, alcohol, and coffee (including decaffeinated coffee, which stimulates acid secretion).
3. Eat three regular meals a day.
4. Avoid diets rich in milk and cream because they are potent acid stimulators.

Medications

1. H_2 receptor antagonist (decrease acid secretion in stomach).
2. Cytoprotective agents (protect mucosal cells from acid of NSAID).
3. Antacids.
4. Anticholinergics (inhibit acid secretion).

5. Combination of antibiotics with bismuth salts (suppress *H. pylori* bacteria).

Duration of Treatment

1. Patient should adhere to the drug program to ensure complete healing of the ulcer.
2. Maintenance doses of H_2 receptor antagonists are usually recommended for 1 year.

Surgical Intervention

1. With the advent of H_2 receptor antagonists, surgical intervention is less common.
2. Surgery is recommended for intractable ulcers, life-threatening hemorrhage, perforation, or obstruction.
3. Surgical procedures include vagotomy, vagotomy with pyloroplasty, or Billroth I or II.

NURSING PROCESS

Assessment

1. Assess patient's pain and methods used to relieve it; take a thorough history.
2. Question whether patient has vomited. Is emesis bright red or coffee ground in appearance?
3. Presence of blood in the stools? Test for occult blood.
4. Usual food habits; smoking; level of tension or nervousness?
5. How does the patient express anger (especially at work and family)?
6. Is there occupational stress or problems in the family?
7. Family history of ulcer disease.
8. Assess vital signs for indicators of anemia (tachycardia, hypotension).
9. Palpate abdomen for localized tenderness.

P

Major Nursing Diagnosis

1. Pain, related to the effect of gastric acid secretion on damaged tissue.
2. Anxiety related to coping with an acute disease.
3. Knowledge and deficit about prevention of symptoms and management of the condition.

Collaborative Problems

1. Hemorrhage: upper gastrointestinal.
2. Perforation.
3. Pyloric obstruction (gastric outlet obstruction).

Planning and Implementation

The major goals may include relief of pain, reduction of anxiety, acquisition of knowledge about management and prevention of ulcer recurrence, and absence of potential complications.

Interventions

RELIEVING PAIN

1. Administer prescribed medications.
2. Avoid aspirin and foods and beverages that contain caffeine (colas, tea, coffee, chocolate).
3. Encourage regularly spaced meals in a relaxed atmosphere.
4. Encourage relaxation techniques and assist to cope with stress and pain and stop smoking.

REDUCING ANXIETY

1. Assess what the patient wants to know about the disease and evaluate level of anxiety; encourage to express fears openly and without criticism.
2. Explain diagnostic tests; administer medications on schedule.
3. Assure patient that nurses are always available to help with problems.
4. Interact in a relaxing manner, help in identifying stressors, and explain effective coping techniques and relaxation methods.

5. Encourage participation of the patient's family in care and give emotional support.

✎ PATIENT EDUCATION AND HEALTH MAINTENANCE: CARE IN THE HOME AND COMMUNITY

Assist the patient in understanding the condition and factors that help or aggravate.

Medication

1. Teach patient what medications are taken at home, including name, dosage, frequency, and possible side effects.
2. Teach patient what drugs to avoid.

Diet

1. Teach patient to be aware of particular foods that are upsetting.
2. Teach to avoid coffee, tea, colas, and alcohol, which have acid-producing potential.
3. Encourage regular meals in a relaxed setting and to avoid overeating.

Smoking

1. Teach patient that smoking may interfere with ulcer healing.
2. Make aware of programs to assist with smoking cessation.

Rest and Stress Reduction

1. Help patient to be aware of sources of stress in family and work environments.
2. Help to identify rest periods during the day.
3. Evaluate need for extended psychological counseling.

Awareness of Complications

Alert patient to signs and symptoms of complications that should be reported.

P

1. Hemorrhage: cool skin, confusion, increased heart rate, labored breathing, blood in stool.
2. Perforation: severe abdominal pain, rigid and tender abdomen, vomiting, elevated temperature, increased heart rate.
3. Pyloric obstruction: nausea, vomiting, distended abdomen, abdominal pain.

Posttreatment Care

1. Teach patient that follow-up supervision is necessary for about 1 year.
2. Teach that the ulcer could recur and to seek medical assistance if symptoms recur.
3. Inform patient and family that surgery is no guarantee of cure.
4. Discuss possible postoperative sequelae, i.e., intolerance to dairy products and sweet foods.

For more information see Chapter 36 in Smeltzer and Bare: *Brunner and Suddarth's Textbook of Medical–Surgical Nursing,* 8th Edition. Philadelphia: Lippincott–Raven, 1996.

PERICARDITIS

Pericarditis refers to an inflammation of the pericardium, the membranous sac enveloping the heart. It may be primary, or develop in the course of a variety of medical and surgical diseases. Some causes include idiopathic, infection (bacterial, viral, or fungal), connective tissue disorders, hypersensitivity states, diseases of adjacent structures, neoplastic disease, radiation therapy, trauma, renal disorder association, and tuberculosis.

CLINICAL MANIFESTATIONS

Often no signs other than fever and production of friction rub.

1. Pain over the precordium or may also be felt beneath the clavicle and in the neck and left scapular region.

2. Pericardial pain is aggravated by breathing, turning in bed, and twisting body.
4. Pain relieved by sitting up.
5. Dyspnea may occur as a result of pericardial compression of the heart's movements.

DIAGNOSTIC EVALUATION

Signs and symptoms and ECG.

MANAGEMENT

The objectives of management are to determine the cause, to administer therapy for the specific cause (when known), and to watch for cardiac tamponade (compression of the heart from fluid in the pericardial sac).

1. Bed rest when cardiac output is impaired, until fever, chest pain, and friction rub have disappeared.
2. Narcotic analgesics for pain relief during the acute phase.
3. Salicylates to relieve pain and hasten reabsorption of fluid in rheumatic pericarditis.
4. Corticosteroids to control symptoms, hasten resolution of the inflammatory process, and prevent recurring pericardial effusion.
5. Penicillin for pericarditis of rheumatic fever.
6. Isoniazid ethambutol, rifampin, and streptomycin for pericarditis of tuberculosis.
7. Amphotericin B for fungal pericarditis.
8. Adrenal steroids for pericarditis from lupus erythematosus.
9. Increase activity gradually as condition improves.

P

NURSING PROCESS

Assessment

1. Assess pain by observation and evaluation while having patient vary positions.
2. Monitor temperature frequently; pericarditis will cause an abrupt onset in a previously afebrile patient.

ASSESSING PERICARDIAL FRICTION RUB

1. Audible on auscultation.
2. Synchronous with the heartbeat.
3. Best heard at the left sternal edge in the fourth intercostal space where the pericardium comes into contact with the left chest wall.
4. Has a scratchy or leathery sound.
5. The rub is louder at the end of expiration and may be best heard in sitting position.
6. Note that a pericardial friction rub is continuous, distinguishing it from a pleural friction rub.

Major Nursing Diagnosis

Pain related to inflammation of the pericardium.

Collaborative Problems

1. Pericardial effusion.
2. Cardiac tamponade.

Planning and Implementation

The major goals may include relief of pain and maintenance and absence of potential complications.

Interventions

RELIEVING PAIN

1. Bed rest or chair rest in a sitting upright and leaning forward position.
2. Resume activities of daily living as the chest pain and friction rub abate.
3. Administer medications; monitor and record response.
4. Resume bed rest if chest pain and friction rub recur.

MONITORING AND MANAGING POTENTIAL COMPLICATIONS

1. Observe for cardiac tamponade indicated by falling arterial pressure; systolic pressure falls while diastolic pressure remains stable; pulse pressure narrows; heart sounds progress from being distant to imperceptible.

2. Observe for neck vein distention and other signs of rising central venous pressure.
3. Notify physician immediately upon observing any of the above symptoms.

PREPARING FOR PERICARDIOCENTESIS

Assure patient and continue to assess and record signs and symptoms.

For more information see Chapter 29 in Smeltzer and Bare: *Brunner and Suddarth's Textbook of Medical–Surgical Nursing*, 8th Edition. Philadelphia: Lippincott–Raven, 1996.

PERICARDITIS, CHRONIC CONSTRICTIVE

Chronic constrictive pericarditis is inflammatory thickening of the pericardium that compresses the heart and prevents it from expanding to normal size. It is caused by longstanding pyogenic infections, postviral infections, tuberculosis, or hemopericardium. Signs and symptoms are predominantly those of congestive heart failure. Dyspnea on exertion is the most prominent symptom. Chronic atrial fibrillation is commonly present. Surgical removal of the tough encasing pericardium (pericardiectomy) is the only treatment of any benefit. The objective of the operation is to release those ventricles from the constrictive and restrictive inflammation.

P

PERIPHERAL ARTERIAL OCCLUSIVE DISEASE

Arterial insufficiency of the extremities is usually found in individuals over 50 years of age, most often in men, and predominantly in the legs. The age of onset and severity is influenced by the type and number of atherosclerotic risk factors present. Obstructive lesions are predominantly confined to segments of the arterial system extending from the aorta, below the renal arteries, to the popliteal artery.

CLINICAL MANIFESTATIONS

Intermittent Claudication

1. Insidious and described as aching, cramping, fatigue, or weakness.
2. Rest pain is persistent, aching, or boring and is usually present in distal extremities.
3. Elevation or horizontal placement of the extremity will aggravate the pain; dependency of the extremity will reduce pain.

Other Manifestations

1. Coldness or numbness in the extremities accompanying intermittent claudication.
2. Extremities may be cool and exhibit pallor on elevation or a ruddy, cyanotic color when in a dependent position.
3. Skin and nail changes, ulcerations, gangrene, and muscle atrophy are present.
4. Bruits may be auscultated.
5. Peripheral pulses may be diminished or absent.
6. Inequality of pulses between extremities or absence of a normally palpable pulse is a reliable sign of occlusion.
7. Nails may be thickened and opaque, and the skin shiny, atrophic, and dry with sparse hair growth.

DIAGNOSTIC EVALUATION

1. Doppler ultrasonic flow studies, angiography, digital subtraction angiography (DSA).
2. Oscillometry, exercise test, plethysmography, lumbar sympathetic block.

MANAGEMENT

1. Maintain meticulous cleanliness of the feet; wash feet daily, dry carefully, and do not rub with a towel.

2. Keep feet warm; protect feet from injury.
3. Wear shoes that provide adequate comfort.
4. Prevent constriction of blood vessels: do not cross legs; avoid any activity that cuts off blood supply to legs and feet.
5. Promote exercise to stimulate circulation and tissue repair.
6. Report redness, blistering, swelling, pain, any peeling or itching.
7. Avoid tobacco in any form, since it aggravates peripheral vascular circulation.
8. Exercise programs combined with weight reduction and cessation of smoking often improve patient activity limitations.
9. Sympathectomy to improve collateral circulation.
10. Vascular grafting or endarterectomy when the limb is at risk for amputation.
11. Percutaneous transluminal angioplasty (PTA) for stenosis or occlusion of the vessel.

POSTOPERATIVE NURSING MANAGEMENT

The primary objective in postoperative management of patients who have had vascular procedures is to maintain adequate circulation through the arterial repair.

P

1. Check pulses of affected extremity and compare with other.
2. Disappearance of a pulse may indicate thrombotic occlusion of the graft; notify surgeon immediately.
3. Monitor color and temperature of extremity and report changes.
4. Monitor urine output, mental status, and pulse rate to permit early recognition and treatment of fluid imbalances.
5. Avoid leg crossing and prolonged extremity dependence.
6. Leg elevation to reduce edema.

For more information see Chapter 31 in Smeltzer and Bare: *Brunner and Suddarth's Textbook of Medical–Surgical Nursing*, 8th Edition. Philadelphia: Lippincott–Raven, 1996.

PERIPHERAL VEINOUS DISEASE

See Vein Disorders

PERITONITIS

Peritonitis is inflammation of the peritoneum. Usually the result of bacterial infection, the organisms coming from disease of the gastrointestinal tract or, in women, the internal reproductive organs. It can also result from external sources such as injury or trauma or an inflammation from an extraperitoneal organ, such as the kidney. The most common bacterial implicated are *Escherichia coli, Klebsiella, Proteus,* and *Pseudomonas.* Other common causes are appendicitis, perforated ulcer, diverticulitis, and bowel perforation. Peritonitis may also be associated with abdominal surgical procedures.

CLINICAL MANIFESTATIONS

Depend on location and extent of inflammation.
1. Diffuse type of pain that becomes constant, localized, and more intense near site of the process.
2. Pain is aggravated by movement.
3. Affected area of the abdomen becomes extremely tender and muscles become rigid.
4. Rebound tenderness and ileus may be present.
5. Temperature and pulse increase; leukocyte count is elevated.

MANAGEMENT

1. Fluid, colloid, and electrolyte replacement is the major focus of medical management.
2. Analgesics for pain; antiemetics for nausea and vomiting.
3. Intestinal intubation and suction to relieve abdominal distention.

4. Oxygen therapy by nasal cannula or mask to improve ventilatory function.
5. Occasionally airway intubation and ventilatory assistance may be required.
6. Massive antibiotic therapy (sepsis is the major cause of death).
7. Surgical objectives include removal of infected material and are directed toward excision, resection, repair, and drainage.
8. Postoperative complications: wound evisceration and abscess.

Nursing Interventions

PERFORMING PAIN ASSESSMENT

1. Assess nature of pain, location in the abdomen, and shifts of pain.
2. Assess vital signs, gastrointestinal function, fluid and electrolyte balance.
3. Administer analgesic medication and position for comfort, i.e., on side with knees flexed.
4. Record intake and output and central venous pressure.
5. Administer and monitor intravenous fluids closely.
6. Observe and record character of any surgical drainage.
7. Observe for decrease in temperature and pulse rate, softening of the abdomen, return of peristaltic sounds, and passing of flatus and bowel movements, which indicate peritonitis is subsiding.
8. Increase food and oral fluids gradually when peritonitis subsides.
9. Observe and record character of drainage from postoperative wound drains if inserted; take care to avoid dislodging drains.
10. Postoperatively, prepare patient and family for discharge; teach care for incision and drains if still in place at discharge.

P

For more information see Chapter 37 in Smeltzer and Bare: *Brunner and Suddarth's Textbook of Medical–Surgical Nursing,* 8th Edition. Philadelphia: Lippincott–Raven, 1996.

PERNICIOUS ANEMIA

See Anemia, Megaloblastic

PHARYNGITIS, ACUTE

Acute pharyngitis (strep throat) is a febrile inflammation caused by a viral organism 70% of the time. Uncomplicated viral infections usually subside promptly within 3 to 10 days after onset. When caused by a bacteria, the most common organism is group A streptococcus. Pharyngitis caused by bacteria is a more severe illness because of dangerous complications, i.e., sinusitis, otitis media, mastoiditis, cervical adenitis, rheumatic fever, and nephritis.

CLINICAL MANIFESTATIONS

1. Fiery, red pharyngeal membrane.
2. Tonsils and lymphoid follicles are swollen and freckled with exudate.
3. Cervical lymph nodes are enlarged and tender.
4. Fever, malaise, and sore throat may be present.
5. Hoarseness, cough, and rhinitis are not uncommon.

DIAGNOSTIC EVALUATION

Throat culture.

MANAGEMENT

1. Antimicrobial agents for bacterial cause: penicillin for group A streptococci and cephalosporins for penicillin allergies or erythromycin resistance.

2. Antibiotics are administered for at least 10 days.
3. Give liquid or soft diet during the acute stage.
4. IV fluids administered if unable to swallow due to sore throat.
5. Encourage to drink if able to swallow (2500 ml each day).

Nursing Interventions

1. Encourage bed rest during febrile stage of illness.
2. Implement secretion precautions to prevent spread of infection.
3. Examine skin once or twice daily for possible rash because acute pharyngitis may precede some other communicable disease.
4. Secure nasal swabbings; throat and blood cultures as needed.
5. Administer warm saline gargles or irrigations to ease pain.
6. Apply ice collar for symptomatic relief.
7. Administer analgesic drugs or antitussive medications.
8. Perform mouth care to prevent fissures of lips and inflammation in the mouth.

P

✎ PATIENT EDUCATION AND HEALTH MAINTENANCE: CARE IN THE HOME AND COMMUNITY

1. Permit resumption of activity gradually.
2. Advise of importance of taking full course of antibiotic therapy.
3. Inform patient and family of possible development of complications, i.e., nephritis and rheumatic fever; onset 2 or 3 weeks after pharyngitis has subsided.
4. Inform patient and family of other potential complications, i.e., peritonsillar abscess, sinusitis, otitis media, mastoiditis, or cervical adenitis.
5. Inform about symptoms to watch for that indicate complications.

For more information see Chapter 23 in Smeltzer and Bare: *Brunner and Suddarth's Textbook of Medical–Surgical Nursing,* 8th Edition. Philadelphia: Lippincott–Raven, 1996.

PHARYNGITIS, CHRONIC

Chronic pharyngitis is common in adults who work or live in dusty surroundings, use the voice to excess, suffer from chronic cough, and habitually use alcohol and tobacco. Three types are recognized: hypertrophic, a general thickening and congestion of the pharyngeal mucous membranes; atrophic, a late stage of type 1; and chronic granular ("clergyman's sore throat"), with numerous swollen lymph follicles of the pharyngeal wall.

CLINICAL MANIFESTATIONS

1. Constant sense of irritation or fullness in the throat.
2. Mucus, which collects in the throat and is expelled by coughing.
3. Difficulty in swallowing.

MANAGEMENT

Treatment is based on symptom relief, avoidance of exposure to irritants, and correction of any upper respiratory, pulmonary, or cardiac condition that might be responsible for chronic cough.

1. Nasal installations or sprays to relieve nasal congestion.
2. Aspirin or acetaminophen to control malaise.
3. Avoid contact with others until fever has subsided completely to prevent infection from spreading.

Nursing Interventions

1. Instruct to avoid the use of alcohol, tobacco, secondhand smoke, and exposure to cold.
2. Avoid environmental/occupational pollutants or minimize through use of disposable masks.

3. Encourage to drink plenty of fluids.
4. Encourage gargling with warm saline to relieve throat discomfort; lozenges to keep the throat moist.

For more information see Chapter 23 in Smeltzer and Bare: *Brunner and Suddarth's Textbook of Medical–Surgical Nursing,* 8th Edition. Philadelphia: Lippincott–Raven, 1996.

PHEOCHROMOCYTOMA

A pheochromocytoma is a tumor that usually is benign and originates from the chromaffin cells of the adrenal medulla. In 80–90% of patients, the tumor arises in the medulla; in the remaining patients it occurs in the extra-adrenal chromaffin tissue located in or near the aorta, ovaries, spleen, or other organs. It occurs at any age, but peak incidence is between 25 and 50 years of age; affects men and women equally, and has familial tendencies. Although uncommon, it is one form of hypertension that is usually cured by surgery; without detection and treatment, it is usually fatal.

CLINICAL MANIFESTATIONS

P

Classic Symptoms

1. Headache.
2. Diaphoresis.
3. Palpitations.
4. Blood pressures as high as 350/200 mmHg.
5. May precipitate life-threatening complications: cardiac dysrhythmias, dissecting aneurysm, stroke, and acute renal failure.
6. Postural hypotension occurs in most untreated cases.

Other Symptoms

1. Tremor.
2. Flushing.

3. Anxiety.
4. Hyperglycemia from epinephrine secretion; insulin may be required.

Symptoms of the Paroxysmal Form of Pheochromocytoma

1. Acute, unpredictable attacks, lasting seconds or several hours, during which patient is extremely anxious, tremulous, and weak.
2. May experience headache, vertigo, blurring of vision, tinnitus, air hunger, and dyspnea.
3. Polyuria, nausea, vomiting, diarrhea, and abdominal pain, and feeling of impending doom evident.
4. Palpitations and tachycardia.

DIAGNOSTIC EVALUATION

Catecholamines in urine (metanephrines [MN] and vanillylmandelic acid [VMA]) and plasma (norepinephrine and epinephrine) offer the most direct and conclusive test.

MANAGEMENT

Nursing Managment

1. Bed rest, head of bed elevated to promote orthostatic decrease in blood pressure.
2. Monitor ECG changes.
3. Careful administration of alpha-adrenergic blocking agents (phentolamine [Regitine]) or smooth muscle relaxants (sodium nitroprusside [Nipride]) to lower blood pressure.

Surgical Mangement

Treatment is surgical removal of the tumor, usually with adrenalectomy. Hypertension usually subsides with treatment.

1. Preliminary preparation includes effective control of blood pressure and blood volume, carried out over 10 days to 2 weeks.

2. Hydrate patient prior to, during, and after surgery.
3. Postoperative corticosteroid replacement required after bilateral adrenalectomy.
4. Patient will be monitored for several days in the Intensive Care Unit with attention given to ECG changes, arterial pressures, fluid and electrolyte balance, and blood glucose levels.
5. Monitor blood pressure. Hypertension can persist or recur if blood vessels have been damaged or if all pheochromocytoma tissue has not been removed.
6. Measure postoperative urine and plasma levels of catecholamines; when levels return to normal, patient may be discharged.

✎ PATIENT EDUCATION AND HEALTH MAINTENANCE: CARE IN THE HOME AND COMMUNITY

1. Encourage patient to schedule follow-up appointments to observe for return of normal blood pressure and serum and urine levels of catecholamines.
2. Give verbal and written instructions on collecting 24-hour urine specimen.
3. Give instructions regarding long-term steroid therapy.
4. Assess compliance to the medication schedule.
5. Assist in dealing with problems that may result from long-term steroid use.
6. Give encouragement and support because patient may remain fearful of repeated attacks.

P

For more information see Chapter 40 in Smeltzer and Bare: *Brunner and Suddarth's Textbook of Medical–Surgical Nursing,* 8th Edition. Philadelphia: Lippincott–Raven, 1996.

PHLEBITIS

See Vein Disorders

PID

See Pelvic Inflammatory Disease

PITUITARY TUMORS

Pituitary tumors are three principle types, representing an overgrowth of eosinophilic cells, basophilic cells, or chromophobic cells (cells with no affinity for either eosinophilic or basophilic stains).

CLINICAL MANIFESTATIONS: EOSINOPHILIC TUMORS

Eosinophilic Tumors Developing Early in Life

1. Gigantism.
2. May be over 7 feet tall and large in all proportions.
3. Weak and lethargic, hardly able to stand.

Eosinophilic Tumors Developing in Adulthood

1. Acromegaly (excessive skeletal growth occurs of the feet, hands, superciliary ridges, molar eminences, nose, and chin).
2. Enlargement of every tissue and organ of the body.
3. Many suffer from severe headaches and visual disturbances because the tumors exert pressure on the optic nerves.
4. May have loss of color discrimination, diplopia (double vision), or blindness of a portion of the field of vision.
5. Decalcification of the skeleton, muscular weakness, and endocrine disturbances, similar to those occurring in hyperthyroidism.

CLINICAL MANIFESTATIONS: BASOPHILIC TUMORS

Cushing's Syndrome

1. Masculinization and amenorrhea in females.
2. Truncal obesity, hypertension, osteoporosis, and polycythemia in males and females.

CLINICAL MANIFESTATIONS: CHROMOPHOBIC TUMORS

Hypopituitarism

1. Inclined to be obese and somnolent.
2. Fine, scanty hair; dry, soft skin; pasty complexion; and small bones.
3. Headaches, loss of libido, and visual defects progressing to blindness.
4. Polyuria, polyphagia, lowering of the basal metabolic rate, and subnormal body temperature.

DIAGNOSTIC EVALUATION

CT scan and MRI.

MANAGEMENT OF ACROMEGALY OR PITUITARY TUMORS

P

1. Surgical removal through a transphenoidal approach is the treatment of choice.
2. Stereotactic radiotherapy to deliver an external beam radiotherapy to the tumor with minimal effect on normal tissue.
3. Radiation therapy and use of bromocriptine (dopamine agonist) and actreotide (somatostatin analogue) inhibit production or release of growth hormone.
4. Hypophysectomy for treatment of primary tumors.

For more information see Chapter 40 in Smeltzer and Bare: *Brunner and Suddarth's Textbook of Medical–Surgical Nursing,* 8th Edition. Philadelphia: Lippincott–Raven, 1996.

PLEURAL EFFUSION

Pleural effusion, a collection of fluid in the pleural space, is rarely a primary disease process but is usually secondary to other diseases. The effusion can be relatively clear fluid, which may be a transudate, an exudate, or it can be blood or pus.

CLINICAL MANIFESTATIONS

Some symptoms are caused by the underlying disease. Pneumonia will cause fever, chills, and pleuritic chest pain. Malignant effusion may result in dyspnea and coughing. The size of effusion will determine the severity of symptoms.

1. Large effusion: shortness of breath, dullness or flatness to percussion over areas of fluid, minimal or absence of breath sounds, and tracheal deviation away from the affected side.
2. Small to moderate effusion: dyspnea may not be present.

DIAGNOSTIC EVALUATION

1. Chest films.
2. Ultrasound.
3. Thoracentesis.
4. Pleural fluid cultures.

MANAGEMENT

The objectives of treatment are to discover the underlying cause to prevent reaccumulation of fluid, and to relieve discomfort and dyspnea. Specific treatment is directed to the underlying cause.

1. Thoracentesis is performed to remove fluid, collect specimen for analysis, and relieve dyspnea.
2. Chest tube and water-seal drainage may be necessary for pneumothorax (sometimes the result of repeated thoracentesis).

3. Drugs instilled into the pleural space to obliterate the space and prevent further accumulation of fluid.
4. Other treatment modalities: radiation of chest wall, surgical pleurectomy, and diuretic therapy.

NURSING INTERVENTIONS

1. Implement the medical regimen. (a) Prepare and position patient for thoracentesis. (b) Offer support throughout the procedure.
2. Assist patient in pain relief. (a) Assist patient to assume positions that are least painful. (b) Administer pain medication as prescribed and needed.
3. Monitor chest tube drainage and water-seal system; record amount of drainage at prescribed intervals.
4. Administer nursing care related to the underlying cause of the pleural effusion.

For more information see Chapter 24 in Smeltzer and Bare: *Brunner and Suddarth's Textbook of Medical–Surgical Nursing,* 8th Edition. Philadelphia: Lippincott–Raven, 1996.

PLEURISY

Pleurisy refers to inflammation of both the visceral and parietal pleurae. The result is severe, sharp, knifelike pain upon inspiration. Pleurisy may develop with pneumonia or upper respiratory tract infection, tuberculosis, a collagen disease; after chest trauma, pulmonary infarction, or embolism; in primary and metastatic cancer; and after thoracotomy.

DIAGNOSTIC EVALUATION

1. Chest films.
2. Sputum culture.
3. Thoracentesis.
4. Pleural fluid exam.

MANAGEMENT

The objectives of management are to discover the underlying condition causing the pleurisy and to relieve the pain.

1. Monitor for signs and symptoms of pleural effusion, i.e., shortness of breath, pain, and decreased excursion of the chest.
2. Administer prescribed analgesics and applications of heat or cold for symptomatic relief.
3. Nonsteroidal anti-inflammatory drugs for pain relief and effective coughing.
4. Procaine intercostal block for severe pain.

NURSING INTERVENTIONS

1. Enhance comfort by turning frequently on affected side to splint chest wall.
2. Teach patient to use hands to splint rib cage while coughing.
3. Provide emotional support and understanding.

For more information see Chapter 24 in Smeltzer and Bare: *Brunner and Suddarth's Textbook of Medical–Surgical Nursing,* 8th Edition. Philadelphia: Lippincott–Raven, 1996.

PNEUMONIA

Pneumonia is an inflammatory process of the lung parenchyma commonly caused by infectious agents. It is classified according to its causative agent. The two major categories are bacterial and atypical. It may also be caused by radiation therapy, ingestion of chemicals, and aspiration. Lobar pneumonia presents as consolidation in one or more lobes. Bronchopneumonia presents as diffuse patches and is more common. Those at risk for pneumonia often have prolonged debilitating diseases, a suppressed immune system from disease or medications, immobility, and other factors that interfere with normal lung drainage. The elderly are also at high risk. Nosocomial pneumonias are caused by *Staphylococcus aureus,* and enteric gram-negative bacilli and fungi. Other pneumonias are caused by *Streptococcus pneumoniae* and viruses.

CLINICAL MANIFESTATIONS: BACTERIAL

1. Sudden chills, rapidly rising fever and profuse perspiration.
2. Stabbing chest pain aggravated by respiration and coughing.
3. Severely ill with marked tachypnea (25–45/min) and dyspnea.
4. Pulse rapid and bounding.
5. A relative bradycardia for the amount of fever suggests viral infection, Mycoplasma infection, or Legionella species.
6. Sputum is purulent, rusty, blood-tinged, viscous, or green relative to etiologic agent.
7. Other signs: fever, crackles, and signs of lobar consolidation.

DIAGNOSTIC EVALUATION

Primarily chest films, blood and sputum cultures.

MANAGEMENT

1. Penicillin G is the antibiotic of choice.
2. Bed rest until infection shows sign of clearing.
3. Oxygen for hypoxemia, arterial blood gases (ABGs).
4. Respiratory support: endotracheal intubation, high inspiratory oxygen concentrations, and mechanical ventilation and positive end expiratory pressure (PEEP).

NURSING PROCESS

Assessment

1. Assess for pain, tachypnea, use of accessory muscles, rapid, bounding pulse, coughing, purulent sputum, and auscultate breath sounds for consolidation.

2. Note changes in temperature and color of secretions.
3. Assess for restlessness and excited delirium in alcoholism.
4. Assess for complications, i.e., continuing or recurring fever, failure to resolve, atelectasis, pleural effusion, cardiac complications, and superinfection.

Major Nursing Diagnosis

1. Ineffective airway clearance related to copious tracheobronchial secretions.
2. Risk for fluid volume deficit related to fever and dyspnea.
3. Knowledge deficit about the treatment regimen and preventive health measures.

Planning and Implementation

The major goals may include improvement of airway patency, obtaining enough rest to conserve energy, maintenance of proper fluid volume, and an understanding of the treatment protocol and preventive measures.

Interventions

IMPROVING AIRWAY PATENCY

1. Encourage high fluid intake (2–3 L/day) to loosen secretions.
2. Provide humidified air, i.e., high-humidity face mask.
3. Encourage to cough and provide chest physiotherapy.
4. Provide nasotracheal suctioning if necessary.
5. Provide appropriate method of oxygen therapy.
6. Monitor effectiveness of oxygen therapy.

PROMOTING FLUID INTAKE

Encourage at least 2–3 liters of fluid per day.

✎ Patient Education and Health Maintenance: Care in the Home and Community

1. Advise to gradually increase activities after fever subsides.
2. Advise that fatigue, weakness, and depression may linger after pneumonia.
3. Encourage breathing exercises to promote expansion and clearing.
4. Encourage follow-up for chest x-rays.
5. Encourage to stop smoking.
6. Instruct to avoid fatigue, sudden changes in temperature, and excessive alcohol intake, which lower resistance to pneumonia.
7. Review principles of adequate nutrition and rest.
8. Recommend influenza vaccine to all patients at risk (elderly, cardiac and pulmonary disease patients).

✿ Gerontologic Considerations

In older patients, or those with COPD, symptoms may develop insidiously. Classic symptoms of cough, chest pain, sputum production, and fever are often absent. Purulent sputum may be the only sign of pneumonia.

Pneumonia may also occur spontaneously or as a complication of a chronic disease. Onset of pneumonia may be signaled by general deterioration, confusion, tachycardia, and increased respiratory rate.

Pulmonary infections are difficult to treat and associated with a higher mortality than in younger patients. Presence of some signs may be misleading; chest radiography may be performed to assist in differentiating diagnosis.

Supportive treatment includes increased fluid intake (with caution regarding fluid overload); oxygen therapy; assistance with deep breathing, coughing, sputum production, and position changes.

Assess the elderly patient for alterations in mental status, prostration, and congestive heart failure.

Vaccination against pneumococcal and influenzae viral infections is recommended for persons over 50 years, nursing home residents, debilitated patients, and those with cardiovascular disease.

PNEUMONIA, ATYPICAL SYNDROMES

Mycoplasmas, fungus, Q fever, Legionnaires' disease, and viruses are included in the atypical pneumonia syndromes. *Mycoplasma pneumoniae* is the most common. It occurs most frequently in older children and young adults and is spread by infected respiratory droplets through person-to-person contact. Patients can be tested for mycoplasma antibodies. It generally has the characteristics of bronchopneumonia.

For more information see Chapter 24 in Smeltzer and Bare: *Brunner and Suddarth's Textbook of Medical–Surgical Nursing,* 8th Edition. Philadelphia: Lippincott–Raven, 1996.

PNEUMOTHORAX AND HEMOTHORAX

Severe chest injuries usually are accompanied by the collection of blood in the chest cavity (hemothorax) because of torn intercostal vessels, laceration of the lungs, or escape of air from the injured lung into the pleural cavity (pneumothorax). Often, both blood and air are found in the chest cavity (hemopneumothorax). Chest injury compresses lung tissue, resulting in interference with normal function.

MANAGEMENT

The goal is evacuation of air or blood from the pleural space while maintaining fluid balance.

1. A large-diameter chest tube is inserted usually in the fourth through sixth intercostal space for hemothorax.

2. A small chest tube is inserted near the second inter-costal space for a pneumothorax.
3. Autotransfusion, if excessive bleeding from chest tube.

TENSION PNEUMOTHORAX

A tension pneumothorax is a life-threatening medical emergency. Air is drawn into the pleural space from the lacerated lung or through a small hole in the chest wall. Air that enters the pleural space is trapped there. A tension (pressure) is built up, producing a collapse of the lung and a shift of the heart and great vessels and trachea toward the unaffected side of the chest.

CLINICAL MANIFESTATIONS

1. Air hunger and agitation.
2. Hypotension, tachycardia, profuse diuresis, and cyanosis.

MANAGEMENT

1. High concentration of oxygen to treat hypoxia.
2. Convert to simple pneumothorax by insertion of a large-bore needle into the pleural space to relieve pressure.
3. Chest tube inserted to remove remaining air and fluid.

P

OPEN PNEUMOTHORAX

Open pneumothorax is an opening in the chest wall large enough to allow air to pass freely in and out of the thoracic cavity with each respiration (sucking wounds). The lung is collapsed; the heart and great vessels are shifted toward the uninjured side with each inspiration and in the opposite direction with expiration (mediastinal flutter).

MANAGEMENT

Emergency Interventions: Stopping the Flow of Air Through the Opening in the Chest Wall

1. Use anything large enough to fill the hole (towel, handkerchief, heel of hand).
2. Have patient inhale and strain against a closed glottis if conscious.
3. When possible, the opening is plugged by sealing with petroleum-impregnated gauze.
4. Apply pressure dressing by circumferential strapping.

Medical Interventions

1. Chest tube to water seal drainage for exit of air and fluid.
2. Antibiotics to combat infection from contamination

For more information see Chapter 24 in Smeltzer and Bare: *Brunner and Suddarth's Textbook of Medical–Surgical Nursing,* 8th Edition. Philadelphia: Lippincott–Raven, 1996.

POLYCYTHEMIA

Polycythemia refers to an increased concentration of red cells. The red cell count is greater than 6 million/mm^3 or the hemoglobin exceeds 18 g/dl.

SECONDARY POLYCYTHEMIA

Secondary polycythemia is caused by excessive production of erythropoietin. This may occur in response to a hypoxic stimulus, as in chronic obstructive pulmonary disease or cyanotic heart disease, or in certain hemoglobinopathies in which the hemoglobin has an abnormally high affinity for oxygen. Management of secondary polycythemia involves treatment of the primary problem.

If the cause cannot be corrected, phlebotomy may be necessary to reduce hypervolemia and hyperviscosity.

POLYCYTHEMIA VERA

Polycythemia vera, or primary polycythemia, is a proliferative disorder of the marrow cells. The bone marrow is intensely cellular, and in the peripheral blood the red count, white count, and platelets are often elevated. Patients typically have a ruddy complexion and hepatosplenomegaly. The symptoms are due to the increased blood volume (headache, dizziness, fatigue, and blurred vision) or to increased blood viscosity (angina, claudication, thrombophlebitis). Bleeding is a complication and pruritus is another common and unexplained problem.

MANAGEMENT

The objective of management is to reduce the high blood viscosity.

1. Phlebotomy is performed repeatedly to keep the hemoglobin within normal range.
2. Radioactive phosphorus or chemotherapeutic agents are used to suppress marrow function (may increase risk of leukemia).
3. Allopurinol is used to prevent gouty attacks, when elevated uric acid level.
4. Antihistamines administered to control pruritus.

For more information see Chapter 32 in Smeltzer and Bare: *Brunner and Suddarth's Textbook of Medical–Surgical Nursing,* 8th Edition. Philadelphia: Lippincott–Raven, 1996.

POLYRADICULONEURITIS

See Guillain-Barré Syndrome

PRIMARY DEGENERATIVE DEMENTIA

See Alzheimer's Disease

PRODUCTIVE COUGH

See Bronchitis, Chronic

PROSTATE CANCER

See Cancer of the Prostate

PROSTATIC HYPERPLASIA, BENIGN

See Benign Prostatic Hyperplasia

PROSTATITIS

Prostatitis is an inflammation of the prostate gland caused by infectious agents (bacteria, fungi, mycoplasma) or by various other problems (e.g., urethral stricture, prostatic hyperplasia). Micro-organisms usually are carried to the prostate from the urethra. Prostatitis may be classified as bacterial or abacterial, depending on the presence or absence of micro-organisms in the prostatic fluid.

CLINICAL MANIFESTATIONS

1. Perineal discomfort, burning, urgency, frequency, and pain with or after ejaculation.

2. Prostatodynia (pain in the prostate) manifested by painful voiding or by perineal pain without evidence of inflammation or bacterial growth in prostatic fluid.

Symptoms of Acute Bacterial Prostatitis

1. Sudden fever and chills.
2. Perineal, rectal, or low back pain.
3. Urinary symptoms of burning, frequency, urgency, nocturia, and dysuria may be evident.
4. Some are asymptomatic.

DIAGNOSTIC EVALUATION

1. History; culture of prostatic fluid or tissue.
2. Histologic examination of tissue; segmental urine culture.

MANAGEMENT

The goal of management is to avoid the complications of abscess formation and septicemia.

1. Broad-spectrum antimicrobial given for 10–14 days.
2. Encourage to remain on bed rest to alleviate symptoms rapidly.
3. Promote comfort with analgesics, antispasmodics, and bladder sedatives, sitz baths, and stool softeners.

P

Management of Chronic Bacterial Prostatitis

Chronic bacterial prostatitis is a major source of relapsing urinary tract infection.

1. Pharmacologic therapy: antimicrobials (trimethoprim-sulfamethoxazole, tetracycline, minocycline, doxycycline).
2. Continuous suppressive treatment with low-dose antimicrobial drugs may be indicated.
3. Comfort measures are the same as acute bacterial prostatitis.

Management of Nonbacterial Prostatitis

Symptomatic relief, e.g., sitz baths, analgesics.

COMPLICATIONS OF PROSTATITIS

1. Urinary retention from prostate swelling.
2. Epididymitis.
3. Bacteremia.
4. Pyelonephritis.

✎ PATIENT EDUCATION AND HEALTH MAINTENANCE: CARE IN THE HOME AND COMMUNITY

1. Instruct to complete prescribed course of antibiotics.
2. Take hot sitz baths (10–20 minutes) several times daily.
3. Encourage fluids to satisfy thirst but not "forced" because effective drug level must be maintained in urine.
4. Avoid foods and drinks that have diuretic action or increase prostatic secretions, i.e., alcohol, coffee, tea, chocolate, cola, and spices.
5. Avoid sexual arousal and intercourse during periods of acute inflammation.
6. Ejaculation by sexual intercourse or masturbation may be beneficial for chronic prostatitis by reducing retention of prostatic fluids.
7. Avoid sitting for long periods to minimize discomfort.
8. Medical follow-up is necessary for at least 6 months to 1 year.

For more information see Chapter 47 in Smeltzer and Bare: *Brunner and Suddarth's Textbook of Medical–Surgical Nursing,* 8th Edition. Philadelphia: Lippincott–Raven, 1996.

PRURITUS

Pruritus (itching) is one of the most common complaints in dermatologic disorders. Although pruritus usually is due to primary skin disease, it may also reflect systemic disease, i.e., diabetes mellitus, blood disorders, or cancer. Pruritus may be caused by certain oral medications, external contact with irritating agents, or prickly heat (miliaria). It may also be a side effect of radiation therapy, a reaction to chemotherapy, or a symptom of infection. It may occur in the elderly from dry skin. Also, itching may be caused by psychologic factors.

CLINICAL MANIFESTATIONS

1. Scratching, often is more severe at night.
2. Excoriations, redness, raised areas on the skin (wheals).
3. Infections, changes in pigmentation.
4. Debilitating itching.

MANAGEMENT

1. The cause of pruritus should be identified and removed.
2. Avoid washing with soap and hot water.
3. Apply cold compress, ice cube, or cool agents that contain soothing menthol and camphor.
4. Bath oils (Lubath Alpha-Keri) prescribed, except for elderly patients or those with impaired balance should not add oil to the bath because of slipping danger.
5. Topical steroids to decrease itching.
6. Oral antihistamines (diphenhydramine [Benadryl]).
7. Tricyclic antidepressants (doxepin [Sinequan]) prescribed when pruritus is of neuropsychogenic origin.

P

NURSING INTERVENTIONS

1. Reinforce reasons for the prescribed therapeutic regimen.
2. Remind to use tepid (not hot) water and to shake off excess water and blot between intertriginous areas with a towel.
3. Avoid rubbing vigorously with towel, which over-stimulates skin, causing more itching.
4. Lubricate skin with an emollient that traps moisture.
5. Advise wearing soft cotton clothing next to skin.

For more information see Chapter 54 in Smeltzer and Bare: *Brunner and Suddarth's Textbook of Medical–Surgical Nursing,* 8th Edition. Philadelphia: Lippincott–Raven, 1996.

PSORIASIS

Psoriasis is a chronic, noninfectious, inflammatory disease of the skin in which the production of epidermal cells occurs at a rate that is approximately 6 to 9 times faster than normal. The basal skin cells divide too quickly, and the newly formed cells become evident as profuse scales or plaques of epidermal tissue. There appears to be a hereditary defect that causes overproduction of keratin. The primary defect is unknown. Periods of emotional stress and anxiety aggravate the condition, and trauma, infections, and seasonal and hormonal changes are trigger factors. Onset may occur at any age but is most common between the ages of 10 and 30 years. Main sites of the body to be affected are the scalp, area over the elbows and knees, lower part of the back, and genitalia. Bilateral symmetry often exists. Psoriasis may be associated with asymmetric rheumatoid factor-negative arthritis of multiple joints. Exfoliative psoriatic state is a complication when the disease progresses to involve the total body surface.

CLINICAL MANIFESTATIONS

Symptoms range from a cosmetic annoyance to a physically disabling and disfiguring affliction.

1. Lesions appearing as red, raised patches of skin covered with silvery scales.
2. Lesions enlarge slowly, and coalesce to form extensive irregularly shaped patches.
3. Patches are dry and may or may not itch.
4. May involve nail pitting, discoloration, crumbling beneath the free edges, and separation of the nail plate.
5. If psoriasis occcurs on the palms and soles, pustular lesions may develop.

Psychologic Considerations

1. May cause despair and frustration; observers may stare, comment, ask embarrassing questions, or even avoid the person.
2. Can eventually exhaust resources, interfere with job, and make life miserable in general.
3. Teenagers are especially vulnerable to psychologic effects.
4. Can cause family disruption because of time-consuming treatments, messy salves, and constant shedding of scales.

DIAGNOSTIC EVALUATION

Confirmed by classic plaque-type lesions.

MANAGEMENT

The goals of management are to slow the rapid turnover of epidermis and to promote resolution of the psoriatic lesions. There is no known cure. Therapeutic approach should be understandable; cosmetically acceptable; not too disruptive of lifestyle.

Topical Therapy

1. Used to slow down the overactive epidermis without affecting other tissues.
2. Medications include tar preparations, anthralin, salicylic acid, and corticosteroids; may require occlusive dressings.

Intralesional Therapy

Intralesional injections of triamcinolone acetonide (Aristocort, Kenalog-10, and Trymex).

Systemic Therapy

1. Systemic cytotoxic preparations, i.e., methotrexate.
2. Monitor laboratory studies to ensure hepatic, hematopoietic, and renal systems are functioning adequately.
3. Avoid drinking alcohol while on methotrexate; increases possibility of liver damage.
4. Oral retinoids (synthetic derivatives of vitamin A and vitamin A acid).

Photochemotherapy

1. Psoralen and ultraviolet A (PUVA) therapy for severely debilitating psoriasis.
2. Associated with long-term risks of skin cancer, cataracts, and premature aging of the skin.
3. Ultraviolet B (UVB) light therapy used to treat generalized plaque, combined with topical coal tar (Goeckerman therapy).

NURSING PROCESS

Assessment

1. Assessment focuses on how the patient is coping with the skin condition, the appearance of "normal" skin, and the appearance of skin lesions.
2. Note major skin manifestations.

3. Examine areas especially affected: elbows, knees, scalp, gluteal cleft, fingers, and toenails (for small pits).

Major Nursing Diagnosis

1. Knowledge deficit of the disease process and treatment.
2. Impaired skin integrity related to lesions and inflammatory response.
3. Body image disturbance related to embarrassment over appearance and self-perception of uncleanliness.

Collaborative Problems

Psoriatic arthritis.

Planning and Implementation

The major goals may include increased understanding of psoriasis and the treatment regimen, achievement of smoother skin with control of lesions, development of self-acceptance, and absence of potential complications.

Interventions

PROMOTING UNDERSTANDING

P

1. Explain with sensitivity that currently there is no cure and lifetime management is necessary; can usually be cleared and controlled.
2. Review pathophysiology of psoriasis and factors that provoke it: any irritation or injury to the skin (cut, abrasion, sunburn), any current illness, emotional stress, unfavorable environment (cold), and any drug.
3. Review treatment regimen to ensure compliance

INCREASING SKIN INTEGRITY

1. Advise not to pick or scratch areas.
2. Encourage to prevent the skin from drying out; dry skin causes psoriasis to worsen.

3. Inform that water should not be too hot, and skin dried by patting with a towel.
4. Teach to use bath oil or emollient cleansing agent for sore and scaling skin.

IMPROVING SELF-CONCEPT AND BODY IMAGE

Introduce coping strategies and suggestions for reducing or coping with stressful situations to facilitate a more positive outlook and acceptance of the disease.

MONITORING AND MANAGING COMPLICATIONS

Psoriatic arthritis: note joint discomfort and evaluate further.

✎ PATIENT EDUCATION AND HEALTH MAINTENANCE: CARE IN THE HOME AND COMMUNITY

1. Advise topical agent anthralin leaves a brownish purple stain; will subside when treatment stops; cover lesions to avoid staining clothing.
2. Advise that topical corticosteroid preparations on face and around eyes predispose to cataract development; use strict guidelines.
3. Provide helpful tips on application of tar preparations.
4. Avoid exposure to sun when undergoing PUVA treatments.
5. Schedule ophthalmic examinations on regular basis.
6. Prevent nausea by taking food with methoxsalen.
7. Use lubricants and bath oils to remove scales and dryness.
8. Women should use contraceptives to prevent the teratogenic effect of PUVA (fetal defects).
9. Encourage belonging to a support group.

For more information see Chapter 54 in Smeltzer and Bare: *Brunner and Suddarth's Textbook of Medical–Surgical Nursing,* 8th Edition. Philadelphia: Lippincott–Raven, 1996.

PULMONARY DISEASE

See Chronic Obstructive Pulmonary Disease

PULMONARY EDEMA, ACUTE

Pulmonary edema is the abnormal accumulation of fluid in the lungs, either in the interstitial spaces or in the alveoli. Fluid leaks through the capillary walls, permeating the airways and giving rise to severe dyspnea. This is a life-threatening condition that requires immediate attention. Noncardiac pulmonary edema has a wide variety of causes: toxic inhalants, drug overdose, and neurogenic pulmonary edema. The most common cause of pulmonary edema is cardiac disease, i.e., atherosclerotic, hypertensive, valvular, myopathic. If appropriate measures are taken promptly, attacks can be aborted and patients can survive this complication.

CLINICAL MANIFESTATIONS

1. A typical attack occurs at night after lying down for a few hours and is usually preceded by increasing restlessness, anxiety, and inability to sleep.
2. Sudden onset of breathlessness and a sense of suffocation, hands become cold and moist, nailbeds become cyanotic, and skin color turns gray.
3. Pulse is weak and rapid; neck veins are distended.
4. Incessant coughing produces increasing quantities of mucoid sputum.
5. As pulmonary edema progresses, anxiety develops into near panic, patient becomes confused, then stuporous.
6. Breathing is noisy and moist, can suffocate with blood-tinged, frothy fluid (can drown in own fluid).

P

DIAGNOSTIC EVALUATION

Clinical manifestations and hemodynamic testing.

MANAGEMENT

Goals of medical management are to reduce total circulating volume and to improve respiratory exchange.

Oxygenation

1. Administer in concentrations adequate to relieve hypoxia and dyspnea.
2. Oxygen by intermittent or continuous positive pressure, if signs of hypoxemia persist.
3. Endotracheal intubation and mechanical ventilation, if respiratory failure occurs.
4. Positive end expiratory pressure (PEEP).
5. Arterial blood gases (ABGs).

Pharmacotherapy

1. Morphine: IV in small doses to reduce anxiety and dyspnea; contraindicated in cerebral vascular accident, chronic pulmonary disease, or cardiogenic shock. Keep naloxone hydrochloride (Narcan) available for excessive respiratory depression.
2. Diuretics: furosemide (Lasix) IV to produce a rapid diuretic effect.
3. Digitalis: to improve contractile force of heart; administer with extreme caution to patients with acute MI.
4. Aminophylline: for wheezing and bronchospasm, continuous IV drip in dosages based on body weight.

Supportive Care

1. Positioning the patient upright, with legs and feet down, preferably with legs dangling over the side of bed, to help reduce venous return to the heart.
2. Reassure patient, touching to offer a sense of concrete reality.

3. Maximize time at the bedside.
4. Give frequent, simple, concise information about what is being done to treat the condition and what the responses to treatment mean.

PREVENTION

1. Recognize early stages, when presenting signs and symptoms are those of pulmonary congestion, i.e., auscultation of lung fields of patients with cardiac disease.
2. Place in an upright position with feet and legs dependent.
3. Eliminate overexertion and emotional stress to reduce left ventricular load.
4. Administer morphine to reduce anxiety, dyspnea, and preload.
5. Long-range approach directed at its precursor, pulmonary congestion.
6. Use measures to prevent congestive heart failure and patient teaching.
7. Advise to sleep with head of bed elevated on 25 cm (10 inch) blocks.
8. Surgical treatment to eliminate or to minimize valvular defects that limit flow of blood into or out of left ventricle.

P

✚ CLINICAL ALERT AND GERONTOLOGIC CONSIDERATIONS

Use extreme caution when administering infusions and transfusions to cardiac patients and elderly persons.

To prevent circulatory overload, administer IV fluids at a slower rate; position patient upright in bed and place under close nursing surveillance. Use IV control devices to restrict volume of fluid that can be delivered.

For more information see Chapter 28 in Smeltzer and Bare: *Brunner and Suddarth's Textbook of Medical–Surgical Nursing,* 8th Edition. Philadelphia: Lippincott–Raven, 1996.

PULMONARY EMBOLISM

Pulmonary embolism refers to the obstruction of one or more pulmonary arteries by a thrombus (or thrombi) that originates somewhere in the venous system or in the right side of the heart, becomes dislodged, and is carried to the lung. It is a common disorder associated with trauma, surgery (orthopedic, pelvic, gynecologic), pregnancy, oral contraceptive use, congestive heart failure, advanced age (over 60), and prolonged immobility. Most thrombi originate in the deep veins of the legs.

CLINICAL MANIFESTATIONS

Symptoms depend on the size of the thrombus and the area of the pulmonary artery occlusion.

1. Chest pain, most common, usually sudden in onset; pleuritic in nature; can be substernal; and may mimic angina pectoris.
2. Dyspnea, second most common symptom.
3. Tachypnea.
4. Fever, tachycardia, apprehension, cough, diaphoresis, hemoptysis, syncope, and sudden death.
5. Multiple small emboli in the terminal pulmonary arterioles simulate symptoms of bronchopneumonia or heart failure.

DIAGNOSTIC EVALUATION

Primarily confirmed with ventilation-perfusion scan, pulmonary angiography.

PREVENTIVE MEASURES

1. Anticoagulant therapy prior to abdominothoracic surgery.
2. Intermittent pneumatic leg compression devices.

EMERGENCY MEDICAL MANAGEMENT

1. Occlusive pulmonary embolism is a true life-threatening emergency; condition tends to deteriorate rapidly.
2. Immediate objective is to stabilize the cardiorespiratory system.
3. Majority of patients who die do so in the first 2 hours after the embolic event.
4. Administer nasal oxygen immediately to relieve hypoxemia, respiratory distress, and cyanosis.
5. Start an infusion to establish IV route for drugs or fluids.
6. Perform pulmonary angiography, hemodynamic measurements, arterial blood gases (ABGs), and perfusion lung scans.
7. Insert indwelling urethral catheter to monitor urinary output.
8. Treat hypotension by infusion of isoproterenol or dopamine.
9. Monitor ECG continuously for right ventricular failure.
10. Administer digitalis glycosides, IV diuretics, and antidysrhythmic agents when appropriate.
11. Draw blood for serum electrolytes, blood urea nitrogen, complete blood count, and hematocrit.
12. Place on a volume-controlled ventilator if clinical assessment and ABGs indicate.
13. Give small doses of IV morphine to relieve anxiety, alleviate chest discomfort, and help tolerate endotracheal tube, and ease adaptation to mechanical ventilator.

P

OTHER INTERVENTIONS

Anticoagulation Therapy

1. Keep the partial thromboplastin time (PTT) 1.5–2 times normal.
2. Heparin is administered for 5–7 days.

3. Begin coumadin during heparin therapy and continue for 3 months.

Thrombolytic Therapy (Urokinase, Streptokinase)

Bleeding is a significant side effect.

Surgical Intervention

1. Thoracotomy, cardiopulmonary bypass technique.
2. Interruption of inferior vena cava.
3. Transvenous catheter embolectomy.

NURSING PROCESS

Assessment

1. Examine for a positive Homans' sign, may or may not indicate impending thrombosis of the leg veins.
2. Key role is to minimize risk of pulmonary embolism and identify those who are at high risk.
3. Suspect pulmonary embolism in conditions predisposing to slowing of venous return.

Interventions

PROVIDING GENERAL CARE

1. Be alert for potential complication of cardiogenic shock or right ventricular failure.
2. Ensure understanding of need for continuous oxygen therapy.
3. Assess frequently for signs of hypoxia.
4. Give nebulizers, incentive spirometry, or postural drainage.

PREVENTING THROMBUS FORMATION

1. Encourage ambulation, and active and passive leg exercises.
2. Move legs in a "pumping" exercise.
3. Advise to avoid prolonged sitting, immobility, tight clothing.
4. Do not permit dangling of legs and feet in a dependent position.

5. Place feet on floor or chair and avoid crossing legs.
6. Do not leave IV catheters in veins for prolonged periods.

MONITORING THROMBOLYTIC AND ANTICOAGULANT THERAPY

1. Bed rest, vital signs every 2 hours, limit invasive procedures.
2. PT or APTT every 3–4 hours after thrombolytic in fusion started to confirm activation of fibrinolytic systems.
3. Perform only essential ABG studies on upper extremities, with digital compression of puncture site for at least 30 minutes.

MINIMIZING CHEST PAIN, PLEURITIC

1. Semi-Fowler's position.
2. Administer analgesics as prescribed for severe pain.

HELPING PATIENT TO COPE WITH ANXIETY

1. Encourage to express feelings and concerns.
2. Answer questions concisely and accurately; explain therapy.
3. Prior to discharge, and at follow-up clinic or home visits, instruct how to prevent recurrence and what signs/symptoms should alert patient to seek medical attention.

Postoperative Nursing Care

1. Measure pulmonary arterial pressure and urinary output.
2. Assess insertion site of arterial catheter for hematoma formation and infection.
3. Maintain blood pressure to ensure profusion of vital organs.
4. Encourage isometric exercises, elastic stockings, and walking when permitted out of bed.
5. Discourage sitting; hip flexion causes compression of large veins in the legs.

✎ Patient Education and Health Maintenance: Care in the Home and Community

1. Look for bruising and bleeding when taking anticoagulants; protect from bumping into objects that can cause bruising.
2. Use a toothbrush with soft bristles.
3. Do not take aspirin or antihistamine drugs while receiving warfarin sodium (Coumadin). Always check with physician before taking any medication including over-the-counter meds.
4. Continue to wear antiembolism stockings as long as directed.
5. Avoid laxatives, which affect vitamin K absorption.
6. Avoid sitting with legs crossed or for prolonged periods.
7. Change position regularly when traveling, walk occasionally, and do active exercises of legs and ankles. Drink plenty of liquids.
8. Report dark, tarry stools immediately.
9. Wear identification stating anticoagulants are being taken.

For more information see Chapter 24 in Smeltzer and Bare: *Brunner and Suddarth's Textbook of Medical–Surgical Nursing,* 8th Edition. Philadelphia: Lippincott–Raven, 1996.

PULMONARY EMPHYSEMA

See Emphysema, Pulmonary

PULMONARY HEART DISEASE (COR PULMONALE)

Cor pulmonale is a condition in which the right ventricle enlarges (with or without failure) as a result of diseases that affect the structure or function of the lung or its vasculature. The most frequent cause is COPD. Other causes are conditions that restrict or compromise ventilatory function (massive obesity), or reduce the pulmonary vascular bed (pulmonary embolus). Certain disorders of the nervous system, respiratory muscles, chest wall, and pulmonary arterial tree may also be responsible for cor pulmonale. Prognosis depends on reversing the hypertensive process.

CLINICAL MANIFESTATIONS

Symptoms are those of the underlying lung disease.

1. COPD, shortness of breath and cough.
2. Right ventricular failure develops (edema of the feet and legs; distended neck veins; enlarged palpable liver; pleural effusion; ascites; and a heart murmur).
3. Headache, confusion, somnolence from carbon dioxide narcosis.

MANAGEMENT

The goals are to improve the patient's ventilation and to treat both the underlying lung disease and the symptoms of heart disease.

1. Give oxygen to reduce pulmonary arterial pressure and pulmonary vascular resistance.
2. Provide continuous (24 hr/day) O_2 therapy for severe hypoxia.
3. Assess arterial blood gases (ABGs).
4. Provide bronchial hygiene, bronchodilators, and chest physical therapy.
5. If respiratory failure occurs, intubation and mechanical ventilation may be necessary.
6. If heart failure occurs, improve hypoxemia and hypercapnia.
7. Reduce peripheral edema and circulatory load on the right side of the heart with bed rest, sodium restriction, and diuretics.
8. Monitor electrocardiogram.
9. Treat respiratory infection (precipitates cor pulmonale).

P

Patient Education and Health Maintenance: Care in the Home and Community

1. Advise patient and family that management is long term and most of care and monitoring is performed at home.
2. Advise to avoid things that irritate airway if COPD exists.
3. Administer continuous oxygen and instruct how to use.
4. Urge to stop smoking.
5. Counsel about nutrition if on a sodium-restricted diet or taking diuretics.
6. Counsel family that restlessness, depression, irritability, or atypical behavior may be encountered with hypoxemia or hypercapnia. Symptoms should decrease as ABG values improve.

 Clinical Alert

If coincident left ventricular failure, supraventricular dysrhythmia, or right ventricular failure occurs and is nonresponsive to other therapy, give digitalis with extreme caution, because pulmonary heart disease appears to enhance susceptibility to digitalis toxicity.

For more information see Chapter 24 in Smeltzer and Bare: *Brunner and Suddarth's Textbook of Medical–Surgical Nursing,* 8th Edition. Philadelphia: Lippincott–Raven, 1996.

PULMONARY HYPERTENSION

Pulmonary hypertension is a condition that is not clinically evident until late in disease progression. The systolic pulmonary arterial pressure exceeds 30 mmHg and the mean pulmonary artery pressure is above 15 mmHg. There are two forms: primary (idiopathic) and secondary. Primary pulmonary hypertension is uncommon;

diagnosis is made by exclusion. The exact cause is unknown. The clinical presentation exists with no evidence of pulmonary and cardiac disease or pulmonary embolism. It occurs most often in women between 20 and 40 years of age and is usually fatal within 5 years of diagnosis.

Secondary pulmonary hypertension is more common and results from existing cardiac or pulmonary disease. The prognosis depends on the severity of the underlying disorder and the changes in the pulmonary vascular bed. The most common cause is pulmonary artery constriction due to hypoxia from COPD.

CLINICAL MANIFESTATIONS

1. Dyspnea, main symptom noticed first with exertion and then rest.
2. Substernal chest pain common.
3. Weakness, fatigability, syncope.
4. Signs of right-sided heart failure (peripheral edema, ascites, distended neck veins, liver engorgement, crackles, heart murmur).
5. Electrocardiogram (ECG) changes (right ventricular hypertrophy).
6. Decreased PaO_2 (hypoxemia).

P

DIAGNOSTIC EVALUATION

1. Chest x-ray.
2. ECG.
3. Cardiac catheterization.
4. Perfusion lung scan.
5. Pulmonary function studies.
6. Lung biopsy.

MANAGEMENT

The objective of treatment is to manage the underlying cardiac or pulmonary condition. For all cases management includes continuous oxygen therapy.

When Caused by Cor Pulmonale

1. Fluid restriction.
2. Cardiac glycosides (digitalis).
3. Rest.
4. Diuretics to decrease fluid accumulation.

When Caused by Primary Pulmonary Hypertension

1. Vasodilators.
2. Anticoagulants, i.e., Coumadin.
3. Heart–lung transplant when not responsive to other therapies.

NURSING INTERVENTIONS

1. Identify those patients who are at high risk for developing pulmonary hypertension (i.e., those with COPD, pulmonary emboli, congenital heart disease, and mitral valve disease).
2. Be alert for signs and symptoms.
3. Administer oxygen therapy appropriately.

For more information see Chapter 24 in Smeltzer and Bare: *Brunner and Suddarth's Textbook of Medical–Surgical Nursing,* 8th Edition. Philadelphia: Lippincott–Raven, 1996.

PYELONEPHRITIS (UPPER URINARY TRACT INFECTION)

Pyelonephritis is a bacterial infection of the renal pelvis, tubules, and interstitial tissue of one or both kidneys. Bacteria reach the bladder via the urethra and ascend to the kidney. It is frequently secondary to urine backup (reflux) into the ureters, usually at the time of voiding. Urinary tract obstruction and renal diseases are other causes. Pyelonephritis may be acute or chronic.

CLINICAL MANIFESTATIONS

1. Chills and fever, flank pain, costovertebral angle tenderness.

2. Leukocytosis, bacteria and white blood cells in the urine, frequent symptoms of lower urinary tract involvement, i.e., dysuria and frequency.
3. In chronic pyelonephritis kidneys become scarred, contracted, and nonfunctioning.

DIAGNOSTIC EVALUATION

1. Intravenous urogram.
2. Ultrasound.
3. Urine culture and sensitivity.

MANAGEMENT

1. Intensive antimicrobial therapy; parenteral therapy until patient is afebrile 24–48 hours; follow with oral agents.
2. Maintain on continuous antimicrobial treatment after initial regimen until there is no evidence of infection, all causative factors have been treated or controlled, and kidney function has stabilized.
3. Monitor with serum creatinine determinations and blood counts for duration of long-term therapy.

For more information see Chapter 43 in Smeltzer and Bare: *Brunner and Suddarth's Textbook of Medical–Surgical Nursing,* 8th Edition. Philadelphia: Lippincott–Raven, 1996.

P

PYELONEPHRITIS, CHRONIC

Repeated bouts of acute pyelonephritis may lead to chronic pyelonephritis (chronic interstitial nephritis). Evidence suggests chronic pyelonephritis is less frequently a cause of chronic renal failure. Complications of chronic pyelonephritis include end-stage renal disease (from progressive loss of nephrons secondary to chronic inflammation and scarring), hypertension, and formation of kidney stones (from chronic infection with urea-splitting organisms, resulting in stone formation).

CLINICAL MANIFESTATIONS

1. Usually has no symptoms of infection unless an acute exacerbation occurs.
2. Fatigue, headache, and poor appetite.
3. Polyuria, excessive thirst, and weight loss.
4. Persistent and recurring infection may produce progressive scarring with renal failure.

DIAGNOSTIC EVALUATION

Intravenous urogram, BUN, creatinine levels, creatinine clearance.

MANAGEMENT

Eradicate Bacteria from Urine

1. Antimicrobial medication based on culture identification.
2. Nitrofurantoin or a combination of sulfamethoxazole and trimethoprim used to suppress bacterial growth.

Carefully Monitor Renal Function

Careful monitoring of renal function related to compromised renal function in excretion of antimicrobial agents.

For more information see Chapter 43 in Smeltzer and Bare: *Brunner and Suddarth's Textbook of Medical–Surgical Nursing,* 8th Edition. Philadelphia: Lippincott–Raven, 1996.

RAYNAUD'S DISEASE

Raynaud's disease is a form of intermittent arteriolar vasoconstriction. The cause is unknown. Episodes may be triggered by emotional factors or by unusual sensitivity to cold. Most common in women between the ages of 16 and 40 years and is seen much more frequently in cool climates and during the winter months. The term *Raynaud's phenomenon* is currently used to refer to localized, intermittent episodes of vasoconstriction of small arteries of the feet and hands, causing color and temperature changes. It is generally unilateral and affects only one or two digits. It is always associated with an underlying systemic disease. The prognosis for Raynaud's disease varies: some patients slowly improve, some grow slowly worse, and others show no change.

CLINICAL MANIFESTATIONS

1. Pallor brought on by sudden vasoconstriction followed by cyanosis followed by vasodilation. The progression follows the characteristic color change—white, blue, and red.
2. Numbness, tingling, and burning pain occur as color changes.
3. Involvement tends to be bilateral and symmetric.

MANAGEMENT

The prime objective in controlling Raynaud's disease is avoiding the particular stimuli that provoke vasoconstriction.

1. Avoid situations that may be upsetting.
2. Reassure that serious sequelae are not usual.

R

3. Avoid smoking.
4. Minimize exposure to cold; remain indoors as much as possible and wear protective clothing when outdoors.
5. Handle sharp objects carefully to avoid injuring the fingers.
6. Prescribed vasodilators, calcium channel blockers, and sympatholytic agents, i.e., procardia, nifedipine, or other rauwolfia derivatives.
7. Caution about postural hypotension (results from drugs and increased by alcohol, exercise, and hot weather).
8. Sympathectomy (interruption of sympathetic nerves by removal of sympathetic ganglia or division of their branches).

For more information see Chapter 31 in Smeltzer and Bare: *Brunner and Suddarth's Textbook of Medical–Surgical Nursing,* 8th Edition. Philadelphia: Lippincott–Raven, 1996.

REGIONAL ENTERITIS (CROHN'S DISEASE)

Regional enteritis commonly occurs in adolescents or young adults, but can appear at any time of life. The most common areas in which it is found are the distal ileum and colon. It can occur anywhere along the gastrointestinal tract. This inflammatory disease process extends through all layers of the bowel wall. Formation of fistulas, fissures, and abscesses occurs as the inflammation extends into the peritoneum. In some cases the intestinal mucosa has a "cobblestone" appearance. As the disease advances, the bowel wall thickens and becomes fibrotic, and the intestinal lumen narrows. The clinical course and symptoms vary. In some, periods of remission and exacerbation occur; in others the disease follows a fulminating course.

CLINICAL MANIFESTATIONS

1. Onset of symptoms is usually insidious, with prominent abdominal pain, and diarrhea unrelieved by defecation.
2. Diarrhea present in 90% of patients.
3. Crampy pains occur after meals; patients tend to limit intake, causing weight loss, malnutrition, and secondary anemia.
4. Chronic diarrhea may occur, resulting in a very uncomfortable person who is thin and emaciated from inadequate food intake and constant fluid loss. The inflamed intestine may perforate and form intra-abdominal and anal abscesses.
5. Fever and leukocytosis occur.
6. Abscesses, fistulas, and fissures are common.

Fulminating Course

Symptoms extend beyond the gastrointestinal tract.

1. Joint problems (arthritis).
2. Skin lesions (erythema nodosum).
3. Ocular disorders (conjunctivitis).
4. Oral ulcers.

DIAGNOSTIC EVALUATION

The most conclusive diagnostic aid is a barium study of the upper gastrointestinal tract that shows the classic "string sign" of the terminal ileum, indicating constriction of segment of intestine.

MANAGEMENT

See management under Ulcerative Colitis.

For more information see Chapter 37 in Smeltzer and Bare: *Brunner and Suddarth's Textbook of Medical–Surgical Nursing,* 8th Edition. Philadelphia: Lippincott–Raven, 1996.

RENAL CANCER

See Cancer of the Kidneys

RENAL FAILURE, ACUTE

Renal failure results when the kidneys are unable to remove the body's metabolic waste and perform their regulatory functions. Acute renal failure (ARF) is a sudden and almost complete loss of kidney function caused by failure of the renal circulation or glomerular or tubular dysfunction. Three major catagories of ARF are prerenal (hypoperfusion of kidney), intrarenal (actual damage to kidney tissue), and postrenal (obstruction to urine flow).

CLINICAL PHASES OF ARF

1. Initiation period begins with the initial insult and ends when oliguria develops.
2. Period of oliguria (urine volume less than 400 ml/24 hr): uremic symptoms first appear.
3. Period of diuresis: gradual increase in urinary output, which signals glomerular filtration has started to recover.
4. Period of recovery: improvement of renal function may take 3–12 months.

RISK FACTORS FOR ARF

1. Hypovolemia.
2. Hypotension.
3. Reduced cardiac output and congestive failure.
4. Obstruction of the kidney or lower urinary tract by tumor.
5. Blood clot or kidney stone.
6. Bilateral obstruction of the renal arteries or veins.

CLINICAL MANIFESTATIONS

1. Anuria, polyuria, or oliguria may occur.
2. Appears critically ill and lethargic with persistent nausea, vomiting, and diarrhea.
3. Skin and mucous membranes are dry; breath may have odor of urine (uremic fetor).
4. Central nervous system manifestations: drowsiness, headache, muscle twitching, and seizures.
5. Urinary output scanty, may be bloody and of low specific gravity.
6. Steady rise in BUN and serum creatinine values noted.
7. Severe hyperkalemia may lead to dysrhythmias and cardiac arrest.
8. Progressive acidosis, increase in serum phosphate concentrations, and low serum calcium levels.
9. Anemia (from blood loss due to uremic gastrointestinal lesions, reduced red cell life span, and reduced erythropoietin production).

MANAGEMENT

The objective of treatment is to restore normal chemical balance and prevent complications so that repair of renal tissue and restoration of renal function can take place. Identify, treat, and eliminate any possible cause.

1. Treat reduced levels of erythropoietin production with parenteral form of erythropoietin (Epogen) to prevent anemia.
2. Dialysis to prevent serious complications of uremia, i.e., hyperkalemia, pericarditis, and seizures: hemodialysis, hemofiltration, or peritoneal dialysis.
3. Monitor for hyperkalemia including serum electrolyte levels, electrocardiographic assessment (peaked T waves).
4. Administer ion exchange resins (sodium polystyrene sulfonate [Kayexalate]) orally or by retention enema.

5. Sorbitol orally or as an enema. Assess for development of fecal impaction.
6. Initiate immediate peritoneal dialysis, hemodialysis, or hemofiltration for patient with a high and rising level of serum potassium.
7. Give IV glucose and insulin or calcium glutamate as an emergency and temporary measure to treat hyperkalemia.
8. Give sodium bicarbonate to promote an elevation of plasma pH.
9. Use sodium bicarbonate with other long-term measures, such as dietary restriction and dialysis.
10. Manage fluid balance based on daily body weight; serial measurements of central venous pressure; serum and urine concentrations; fluid losses; blood pressure; and clinical status.
11. Use flowchart to record pertinent information to indicate degree to which condition is improving or deteriorating.
12. Use parenteral and oral intake and output of urine, gastric drainage, stools, wound drainage, and perspiration as basis for fluid replacement.
13. Weigh daily.
14. Auscultate lungs for signs of moist crackles.
15. Assess for generalized edema by examining presacral and pretibial areas several times daily.
16. Restore adequate blood flow to kidneys by intravenous fluids and medications, i.e., mannitol, furosemide, or ethacrynic acid.
17. Infuse albumin if acute renal failure is caused by hypovolemia secondary to hypoproteinemia.
18. Treat shock and infection, if present.
19. Monitor arterial blood gases when severe acidosis is present.
20. Institute appropriate ventilatory measures if respiratory problems develop (may require sodium bicarbonate therapy or dialysis).
21. Control elevated serum phosphate concentration with phosphate-binding agents (aluminum hydroxide).

22. Limit dietary protein to approximately 1 g/kg during oliguric phase to minimize protein breakdown and to prevent accumulation of toxic end products.
23. Meet caloric requirements with high-carbohydrate feedings.
24. Restrict foods and fluids containing potassium and phosphorus (bananas, citrus fruits and juices, coffee); restrict potassium intake to 40–60 mEq/day.
25. Restrict sodium to 2 g/day (may require total parenteral nutrition).
26. Evaluate blood chemistry to determine the amounts of sodium, potassium, and water needed for replacement during oliguric phase.
27. After the diuretic phase, place on a high-protein, high-calorie diet and encourage to resume activities gradually.

Nursing Interventions

1. Direct attention to patient's primary disorder; monitor for complications.
2. Participate in emergency treatment of fluid and electrolyte imbalances.
3. Assess patient's progress and response to treatment.
4. Provide physical and emotional support.
5. Keep patient's family informed about condition, assist in understanding the treatments, and provide psychologic support.
6. Continue to include in the plan of care those nursing measures indicated for the patient's primary disorder (e.g., burns, shock, trauma, obstruction of the urinary tract).

MONITORING FLUID AND ELECTROLYTES

1. Screen parenteral fluids, all oral intake, and all medications carefully to ensure that hidden sources of potassium are not inadvertently administered or consumed.
2. Monitor cardiac function and musculoskeletal status closely for changes suggestive of hyperkalemia.

3. Monitor fluid status by careful attention to fluid intake, urine output, changes in body weight, presence of edema, distention of jugular veins, alterations in heart sounds and breath sounds, and increasing difficulty in breathing.
4. Report immediately to physician indicators of deterioration of fluid and electrolyte status: prepare for emergency treatment, including use of glucose and insulin, calcium gluconate, or cation-exchange resins (Kayexalate) to treat hyperkalemia, and initiation of hemodialysis, peritoneal dialysis, or hemofiltration to correct fluid and electrolyte disturbances.

REDUCING METABOLIC RATE

1. Reduce exertion and metabolic rate during most acute stage with bed rest.
2. Prevent or treat fever and infection promptly.

PROMOTING PULMONARY FUNCTION

1. Assist patient to turn, cough, and take deep breaths frequently.
2. Encourage and assist to move and turn.

AVOIDING INFECTION

1. Practice asepsis with invasive lines and catheters.
2. Avoid an indwelling catheter if possible.

PROVIDING SKIN CARE

1. Give meticulous skin care.
2. Massage bony prominences, turn frequently, bathe with cool water for comfort, and prevent skin breakdown.

Dialysis Support

1. Assist, explain, and support patient and family; do not ignore psychologic needs and concerns.
2. Explain rationale of treatment to patient and family.
3. Repeat explanation and clarify questions after physician teaching.

4. Encourage family members to touch and talk to patient during dialysis.
5. Continually assess patient for complications and their precipitating cause.

✿ GERONTOLOGIC CONSIDERATIONS

Mortality rate is slightly higher. Etiology of ARF includes prerenal causes, e.g., dehydration, and intrarenal causes, e.g., nephrotoxic agents (medications [NSAIDS], contrast agents or media).

Diabetes mellitus increases contrast agent–induced renal failure because of preexisting renal insufficiency and imposed fluid restriction.

For more information see Chapter 43 in Smeltzer and Bare: *Brunner and Suddarth's Textbook of Medical–Surgical Nursing,* 8th Edition. Philadelphia: Lippincott–Raven, 1996.

RENAL FAILURE, CHRONIC (END-STAGE RENAL DISEASE)

Chronic renal failure or end-stage renal disease (ESRD) is a progressive, irreversible deterioration in renal function in which the body's ability to maintain metabolic and fluid and electrolyte balance fails, resulting in uremia. It may be caused by chronic glomerulonephritis; pyelonephritis; uncontrolled hypertension; hereditary lesions such as in polycystic disease; vascular disorders; obstruction of the urinary tract; renal disease secondary to systemic disease (diabetes); infections; drugs; or toxic agents. Environmental and occupational agents that have been implicated in chronic renal failure include lead, cadmium, mercury, and chromium. Dialysis or kidney transplantation eventually becomes necessary for patient survival.

R

CLINICAL MANIFESTATIONS

Patients will exhibit a number of signs and symptoms; severity is dependent on degree of renal impairment, other underlying conditions, and patient age.

1. Cardiovascular manifestations: hypertension, congestive heart failure, pulmonary edema, pericarditis.
2. Dermatologic symptoms: severe itching (pruritus); uremic frost uncommon because of early and aggressive treatment.
3. Gastrointestinal symptoms: anorexia, nausea, vomiting, and hiccups, decreased salivary flow, thirst, a metallic taste in the mouth, loss of smell and taste, and parotitis or stomatitis.
4. Neuromuscular changes: altered level of consciousness, mental confusion, inability to concentrate, muscle twitching and seizures.
5. Hematologic changes: bleeding tendencies.
6. Fatigue and lethargy, headache, general weakness.
7. Patient gradually becomes more and more drowsy; respirations become Kussmaul in character; and deep coma develops, often with convulsions (myoclonic jerks) or muscle twitchings.

MANAGEMENT

The goal of management is to retain kidney function and maintain homeostasis for as long as possible. All factors that contribute to ESRD and those that are reversible (e.g., obstruction) are identified and treated.

1. Dietary intervention needed with careful regulation of protein intake, fluid intake to balance fluid losses, sodium intake, and some restriction of potassium.
2. Ensure adequate calorie intake and vitamin supplementation.
3. Restrict protein because of impaired renal clearance of urea, creatinine, uric acid, and organic acids. Allowed protein must be of high biologic value: dairy products, eggs, meats.

4. Fluid allowance is 500–600 ml of fluid or more than the 24-hour urine output.
5. Treat hyperphosphatemia and hypocalcemia with aluminum-based antacids or calcium carbonate; both must be given with food.
6. Supply calories with carbohydrates and fats to prevent wasting.
7. Give vitamin supplementation.
8. Manage hypertension by intravascular volume control and antihypertensive medication.
9. Treat congestive heart failure and pulmonary edema with fluid restriction, low sodium diet, diuretics, inotropic agents (e.g., digitalis or dobutamine), and dialysis.
10. Treat metabolic acidosis if necessary with sodium bicarbonate supplements or dialysis.
11. Treat hyperkalemia with dialysis; monitor medications for potassium content; place on potassium-restricted diet; administer Kayexelate as needed.
12. Observe for early evidence of neurologic abnormalities (e.g., slight twitching, headache, delirium, or seizure activity).
13. Protect from injury with padded bed side rails.
14. Record onset of seizures, type, duration, and general effect on patient; notify physician immediately.
15. Give intravenous diazepam (Valium) or phenytoin (Dilantin) to control seizures.
16. Treat anemia with recombinant human erythropoietin (Epogen): Monitor patient's hematocrit frequently. Adjust heparin as necessary to prevent clotting of the dialysis lines during treatments.
17. Monitor serum iron and transferrin levels to assess iron states (iron is necessary for adequate response to erythropoietin).
18. Monitor blood pressure and serum potassium levels.
19. Refer patient to a dialysis and transplantation center early in the course of progressive renal disease.
20. Initiate dialysis when patient cannot maintain a reasonable lifestyle with conservative treatment.

R

NURSING PROCESS

Major Nursing Diagnosis

1. Fluid volume excess related to decreased urine output, dietary excesses, and retention of sodium and water.
2. Altered nutrition; less than body requirements related to anorexia, nausea, vomiting, dietary restrictions, and altered oral mucous membranes.
3. Knowledge deficit regarding condition and treatment regimen.
4. Activity intolerance related to fatigue, anemia, retention of waste products, and dialysis procedure.
5. Self-esteem disturbance related to dependency, role changes, change in body image, and physiologic sexual dysfunction.

Interventions

1. Assess fluid status and identify potential sources of imbalance.
2. Implement a dietary program to ensure proper nutritional intake within the limits of the treatment regimen.
3. Provide explanations and information to the patient and family concerning ESRD, treatment options, and potential complications.
4. Provide emotional support to patient and family.

✎ PATIENT EDUCATION AND HEALTH MAINTENANCE: CARE IN THE HOME AND COMMUNITY

1. Provide ongoing education and reinforcement of previous teaching.
2. Monitor the patient's progress and compliance with the treatment regimen.
3. Provide a nutritional consult.
4. Teach patient and family what problems to report: worsening signs of renal failure, signs of hyperkalemia.

5. Provide medication teaching.
6. Teach patient how to assess vascular access for patency; precautions, i.e., no venipunctures or blood pressure on access arm.
7. Provide assistance and support to patient and family in dealing with dialysis and its long-term implications.

✪ Gerontologic Considerations

Changes in kidney function with normal aging increase susceptibility to kidney dysfunction and renal failure.
Alterations in renal blood flow, glomerular filtration, and renal clearance increase the risk of drug-associated changes in renal function; take precautions with the administration of all medications.

Incidence of systemic diseases, e.g., cardiac failure and diabetes, predisposes to renal disease.
The kidney is less able to respond to fluid and electrolyte changes; recognize and treat problems quickly to avoid kidney damage.

Use precautions when elderly patient must undergo extensive diagnostic tests, or when new medications (e.g., diuretics) are added, to prevent dehydration leading to acute renal failure.

The elderly patient may develop nonspecific and atypical signs of disturbed renal function and fluid and electrolyte imbalances.

For more information see Chapter 43 in Smeltzer and Bare: *Brunner and Suddarth's Textbook of Medical–Surgical Nursing*, 8th Edition. Philadelphia: Lippincott–Raven, 1996.

R

RESPIRATORY DISTRESS

See Adult Respiratory Distress Syndrome

RHEUMATIC DISEASE

See Osteoarthritis

RHEUMATIC ENDOCARDITIS

See Endocarditis, Rheumatic

RHEUMATOID ARTHRITIS

See Arthritis, Rheumatoid

RUP·TURED DISC

See Herniation or Rupture of an Intervertebral Disc

SCALDED SKIN SYNDROME

See Toxic Epidermal Necrolysis

SEBORRHEIC DERMATOSES

Seborrhea is an excessive production of sebum. Seborrheic dermatitis is a chronic inflammatory disease of the skin with a predilection for areas that are well supplied with sebaceous glands or lie between folds of the skin, where the bacterial count is high. Seborrheic dermatitis has a genetic predisposition; hormones, nutritional status, infection, and emotional stress influence its course. There are remissions and exacerbations of this condition.

CLINICAL MANIFESTATIONS

Two forms can occur: an oily form and a dry form; either form may start in childhood with fine scaling of scalp or other areas.

S

1. Oily form appears moist: patches of sallow, greasy-appearing skin, with or without scaling, and slight erythremia; small pustules or papulopustules on trunk, resembles acne.
2. Dry form consists of flaky desquamation of the scalp (dandruff).
3. Mild forms of both are asymptomatic.
4. When scaling is present, it is often accompanied by pruritus, leading to scratching and secondary complications, i.e., infection and excoriation.

MANAGEMENT

Because there is no known cure for seborrhea the objective of therapy is to control the disorder and allow the skin to repair itself.

1. Topical corticosteroid cream to body and face
2. Ensure maximum aeration of skin and carefully cleanse areas where there are creases or folds to avoid Candida yeast infection.
3. Shampoo daily or at least three times weekly with medicated shampoos. Use two or three different types of shampoo in rotation to prevent the seborrhea from becoming resistant to a particular shampoo.

Nursing Interventions

1. Advise to remove external irritants and to avoid excess heat and perspiration; rubbing and scratching prolong the disorder.
2. Avoid secondary infections: air skin; keep skin folds clean and dry.
3. Instruct on use of medicated shampoo.
4. Caution patient that seborrheic dermatitis is a chronic problem that tends to wax and wane. The goal is to keep it under control.
5. Encourage to adhere to treatment program.
6. Treat patients with sensitivity and an awareness of their need to express their feelings when they become discouraged by the effect on body image.

For more information see Chapter 54 in Smeltzer and Bare: *Brunner and Suddarth's Textbook of Medical–Surgical Nursing,* 8th Edition. Philadelphia: Lippincott–Raven, 1996.

SECONDARY POLYCYTHEMIA

See Polycythemia

SEIZURES

See Epilepsies

SENILE DEMENTIA OF THE ALZHEIMER TYPE

See Alzheimer's Disease

SHOCK, CARDIOGENIC

Cardiogenic shock occurs when the heart's ability to pump blood is impaired. The result is a marked reduction in cardiac output with inadequate tissue perfusion to the vital organs (heart, brain, kidneys). Causes of cardiogenic shock are either of a coronary or noncoronary etiology. Coronary cardiogenic shock is more common and is seen most often in patients with myocardial infarction. Noncoronary causes include cardiac tamponade, pulmonary embolism, cardiomyopathy, valvular damage, and dysrhythmias.

CLINICAL MANIFESTATIONS

Dysrhythmias are common and result from a decrease in oxygen to the myocardium.

Classic Signs

1. Low blood pressure, rapid and weak pulse.
2. Cerebral hypoxia manifested by confusion and agitation.
3. Decreased urinary output, and cold, clammy skin.

MEDICAL MANAGEMENT

The goals of medical treatment include limiting further myocardial damage, preserving the healthy myocardium, and improving the heart's ability to pump effectively.

1. First-line treatment of cardiogenic shock: supplying supplemental oxygen, controlling chest pain, administering vasoactive drugs, and selective fluid support.
2. Treat oxygenation needs of heart muscle.
3. Hemodyanamic monitoring.
4. Drug therapy, e.g., dopamine, nitroglycerine, dobutamine, and various antidysrhythmics.
5. Mechanical support, e.g., intra-aortic balloon counterpulsation (IABC).
6. Coronary cardiogenic shock: thrombolytic therapy, angioplasty, or coronary artery bypass graft surgery.
7. Noncoronary cardiogenic shock: cardiac valve replacement or correction of a dysrhythmia.

NURSING MANAGEMENT

Prevention

1. Identify patients at risk early.
2. Promote adequate oxygenation of the heart muscle and decrease cardiac workload.

Hemodynamic Monitoring

1. Monitor patient's hemodynamic and cardiac status, e.g., arterial lines and ECG.
2. Anticipate need for medications, IV fluids, and other equipment.
3. Document and report promptly changes in hemodynamic, cardiac, and pulmonary status.

Fluids Administration

Provide for safe and accurate administration of intravenous fluids and medications.

IABC

Provide ongoing timing adjustments of the balloon pump for maximum effectiveness.

Safety and Comfort

Take an active role in assuring patient's safety, physical comfort, and reducing anxiety.

For more information see Chapter 15 in Smeltzer and Bare: *Brunner and Suddarth's Textbook of Medical–Surgical Nursing,* 8th Edition. Philadelphia: Lippincott–Raven, 1996.

SHOCK, HYPOVOLEMIC

Hypovolemic shock is a condition in which there is loss of effective circulating blood volume. It is the most common type of shock. Hypovolemic shock is caused by external fluid losses from hemorrhage; internal fluid shifts, i.e., severe dehydration, severe edema, or ascites; fluid losses from prolonged vomiting or diarrhea.

CLINICAL MANIFESTATIONS

1. Fall in venous pressure; rise in peripheral resistance; tachycardia.
2. Cold, moist skin; pallor; thirst; diaphoresis.
3. Altered sensorium; oliguria; metabolic acidosis; and hyperpnea.
4. Most dependable criterion is level of arterial blood pressure.

MEDICAL MANAGEMENT

The goals of treatment are to restore intravascular volume, redistribute fluid volume, and correct the underlying cause.

Fluid and Blood Replacement

1. Give Ringer's lactate, colloids, and 0.9% NACL to restore intravascular volume.
2. Blood products used only if other alternatives are unavailable or blood loss is extensive and rapid; consider autotransfusion methods for closed cavity hemorrhage.

Redistribution of Fluids

1. Positioning of patient properly to assist in fluid redistribution (modified Trendelenburg).
2. Military antishock trousers (MAST) used in extreme emergency situations where bleeding cannot be controlled.

Treatment of Underlying Cause

1. Stop the bleeding if hemorrhaging, i.e., application of pressure or surgery.
2. Treat diarrhea or vomiting with medications.

Medications

1. Use same medications given in cardiogenic shock.
2. Type of medication depends on the underlying cause.

NURSING MANAGEMENT

Primary Prevention

1. Closely monitor patients who are at risk for fluid deficits.
2. Assist with fluid replacement before intravascular volume is depleted.

General Nursing Measures

1. Assure safe administration of prescribed fluids/medications and document effects.
2. Monitor/report signs of complications and side effects of treatment.

Administering Blood Transfusions

Monitor patient closely for adverse effects.

Fluid Replacement Complications

Monitor for cardiovascular overload and pulmonary edema, e.g., hemodynamic pressure monitoring, vital signs, arterial blood gases, fluid intake and output.

Oxygen

Reduce fear and anxiety about the need for oxygen mask by giving patient explanation and frequent reassurance.

For more information see Chapter 15 in Smeltzer and Bare: *Brunner and Suddarth's Textbook of Medical–Surgical Nursing,* 8th Edition. Philadelphia: Lippincott–Raven, 1996.

SHOCK, SEPTIC

Septic shock is the most common type of distributive shock and is caused by widespread infection (gram-negative bacteria, most common). Other infectious agents such as gram-positive bacteria and viruses can also cause septic shock. Conditions placing patients at risk for septic shock are immunosuppression, extremes of age (<1 year and >65 years), malnourishment, chronic illness, and invasive procedures.

CLINICAL MANIFESTATIONS

First Phase: Hyperdynamic or "Warm" Phase

1. High cardiac output with vasodilation.
2. Hyperthermia with warm flushed skin.
3. Heart and respiratory rates elevated.
4. Urinary output may increase or remain normal.
5. Gastrointestinal status compromised, e.g., nausea, vomiting, or diarrhea.

Later Phase: Hypodynamic or "Cold" Phase

1. Low cardiac output with vasoconstriction.
2. Blood pressure drops.
3. Skin cool and pale.
4. Temperature normal or below.
5. Heart and respiratory rates remain rapid.
6. Anuria and multiple organ failure may occur.

MEDICAL MANAGEMENT

1. Identify and eliminate the cause of infection.

S

2. Collect specimens of urine, blood, sputum, and wound drainage.
3. Start broad-spectrum antibiotics immediately.
4. Eliminate potential routes of infection (reroute IV lines if necessary).
5. Drain abscesses and debride necrotic areas.
6. Institute fluid replacement.
7. Provide aggressive nutritional supplementation (high protein). Enteral feedings preferred.

NURSING MANAGEMENT

1. Carry out all invasive procedures with correct aseptic technique and follow with careful handwashing.
2. Monitor for signs of infection, i.e., IV lines, arterial and venous puncture sites, surgical incisions, trauma wounds, urinary catheters, and pressure ulcers.
3. Identify patients at risk for sepsis and septic shock.
4. Reduce patient's temperature by administering salicylates, ice bags, and hypothermia blankets; monitor closely for shivering.
5. Administer prescribed IV fluids and medications.
6. Monitor blood levels (antibiotic levels, BUN, creatinine, white blood count) and report.
7. Monitor hemodynamic status, fluid intake and output, and nutritional status.
8. Monitor daily weights and serum albumin levels for daily protein requirements.

✪ GERONTOLOGIC CONSIDERATIONS

Septic shock may be manifested in atypical or confusing clinical signs. Suspect septic shock in any elderly person who develops an unexplained acute confused state, tachypnea, or hypotension.

For more information see Chapter 15 in Smeltzer and Bare: *Brunner and Suddarth's Textbook of Medical–Surgical Nursing,* 8th Edition. Philadelphia: Lippincott–Raven, 1996.

SIADH (SYNDROME OF INAPPROPRIATE ANTIDIURETIC HORMONE SECRETION)

The syndrome of inappropriate antidiuretic hormone secretion (SIADH) refers to excessive ADH secretion from the pituitary gland. Patients with this disorder cannot excrete or dilute urine. They retain fluids and develop a sodium deficiency (dilutional hyponatremia). SIADH is often of nonendocrine origin. The syndrome may occur in patients with bronchogenic carcinoma in which malignant lung cells synthesize and release ADH. Other causes include severe pneumonia, pneumothorax, other disorders of the lungs, and malignant tumors that affect other organs. Disorders of the central nervous system (head injury, tumor, or meningitis) are thought to produce SIADH by direct stimulation of the pituitary gland. Some medications (vincristine, phenothiazines, tricyclic antidepressants) have been implicated in SIADH.

MANAGEMENT

This syndrome is generally managed by eliminating the underlying cause if possible and restricting the patient's fluid intake.

Use diuretics with fluid restriction for severe hyponatremia.

Nursing Interventions

1. Monitor closely fluid intake and output, daily weight, urine and blood chemistries, and neurologic status.
2. Assist patient to deal with this disorder by providing supportive measures and explanations of procedures and treatments.

For more information see Chapter 40 in Smeltzer and Bare: *Brunner and Suddarth's Textbook of Medical–Surgical Nursing,* 8th Edition. Philadelphia: Lippincott–Raven, 1996.

SICKLE-CELL ANEMIA

See Anemia, Sickle-Cell

SKIN CANCER

See Cancer of the Skin

SLE

See Systemic Lupus Erythematosus

SMALL-BOWEL OBSTRUCTION

See Bowel Obstruction, Small

SPINAL CORD INJURY

Spinal cord injury is a major health problem with an estimated 10,000 new injuries occurring each year. Half of these injuries result from motor vehicle accidents; most of the others occur from falls, sporting, and industrial accidents, and gunshot wounds. Two-thirds of the victims are 30 years of age or younger. There is a high frequency of associated injuries and medical complications. The vertebrae most frequently involved in spinal cord injuries are the 5th, 6th, and 7th cervical, the 12th thoracic, and the 1st lumbar. These vertebrae are the most susceptible because there is a greater range of mobility in the vertebral column in these areas. Damage to the spinal cord ranges from transient concussion (recovers fully) to contusion, laceration, and compression of the cord substance (either alone or in combination), to complete transection of the cord (paralysis below the level of injury).

CLINICAL MANIFESTATIONS

The consequences of spinal cord injury depend on the level of injury of the cord. Type of injury refers to the extent of injury to the spinal cord itself.

Neurologic Level

Refers to that lowest level at which sensory and motor functions are normal.

1. Total sensory and motor paralysis below the neurologic level.
2. Loss of bladder and bowel control (usually with urinary retention and bladder distention).
3. Loss of sweating and vasomotor tone below the neurologic level.
4. Marked reduction of blood pressure from loss of peripheral vascular resistance.

Respiratory Problems

1. Related to compromised respiratory function; severity depends on level of injury.
2. Acute respiratory failure is the leading cause of death in high cervical cord injury.

DIAGNOSTIC EVALUATION

Detailed neurologic examination, radiographic examinations (lateral cervical spine x-rays and CT scanning).

EMERGENCY MANAGEMENT

1. Immediate management of the patient at the scene of the accident is critical. Improper handling can cause further damage and loss of neurologic function.
2. Consider any victim of a motor vehicle or driving accident, a contact sports injury, falls, or any direct trauma to the head and neck as a spinal cord injury until ruled out.

MANAGEMENT OF SPINAL CORD INJURIES (ACUTE PHASE)

The goals of management are to prevent further spinal cord injury and to observe for symptoms of progressive neurologic deficits.
Resuscitate as necessary and maintain oxygenation and cardiovascular stability.

Pharmacotherapy

Administer high-dose steroids (methylprednisolone) to counteract cord edema.

Respiratory Measures

1. Administer oxygen to maintain a high arterial PO_2.
2. Practice extreme care to avoid flexing or extending the neck if endotracheal intubation is necessary.
3. Consider diaphragm pacing (electrical stimulation of the phrenic nerve) for patients with a high cervical lesion.

Skeletal Reduction and Traction

1. Spinal cord injury requires immobilization, reduction of dislocations, and stabilization of the vertebral column.
2. Reduce the cervical fracture and align the cervical spine with a form of skeletal traction, i.e., skeletal tongs/calipers or the halo-vest technique.
3. Hang weights freely so as not to interfere with the traction.

SURGICAL INTERVENTION: LAMINECTOMY

Indicated when:

1. Deformities cannot be reduced by traction.
2. There is significant instability of the cervical spine.
3. The injury is in the thoracic or lumbar regions.
4. Neurologic status is deteriorating to reduce the spinal fracture or dislocation or decompress the cord.

COMPLICATIONS OF SPINAL INJURY: SPINAL SHOCK

Spinal shock represents a sudden depression of reflex activity in the spinal cord (areflexia) below the level of injury. In this condition, the muscles innervated by the part of the cord segment situated below the level of the lesion become completely paralyzed and flaccid, and the reflexes are absent. Blood pressure falls, and parts of the body below the level of the cord lesion are paralyzed and without sensation.

1. Use intestinal decompression to treat bowel distention and paralytic ileus caused by depression of reflexes.
2. Provide close observation to patient who does not perspire on paralyzed portion of body and for early detection of an abrupt onset of fever.
3. Support and maintain body defenses until the spinal shock abates and the system has recovered from the traumatic insult (3–6 weeks).
4. Pay special attention to the respiratory system (may not be enough intrathoracic pressure to cough effectively).
5. Implement chest physical therapy and suctioning to help clear pulmonary secretions.
6. Monitor for respiratory complications (respiratory failure; pneumonia).
7. Monitor for autonomic hyperreflexia (characterized by pounding headache, profuse sweating, nasal congestion, piloerection [gooseflesh], bradycardia, and hypertension).
8. Maintain constant surveillance for signs and symptoms of pressure ulcers and infection (urinary; respiratory; local infection at the pin sites).
9. Observe for deep vein thrombosis (DVT), a complication of immobility, i.e., pulmonary embolism (PE). Symptoms include pleuritic chest pain, anxiety, shortness of breath, and abnormal blood gas values.

10. Assess thigh and calf measurements daily.
11. Initiate low-dose anticoagulation therapy to prevent DVT and PE.
12. Use thigh-high elastic stockings or pneumatic compression devices.

NURSING PROCESS

Assessment

1. Observe breathing pattern; assess strength of cough; auscultate lungs.
2. Monitor constantly for any changes in motor or sensory function and symptoms of progressive neurologic damage.
3. Determine motor and sensory function by careful neurologic examination; record these findings so changes in or progression from the baseline can be evaluated accurately.
4. Test motor ability by asking patient to spread fingers, squeeze examiner's hand, and move toes or turn the feet.
5. Evaluate sensation by pinching the skin or pricking it with the broken end of a cotton swab, starting at shoulder and working down both sides. Ask patient where sensation is felt.
6. Report immediately any decrease in neurologic function.
7. Assess for the presence of spinal shock.
8. Palpate bladder for signs of urinary retention and overdistention.
9. Assess for gastric dilatation and ileus due to atonic bowel.
10. Monitor temperature (hypothermia may result due to autonomic disruption).

Major Nursing Diagnosis

1. Ineffective breathing patterns related to weakness/paralysis of abdominal and intercostal muscles and inability to clear secretions.

2. Impaired physical mobility related to motor and sensory impairment.
3. Risk for impaired skin integrity related to immobility, sensory loss.
4. Urinary retention related to inability to void spontaneously.
5. Constipation related to presence of atonic bowel as a result of autonomic disruption.
6. Pain and discomfort related to treatment and prolonged immobility.

Collaborative Problems

1. Deep vein thrombosis.
2. Orthostatic hypotension.
3. Autonomic hyperreflexia.

Planning and Implementation

The goals may include improvement of breathing pattern, improvement of mobility, maintenance of skin integrity, relief of urinary retention, improvement of bowel function, promotion of comfort, and absence of complications.

Interventions

PROMOTING ADEQUATE BREATHING

1. Detect possible impending respiratory failure by observing patient, measuring vital capacity, and monitoring arterial blood gas values.
2. Prevent retention of secretions and resultant atelectasis with early and vigorous attention to clearing bronchial and pharyngeal secretions.
3. Employ suctioning with caution. This procedure can stimulate the vagus nerve, producing bradycardia, resulting in cardiac arrest.
4. Initiate chest physical therapy for ineffective cough.
5. Supervise breathing exercises that increase strength and endurance of inspiratory muscles, particularly the diaphragm.
6. Ensure proper humidification and hydration to thin secretions.

S

7. Assess for signs of respiratory infection: cough, fever, and dyspnea.
8. Discourage smoking.

IMPROVING MOBILITY

1. Maintain proper body alignment; place in dorsal or supine position.
2. Turn patient every 2 hours; monitor for hypotension in patients with lesions above the midthoracic level.
3. Do not turn patient if not on a turning frame unless physician has indicated that it is safe to do so.
4. Give passive range-of-motion exercises within 48–72 hours after injury to avoid complications, i.e., contractures and atrophy.
5. Provide a full range of motion at least 4–5 times daily to toes, metatarsals, ankles, knees, and hips.

MAINTAINING SKIN INTEGRITY

1. Change patient's position every 2 hours and inspect the skin.
2. Assess for redness or breaks in skin over pressure points; check perineum for soilage; observe catheter for adequate drainage; assess general body alignment and comfort.
3. Wash skin every few hours with a mild soap, rinse well, and blot dry. Keep pressure-sensitive areas well lubricated and soft with bland cream or lotion; gently perform massage with a circular motion.
4. Teach patient danger of pressure ulcers and encourage to participate in preventive measures.

PROMOTING URINARY ELIMINATION

1. Perform intermittent catheterization to avoid overstretching the bladder and infection; if not feasible, insert indwelling catheter.
2. Show family members how to catheterize and encourage them to participate in this facet of care.
3. Teach patient to record fluid intake, voiding pattern,

amounts of residual urine after catheterization, quality of urine, and any unusual feelings that may be occurring.

IMPROVING BOWEL FUNCTION

1. Monitor patient's reactions to gastric intubation.
2. Give a high-calorie, high-protein, and high-fiber diet with amount of food gradually increased after bowel sounds resume.
3. Administer prescribed stool softener to counteract effects of immobility and pain medications.

PROVIDING COMFORT

1. Assess patient's skull for signs of infection, including drainage around the tongs.
2. Check back of head periodically for signs of pressure and massage at intervals, taking care not to move the neck.
3. Shave hair around tongs to facilitate inspection; avoid probing under encrusted areas.
4. Reassure patient in halo traction that adaption to steel frame (caged in and noises) will occur.
5. Cleanse pin sites daily and observe for redness, drainage, and pain; observe for loosening.
6. Inspect skin under halo vest for excessive perspiration, redness, and skin blistering, especially on the bony prominences.
7. Open vest at the sides to allow the patient's torso to be washed; do not allow vest to become wet; do not use powder inside vest.

Monitoring and Managing Potential Complications

THROMBOPHLEBITIS

Refer to the management heading for care.

ORTHOSTATIC HYPOTENSION

Reduce frequency of hypotensive episodes by providing vasopressor medications, thigh-high elastic stockings, adequate time for slow position change, and tilt tables.

AUTONOMIC HYPERREFLEXIA

1. Remove the triggering stimulus.
2. Place immediately in a sitting position to lower blood pressure.
3. Empty bladder immediately, i.e., catheterize.
4. Examine rectum for fecal mass after the symptoms subside.
5. Give a ganglionic blocking agent (Apresoline) if the above measures do not relieve hypertension and excruciating headache.
6. Instruct patient in prevention and management measures.

✎ PATIENT EDUCATION AND HEALTH MAINTENANCE: CARE IN THE HOME AND COMMUNITY

1. Shift emphasis from ensuring patient is stable and free of complications to specific assessment and planning for independence and skills necessary for activities of daily living.
2. The nurse is in the key position to coordinate the management team and serve as the liaison with rehabilitation centers and home care agencies.
3. Provide assistance in dealing with the psychological impact of the spinal cord injury and its consequences.

For more information see Chapter 60 in Smeltzer and Bare: *Brunner and Suddarth's Textbook of Medical–Surgical Nursing,* 8th Edition. Philadelphia: Lippincott–Raven, 1996.

SQUAMOUS CELL CANCER

See Cancer of the Skin

STENOSIS, AORTIC

See Aortic Stenosis

STENOSIS, MITRAL

See Mitral Stenosis

STOMACH DISORDERS

See Gastritis

STONES, URINARY

See Urolithiasis

STREP THROAT

See Pharyngitis, Acute

STRESS ULCER

Stress ulcer is a term given to acute mucosal ulceration of the duodenal or gastric area that occurs following physiologically disturbing conditions such as burns, shock, severe sepsis, and multiple organ trauma. Fiberoptic endoscopy within 24 hours of injury shows shallow erosions of the stomach wall; by 72 hours multiple gastric erosions are observed, and as the stressful condition continues, the ulcers spread. When the patient recovers, the lesions are reversed; this pattern is typical of stress ulceration.

MANAGEMENT

Antacids

1. Basis for treatment.
2. Antacids may be given through a nasogastric tube.

3. Cimetidine (Tagamet) or ranitidine (Zantac) therapy in addition to antacids may be used.

For more information see Chapter 36 in Smeltzer and Bare: *Brunner and Suddarth's Textbook of Medical–Surgical Nursing,* 8th Edition. Philadelphia: Lippincott–Raven, 1996.

STROKE

See Cerebral Vascular Accident

SYNDROME OF INAPPROPRIATE ANTIDIURETIC HORMONE SECRETION

See SIADH

SYSTEMIC LUPUS ERYTHEMATOSUS

Lupus erythematosus (LE) is a chronic, inflammatory autoimmune disease that takes three basic forms: discoid lupus involves the skin; the lupus may be chemically or drug induced; and systemic lupus erythematosus (SLE) involves major organ systems. Women tend to be affected nine times more frequently than men; the average age at onset is 30 years, with predominance in nonwhites. A genetic link has not been found. There is a familial association that suggests that a genetic predisposition may be related to environmental factors or susceptibility to certain viruses. Certain drugs and foods (alfalfa sprouts) seem to trigger the onset of symptoms or aggravate an existing disease. A hormonal abnormality is a possible risk factor because an increased incidence has been noted during the childbearing years. Ultraviolet radiation is also a possible risk factor.

CLINICAL MANIFESTATIONS

1. Onset insidious or acute. May be undiagnosed for many years.
2. Clinical course is one of exacerbations and remissions. Features include nephritis, cardiopulmonary disease, skin rashes, and more indirect evidence of systemic inflammation (fever, fatigue, and weight loss).
3. Musculoskeletal system: arthralgias and arthritis (synovitis) are common presenting features. Joint swelling, tenderness, and pain on movement are common, accompanied by morning stiffness.
4. Several different types of skin manifestations, i.e., subacute cutaneous lupus erythematosus (SCLE), and discoid lupus erythematosus (DLE).
5. Butterfly rash across the bridge of the nose and cheeks, occurring in less than 50% of patients, may be precursor to systemic involvement.
6. Lesions worsen during exacerbations ("flares") and may be provoked by sunlight or artificial ultraviolet light.
7. Oral ulcers may involve buccal mucosa or hard palate.
8. Pericarditis is the most common clinical cardiac manifestation.
9. Pleuritis or pleural effusions.
10. Papular, erythematous, and purpuric lesions on fingertips, elbows, toes, and extensor surfaces of forearms or lateral sides of hands and may progress to necrosis.
11. Lymphadenopathy occurs in 50% of all SLE patients.
12. Renal involvement (glomeruli) occurs in about 50%.
13. Varied and frequent neuropsychiatric presentations, generally demonstrated by subtle changes in behavior patterns. Depression and psychosis are frequent.

DIAGNOSTIC EVALUATION

Diagnosis is based on a complete history and analysis of blood work; no single laboratory test confirms SLE.

MANAGEMENT

Treatment includes management of acute and chronic disease.

1. Prevent progressive loss of organ function, reduce the likelihood of acute disease, minimize disease-related disabilities, and prevent complications from therapy.
2. Use nonsteroidal anti-inflammatory drugs (NSAIDs) with corticosteroids to minimize corticosteroid requirements.
3. Use corticosteroids topically for cutaneous manifestations.
4. Use bolus IV administration as an alternative to traditional high-dose oral use.
5. Manage cutaneous, musculoskeletal, and mild systemic features of SLE with antimalarial drugs.
6. Immunosuppressive agents (experimental) reserved for serious forms of SLE.

Nursing Assessment

1. Perform a thorough, systematic physical assessment, inspecting skin for erythematosus rashes.
2. Observe cutaneous erythematosus plaques with an adherent scale on scalp, face, or neck.
3. Note areas of hyperpigmentation or depigmentation depending on the phase and type of the disease.
4. Question patient about skin changes, specifically about sensitivity to sunlight or artificial ultraviolet light.
5. Inspect scalp for alopecia.
6. Examine mouth and throat for ulcerations.
7. Check for presence of pericardial friction rub and abnormal lung sounds (pleural effusion).

8. Assess for vascular involvement, i.e., papular erythematosus, and purpuric lesions.

9. Observe for signs of musculoskeletal involvement, i.e., joint swelling, tenderness, warmth, pain on movement, and stiffness. Joint involvement often symmetric.

10. Observe for edema and hematuria, indicative of renal involvement.

11. Facilitate interactions with patient and family to provide further evidence of systemic involvement.

12. Direct neurologic assessment at identifying and describing central nervous system involvement.

13. Question family members regarding behavioral changes, neuroses, or psychoses.

14. Note signs of depression, reports of seizures, chorea, or other CNS manifestations.

15. Assess knowledge of disease process and self-management.

16. Assess patient's perception of and coping with fatigue, body image, and other problems caused by disease.

The nursing care of the patient with SLE is generally the same as the basic care plan for the patient with rheumatic disease.

For more information see Chapter 52 in Smeltzer and Bare: *Brunner and Suddarth's Textbook of Medical–Surgical Nursing.* 8th Edition. Philadelphia: Lippincott–Raven, 1996.

S

T&A

See Tonsillitis and Adenoiditis

TB

See Tuberculosis

TEN

See Toxic Epidermal Necrolysis

TENSION HEADACHE

See Headache

TENSION PNEUMOTHORAX

See Pneumothorax

TESTICULAR CANCER

See Cancer of the Testis

THROAT CANCER

See Cancer of the Throat

THROMBI

See Pulmonary Embolism

THROMBOANGIITIS OBLITERANS

See Buerger's Disease

THROMBOCYTOPENIA

Thrombocytopenia is the most common cause of abnormal bleeding. It can result either from decreased production of platelets by the bone marrow or from increased peripheral destruction. Causes include failure of production, e.g., certain anemias, septicemia, and cytotoxic medications; increased destruction, e.g., idiopathic thrombocytopenia purpura, lupus erythematosus, malignant lymphoma, medications (digoxin, phenytoin, aspirin), and postviral infections; increased utilization, e.g., disseminated intravascular coagulopathy (DIC).

DIAGNOSTIC EVALUATION

1. Bone marrow studies, if platelet deficiency is secondary to an underlying disease.
2. Increased megakaryocytes and normal platelet production in bone marrow, when peripheral destruction is the cause.

CLINICAL MANIFESTATIONS

1. Bleeding and petechiae (platelet count below 50,000/mm^3).
2. Nosebleeds, excessive menstrual bleeding, and hemorrhage occur after surgery or dental extractions (platelet count below 20,000/mm^3).

T

3. Spontaneous fatal central nervous system hemorrhage or gastrointestinal hemorrhage (platelet count below 5000/mm^3).

MANAGEMENT

1. The management for secondary thrombocytopenia is usually treatment of the underlying disease.
2. Platelet transfusions to raise platelet count.

For more information see Chapter 32 in Smeltzer and Bare: *Brunner and Suddarth's Textbook of Medical–Surgical Nursing,* 8th Edition. Philadelphia: Lippincott–Raven, 1996.

THYROID CANCER

See Cancer of the Thyroid

THYROID STORM (THYROTOXIC CRISIS)

Thyroid storm (thyrotoxic crisis) is a form of severe hyperthyroidism, usually of abrupt onset and characterized by high fever (hyperpyrexia), extreme tachycardia, and altered mental state, which frequently appears as delirium. Thyroid storm is a life-threatening condition that is usually precipitated by stress such as injury, infection, nonthyroid surgery, thyroidectomy, tooth extraction, insulin reaction, diabetic acidosis, pregnancy, digitalis intoxication, abrupt withdrawal of antithyroid drugs, or vigorous palpation of the thyroid. These factors will precipitate thyroid storm in the partially controlled or completely untreated hyperthyroid patient. A patient with thyroid storm or crisis is critically ill. Untreated thyroid storm is almost always fatal, but with proper treatment the mortality rate can be reduced substantially.

CLINICAL MANIFESTATIONS

1. Tachycardia (over 130 beats/min).
2. Temperature above 37.7°C (101°F).
3. Exaggerated symptoms of hyperthyroidism.
4. Disturbances of a major system, e.g., gastrointestinal (weight loss, diarrhea, abdominal pain), neurologic (psychoses, somnolence, coma), or cardiovascular (edema, chest pain, dyspnea, palpitations).

MANAGEMENT

The immediate objective is to reduce body temperature and heart rate and prevent vascular collapse.

1. Employ hypothermia mattress or blanket, ice packs, cool environment, hydrocortisone, and acetaminophen.
2. Administer humidified oxygen to improve tissue oxygenation and meet high metabolic demands.
3. Monitor respiratory status with arterial blood gases or pulse oximetry.
4. Administer IV fluids containing dextrose to replace liver glycogen stores.
5. Give hydrocortisone to treat shock or adrenal insufficiency.
6. Give propylthiouracil (PTU) to impede formation of thyroid hormone.
7. Administer iodine to decrease output of T4 from thyroid gland.
8. Give sympatholytic agents for cardiac problems.

Nursing Interventions

Provide astute observation and aggressive and supportive nursing care during and after acute stage of illness.

 CLINICAL ALERT

Salicylates are not used in the management of thyroid storm because they displace thyroid hormone from binding proteins and worsen the hypermetabolism.

For more information see Chapter 40 in Smeltzer and Bare: *Brunner and Suddarth's Textbook of Medical–Surgical Nursing,* 8th Edition. Philadelphia: Lippincott–Raven, 1996.

THYROIDITIS

Thyroiditis is inflammation of the thyroid and can be acute, subacute, or chronic in nature. Each type of thyroidism is characterized by inflammation, fibrosis, or lymphocytic infiltration of the thyroid gland. Acute thyroiditis is a rare disorder caused by infection of the thyroid gland. The most common cause is *Staphylococcus aureus.* Other causes are bacteria, fungi, mycobacteria, or parasites. Subacute may be granulomatosis thyroiditis (de Quervain's thyroiditis) or painless thyroiditis (silent thyroiditis or subacute lymphocytic thyroiditis). This form occurs in the postpartum period and is thought to be an autoimmune reaction.

CLINICAL MANIFESTATIONS

Acute Thyroiditis

1. Anterior neck pain and swelling, fever, dysphagia, and dysphonia.
2. Pharyngitis or pharyngeal pain often present.
3. Warmth, erythema, and tenderness of the thyroid gland.

Subacute Thyroiditis

1. Thyroid enlarges symmetrically and occasionally is painful.
2. Overlying skin is often reddened and warm.
3. Swallowing may be difficult and uncomfortable.
4. Irritability, nervousness, insomnia, and weight loss, which are manifestations of hyperthyroidism, are common.
5. Chills and fever may be experienced.

MANAGEMENT

Acute Thyroiditis

1. Antimicrobial agents and fluid replacement.
2. Surgical incision and drainage if abscess is present.

Subacute Thyroiditis

1. Control the inflammation.
2. Nonsteroidal anti-inflammatory agents (NSAIDs) to relieve neck pain.
3. Beta-blocking agents to control symptoms of hyper-thyroidism.
4. Oral corticosteroids to relieve pain and reduce swelling; do not usually affect the underlying cause.

For more information see Chapter 40 in Smeltzer and Bare: *Brunner and Suddarth's Textbook of Medical–Surgical Nursing,* 8th Edition. Philadelphia: Lippincott–Raven, 1996.

THYROIDITIS, CHRONIC (HASHIMOTO'S THYROIDITIS)

Chronic thyroiditis occurs most frequently in women 30–50 years of age, and is termed Hashimoto's disease. Diagnosis is based on the histologic appearance of the inflamed gland. The chronic forms are usually accompanied by pain, pressure symptoms, or fever, and thyroid activity is usually normal or low. Cell-mediated immunity plays a significant role in the pathogenesis of thyroiditis. A genetic predisposition also seems to be significant in its etiology. If untreated, the disease slowly progresses to hypothyroidism.

MANAGEMENT

The objective of treatment is to reduce the size of the thyroid gland and prevent myxedema.

1. Thyroid hormone therapy is prescribed to reduce thyroid activity and production of thyroglobulin.

2. Give thyroid hormone, if hypothyroid symptoms are present.
3. Surgery if pressure symptoms persist.

For more information see Chapter 40 in Smeltzer and Bare: *Brunner and Suddarth's Textbook of Medical–Surgical Nursing,* 8th Edition. Philadelphia: Lippincott–Raven, 1996.

THYROTOXIC CRISIS

See Thyroid Storm

TIA

See Transient Ischemic Attack

TIC DOULOUREUX

See Trigeminal Neuralgia

TONSILLITIS AND ADENOIDITIS

The tonsils frequently serve as the site of acute infection. Group A Streptococcus is the most common organism associated with tonsillitis and adenoiditis. Chronic tonsillitis is less common and may be mistaken for other disorders such as allergy, asthma, and sinusitis. Infection of the adenoids frequently accompanies acute tonsillitis.

CLINICAL MANIFESTATIONS

1. Tonsillitis: sore throat, fever, snoring, and difficulty in swallowing.
2. Adenoid hypertrophy: mouth breathing, earache, draining ears, frequent head colds, bronchitis, foul-smelling breath, voice impairment, and noisy respiration.

3. Nasal obstruction (unusually enlarged adenoids).
4. Acute otitis media; caused from extension of infection. Potential complication: spontaneous rupture of eardrums causing acute mastoiditis.
5. Infection in middle ear, e.g., chronic, low-grade process that eventually causes permanent deafness.

DIAGNOSTIC EVALUATION

Primarily repeated history of sore throat; throat cultures.

MANAGEMENT

Tonsillectomy and Adenoidectomy (T&A)

1. Tonsillectomy usually not performed unless medical treatment is unsuccessful and there is severe hypertrophy or peritonsillar abscess that occludes the pharynx, making swallowing difficult and endangering the airway.
2. Appropriate antibiotic therapy is initiated for both T&A.

Nursing Interventions: Postoperative

1. Observe for hemorrhage in immediate postoperative and recovery period.
2. Position patient prone with head turned to the side to allow for drainage from mouth and pharynx.
3. Remove oral airway after swallowing reflex has returned.
4. Apply ice collar to neck, and provide a basin and tissues for expectoration of blood and mucus.
5. Give continuous nursing observation and postoperative care as required if suture or ligation necessary for bleeding vessel.
6. Give water and cracked ice as desired if there is no bleeding.
7. Instruct patient to refrain from too much talking and coughing, can produce throat pain.

T

PATIENT EDUCATION AND HEALTH MAINTENANCE: CARE IN THE HOME AND COMMUNITY

1. Ensure patient and family understand the signs and symptoms of hemorrhage (usually occurs in first 12–24 hours).
2. Report any bleeding to physician; delayed hemorrhage may occur up to a week after surgery.
3. Give alkaline mouth washes/warm saline rinses for thick mucus.
4. Dietary management: liquid or semiliquid diet for several days; sherbet and gelatin desserts; avoid spicy, hot, cold, acidic, or rough foods; and restrict milk and milk products.

✚ CLINICAL ALERT

Notify surgeon immediately if patient vomits large amounts of blood or spits bright blood at frequent intervals, or if pulse rate and temperature rise and patient is restless.

For more information see Chapter 23 in Smeltzer and Bare: *Brunner and Suddarth's Textbook of Medical–Surgical Nursing,* 8th Edition. Philadelphia: Lippincott–Raven, 1996.

TOXIC EPIDERMAL NECROLYSIS

Toxic epidermal necrolysis (TEN) is a severe, potentially fatal skin disease. Etiology is unknown, but is probably linked to the immune system as a reaction to medications or possibly secondary to a viral infection. The total body surface may be involved with widespread areas of erythema and blisters.

CLINICAL MANIFESTATIONS

1. Initial signs: conjunctival burning or itching, cutaneous tenderness, fever, headache, extreme malaise, and myalgias.
2. Followed by rapid onset of erythema, involving the skin surface and mucous membranes; large, flaccid bullae in some areas; in other areas large sheets of epidermis are shed, exposing underlying dermis; fingernails, toenails, eyebrows, and eyelashes may all shed along with surrounding epidermis.
3. Excruciatingly tender skin, and loss of skin leads to weeping surface similar to that of a total-body second-degree burn; condition may be referred to as scalded skin syndrome.

DIAGNOSTIC EVALUATION

Frozen histologic studies of skin cells; cytodiagnosis of cells of a denuded area; immunofluorescent studies for atypical epidermal autoantibodies.

MANAGEMENT

The goals of treatment include control of fluid and electrolyte balance, prevention of sepsis, and prevention of ophthalmic complications. Mainstay of treatment is supportive care.

1. Discontinue immediately all nonessential medications
2. Treat in a regional burn center.
3. Perform surgical debridement or hydrotherapy initially to remove involved skin.
4. Take cultures of nasopharynx, eyes, ears, blood, urine, skin, and unruptured blisters to identify pathogens.
5. Give prescribed IV fluids to maintain fluid and electrolyte balance.
6. Fluid replacement by nasogastric tube, and orally.
7. Systemic corticosteroids, early in the disease process.

T

8. Protect skin with topical agents.
9. Topical antibacterial and anesthetic agents to prevent wound sepsis.
10. Temporary biologic dressings (pig skin, amniotic membrane) or plastic semipermeable dressing (Vigilon).

NURSING PROCESS

Assessment

1. Inspect appearance and extent of involvement of skin. Monitor skin seepage for amount, color, and odor.
2. Inspect oral cavity for blistering and erosive lesions daily. Determine patient's ability to drink fluids.
3. Assess eyes daily for itching, burning, and dryness.
4. Monitor vital signs with special attention given to fever and respiratory status.
5. Monitor urine volume, specific gravity, and color.
6. Inspect IV insertion sites for local signs of infection.
7. Record daily weight.
8. Question patient about fatigue and pain levels.
9. Assess coping mechanisms; identify new effective coping skills.

Major Nursing Diagnosis

1. Impaired tissue integrity (oral, eye, and skin) related to epidermal shedding.
2. Fluid volume deficit and electrolyte losses related to loss of fluids from denuded skin.
3. Risk for altered body temperature (hypothermia) related to heat loss, secondary to skin loss.
4. Pain related to denuded skin, oral lesions, and possible infection.
5. Anxiety related to the physical appearance of the skin and prognosis.

Collaborative Problems

1. Sepsis.
2. Conjunctival retraction, scars, and corneal lesions.

Planning and Implementation

The major goals may include achievement of skin and oral tissue healing, attainment of fluid balance, prevention of heat loss, relief of pain, reduction of anxiety, and absence of complications.

Interventions

MAINTAINING SKIN AND MUCOUS MEMBRANE INTEGRITY

1. Place on a circular turning frame to prevent skin denudement.
2. Apply prescribed topical agents that reduce wound bacteria.
3. Apply warm compresses gently, if prescribed, to denuded areas.
4. Use topical antibacterial agent in conjunction with hydrotherapy; monitor treatment and encourage the patient to exercise extremities during hydrotherapy.
5. Perform oral hygiene carefully. Use prescribed mouthwashes frequently to rid mouth of debris, sooth ulcerative areas, and control odor. Inspect oral cavity frequently, note changes, and report. Apply petrolatum to lips.

ATTAINING FLUID BALANCE

1. Observe for signs of hypovolemia, i.e., vital signs, urine output, and sensorium.
2. Evaluate laboratory tests and report abnormal results.
3. Weigh patient daily.
4. Provide fluid replacement.
5. Provide enteral nourishment.
6. Record intake and output and daily calorie count.

T

PREVENTING HYPOTHERMIA

1. Maintain patient's comfort and body temperature with cotton blankets, ceiling-mounted heat lamps, or heat shields.
2. Work rapidly and efficiently when large wounds are exposed for wound care in order to minimize shivering and heat loss.
3. Monitor temperature carefully.

RELIEVING PAIN

1. Assess for presence and character of pain, behavioral responses, and factors that influence the pain.
2. Administer prescribed analgesics, and observe for pain relief, side effects.
3. Administer analgesics before painful treatments.
4. Provide proper explanations and speak soothingly to the patient during treatments to allay anxiety that may intensify pain.
5. Provide measures to promote rest and sleep; emotional support and reassurance to achieve pain control.
6. Teach self-management techniques for pain relief, such as progressive muscle relaxation and imagery.

REDUCING ANXIETY

1. Assess emotional state, i.e., anxiety, fear of dying, and depression; reassure these reactions are normal.
2. Give support, honesty, and hope that the situation can improve.
3. Encourage patients to express their feelings to someone they trust.
4. Listen to their concerns; be available with skillful, compassionate care.
5. Provide emotional support during the long recovery period with psychiatric nurse, chaplain, psychologist, or psychiatrist.

MONITORING AND MANAGING POTENTIAL COMPLICATIONS

1. Sepsis: monitor vital signs and note adverse changes related to body systems infection; maintain universal precautions at all times.
2. Conjunctival retraction, scars, and corneal lesions: inspect eyes for progression of TEN to keratoconjunctivitis; administer eye lubricant; use eye patches; avoid rubbing eyes; document and report progression of symptoms.

For more information see Chapter 54 in Smeltzer and Bare: *Brunner and Suddarth's Textbook of Medical–Surgical Nursing,* 8th Edition. Philadelphia: Lippincott–Raven, 1996.

TOXIC SHOCK SYNDROME

Toxic shock syndrome (TSS) is caused by the bacterium *Staphylococcus aureus* and usually occurs in menstruating women. About 45% of cases are not related to menstruation. Risk factors include menstruation, chronic vaginal infection, pelvic infection, lung abscess, surgical wound infection, soft tissue infection, postpartum and gynecological infection, use of IV drugs and superabsorbent tampons. Barrier methods of contraception, e.g., sponge and diaphragm, have also been implicated.

CLINICAL MANIFESTATIONS

1. Sudden fever (38.9°C [102°F]), vomiting, diarrhea, myalgia, hypotension, chills, malaise, headache, palmar erythema, and signs suggesting early septic shock.
2. Red, macular rash similar to sunburn often occurs: may become scaly or peel in 7–10 days.
3. Decreased urine output, and blood urea nitrogen level (BUN) increases, resulting in disorientation.
4. Leukocytosis and elevated bilirubin, BUN, and creatinine.

5. Uncontrollable hypotension; clinical picture of shock.
6. Disseminated intravascular coagulopathy (DIC).
7. Respiratory distress may develop from pulmonary edema.
8. Adult respiratory distress syndrome (ARDS) occurs (outlook becomes grave).
9. Inflammation of mucous membranes.
10. About 2–3% die of complications.

DIAGNOSTIC EVALUATION

Cultures of blood, urine, throat, vagina, and possibly cervix.

MANAGEMENT

Patient placed on bed rest and the treatment plan is directed primarily at controlling the infection with antibiotics and restoration of circulating blood volume.

1. Institute oxygen therapy if there is respiratory distress.
2. Give sodium bicarbonate if signs of acidosis appear.
3. Calcium is prescribed for hypocalcemia.
4. Hemodynamic monitoring, intravenous dopamine, and military antishock trousers (MAST) are used to manage shock.
5. Listen to and support patient's emotional and psychological concerns.

NURSING PROCESS

Assessment

Direct nursing history toward determining whether patient used tampons recently, type used, how long tampon was retained before changing it, and whether any problems were noted when inserting the tampon, which may have injured the vaginal tissue.

Major Nursing Diagnosis

1. Anxiety related to the severity and suddenness of the symptoms and to concerns about recovery.
2. Fluid volume deficit related to vomiting and diarrhea.
3. Fatigue related to severity of illness and of shock, prolonged immobility, excessive nutritional demands, and stress.
4. Knowledge deficit about risk factors and behaviors.

Collaborative Problems

1. Septic shock.
2. DIC.

Planning and Implementation

The major goals may include reduction of anxiety and emotional stress, absence of vomiting and diarrhea, acquisition of relevant knowledge, and prevention of potential complications.

Interventions

RELIEVING ANXIETY

1. Provide emotional support and reassurance to reduce anxiety and apprehension.
2. Keep patient and family informed about diagnostic procedures and treatments.
3. Give opportunity for self-care and decision making when able.

IMPROVING FLUID VOLUME STATUS

1. Monitor intake and output; assess for fluid deficit.
2. Administer IV and oral fluids as prescribed; note changes.
3. Administer antiemetics and antidiarrheal agents if necessary.
4. Give comfort measures, e.g., oral hygiene.

T

DECREASING FATIGUE

1. Assist with self-care efforts to increase stamina.
2. Counteract weight loss with nutritious diet.
3. Monitor weight and caloric intake; give dietary supplements.
4. Plan an exercise activity program to build stamina.

MONITORING AND MANAGING COMPLICATIONS

1. Monitor and document vital signs and blood gas levels.
2. Culture body excretions to determine antibiotic therapy.
3. Note skin changes, hydration, and kidney function.
4. Be observant for DIC symptoms: hematomas; petechiae; oozing from needle puncture sites; cyanosis; and coolness of nose, fingertips, and toes.
5. Be alert for changes indicative of severe shock.

✎ PATIENT EDUCATION AND HEALTH MAINTENANCE: CARE IN THE HOME AND COMMUNITY

1. Recommend that superabsorbent tampons not be used. If tampons used, should be changed frequently (every 4 hours). Insert carefully to avoid abrasions (applicators with rough edges should be avoided).
2. Do not leave a diaphragm in place longer than 8–10 hours.
3. Discourage tampons if patient has had TSS.
4. Discourage use of diaphragm or sponge during menses or in the first 3 months postpartum.
5. Teach that risk of developing TSS is increased at any time a woman bleeds vaginally, i.e., during menses and postpartum.

For more information see Chapter 45 in Smeltzer and Bare: *Brunner and Suddarth's Textbook of Medical–Surgical Nursing,* 8th Edition. Philadelphia: Lippincott–Raven, 1996.

TRANSIENT ISCHEMIC ATTACK (TIA)

A TIA is a temporary episode of neurologic dysfunction commonly manifested by a sudden loss of motor, sensory, or visual function. It may last a few seconds or minutes but no longer than 24 hours. Complete recovery usually occurs between attacks. A TIA may serve as a warning of impending stroke, which often occurs the first month after the first attack. The cause is a temporary impairment of blood flow to a specific region of the brain. Reasons may include atherosclerosis of the vessels supplying the brain, obstruction of cerebral microcirculation by a small embolus, a fall in cerebral perfusion pressure, and cardiac dysrhythmias.

CLINICAL MANIFESTATIONS

1. Amaurosis fugax (fleeting blindness) occurring without warning. Sudden, painless loss of vision of one eye or dimming or graying out of the field of vision of one eye.
2. If ischemia occurs in the vertebral basilar system, vertigo, diplopia, disturbances of consciousness, and various signs of motor and sensory impairment may be exhibited.

DIAGNOSTIC EVALUATION

1. Carotid phonoangiography provides auscultation, direct visualization, and photographic recording of carotid bruits.
2. Oculoplethysmography (OPG) measures pulsation and blood flow through the ophthalmic artery.
3. Carotid angiography visualizes intracranial and cervical vessels.
4. Digital subtraction angiography is used to define carotid artery obstruction.

T

MANAGEMENT

1. Place on anticoagulant therapy to prevent future attacks if not a candidate for surgical intervention.
2. Give platelet-inhibiting drugs (aspirin) to decrease the occurrence of cerebral infarction.
3. Common surgical intervention procedures are endarterectomy and angioplasty.

Interventions for Carotid Endarterectomy

1. Keep flow sheet to maintain close assessment of patient's neurologic status.
2. Be aware of primary complications of carotid endarterectomy: stroke, cranial nerve injuries, infection or hematoma of the wound, and carotid artery disruption.
3. Maintain adequate blood pressure levels in immediate postoperative period.
4. Avoid hypotension to prevent cerebral ischemia and thrombosis.
5. Prevent excessive hypertension, which may precipitate cerebral hemorrhage; use sodium nitroprusside.
6. Assess for difficulty in swallowing, hoarseness, or other signs of cranial nerve dysfunction; have a tracheostomy set available.
7. Monitor cardiac status closely because of high incidence of coronary artery disease.
8. Be aware of long-term complications: recurrent stroke and myocardial infarction.

For more information see Chapter 59 in Smeltzer and Bare: *Brunner and Suddarth's Textbook of Medical–Surgical Nursing,* 8th Edition. Philadelphia: Lippincott–Raven, 1996.

TRIGEMINAL NEURALGIA (TIC DOULOUREUX)

Trigeminal neuralgia is a condition of the fifth cranial nerve characterized by paroxysms of pain similar to an electric shock in the area innervated by one or more branches of the trigeminal nerve. Each pain episode can be described as stabbing, lasting from a few seconds to minutes, and producing contraction of some of the facial muscles, i.e., sudden closing of the eye or a twitch of the mouth; hence the name tic douloureux (painful twitch). The cause is not certain. Chronic compression or irritation of the trigeminal nerve or degenerative changes in the gasserian ganglion are suggested causes. Early attacks, appearing most often in the fifth decade of life, are usually mild and brief. Pain-free intervals may be measured in terms of minutes, hours, days, or longer. With advancing years, the painful episodes tend to become more and more frequent and agonizing. The patient lives in constant fear of attacks.

CLINICAL MANIFESTATIONS

1. Pain is felt in the skin, not in the deeper structures, more severe at the peripheral areas of distribution of affected nerve, notably over the lip, chin, nostrils, and in the teeth.
2. Paroxysms are aroused by any stimulation of terminals of the affected nerve branches, i.e., washing the face, shaving, brushing the teeth, eating, and drinking.
3. Draft of cold air and direct pressure against the nerve trunk may also cause pain.
4. Trigger points are certain areas where the slightest touch immediately starts a paroxysm.

T

DIAGNOSTIC EVALUATION

Characteristic behavior avoiding stimulating trigger point areas, e.g., trying not to touch or wash the faces, shave, chew, or anything else that might cause an attack.

MANAGEMENT

Pharmacologic Treatment

1. Anticonvulsive agents carbamazepine (Tegretol) and phenytoin (Dilantin) reduce transmission of impulses at certain nerve terminals, relieve pain in most patients.
2. Give Tegretol with meals, in doses gradually increased until relief is obtained.
3. Observe for side effects including nausea, dizziness, drowsiness, and hepatic dysfunction.
4. Monitor patient for bone marrow depression during long-term drug therapy.
5. Recognize phenytoin side effects, i.e., nausea, dizziness, somnolence, ataxia, and skin allergies.

Alcohol injection

1. Injection of gasserian ganglion and peripheral branches of the trigeminal nerve.
2. Relieves pain for several months.
3. Pain returns after the nerve regenerates.

Percutaneous Radiofrequency Trigeminal Gangliolysis

Percutaneous radiofrequency interruption of the gasserian ganglion is the surgical procedure of choice (small unmyelinated and thinly myelinated fibers that conduct pain are thermally destroyed).

Microvascular Decompression of the Trigeminal Nerve

1. An intracranial approach (craniotomy) to decompress the trigeminal nerve.
2. This procedure relieves facial pain while preserving normal sensation.

NURSING INTERVENTIONS

1. Recognize in preoperative management that certain factors may aggravate excruciating facial pain. Lessen these discomforts by using cotton pads and room-temperature water to wash face.
2. Instruct patient to rinse mouth after eating when tooth brushing causes pain.
3. Perform personal hygiene during pain-free intervals.
4. Advise to take food and fluids at room temperature, to chew on unaffected side, and ingest all foods when maintenance of nutrition is a problem.
5. Recognize anxiety, depression, and insomnia often accompany chronic painful conditions and use appropriate interventions and referrals.

For more information see Chapter 60 in Smeltzer and Bare: *Brunner and Suddarth's Textbook of Medical–Surgical Nursing,* 8th Edition. Philadelphia: Lippincott–Raven, 1996.

TSS

See Toxic Shock Syndrome

TUBERCULOSIS

Tuberculosis (TB) is an infectious disease primarily caused by *Mycobacterium tuberculosis.* It usually involves the lungs, but may spread to almost any part of the body, including the meninges, kidney, bones, and lymph nodes. The initial infection usually occurs 2–10 weeks after exposure. The person may then develop active disease because of a compromised or inadequate immune system response. The activity process may be prolonged and characterized by long remissions when the disease is arrested, only to be followed by periods of renewed activity. TB is a worldwide public health problem. Mortality and morbidity rates continue to rise.

TRANSMISSION AND RISK FACTORS

TB is transmitted from a person with active pulmonary disease who expels the organisms while talking, coughing, sneezing, or singing. A susceptible person inhales the droplets and becomes infected.

High Risk for Infection

Those at high risk for acquiring the infection include:

1. Persons in close contact with someone who has active TB.
2. IV drug users and alcoholics.
3. Persons living in overcrowded, substandard housing.
4. Immunocompromised persons, e.g., elderly, patients with cancer, those on corticosteroid therapy or infected with HIV.
5. Persons with preexisting medical conditions, e.g., diabetes, chronic renal failure, silicosis, malnourishment.
6. Immigrants from countries with a high incidence of TB, e.g., Haiti, southeast Asia.
7. Persons who are medically undeserved, e.g., homeless, impoverished, ethnic and racial minorities, children, and young adults.
8. Persons who are institutionalized, e.g., long-term care, psychiatric, prison inmates.
9. Health care workers.

CLINICAL MANIFESTATIONS

1. Insidious onset.
2. Present with low-grade fever, fatigue, anorexia, weight loss, night sweats, chest pain, and persistent cough.
3. Cough, initially nonproductive, may progress to mucopurulent sputum with hemoptysis.

DIAGNOSTIC EVALUATION

Initially: TB skin test, sputum culture, chest x-ray.

MANAGEMENT

The goals of management are to relieve pulmonary and systemic symptoms; to return the patient to health, work, and family life as quickly as possible; and to prevent transmission of the infection.

Chemotherapy

1. Therapy for 6–12 months.
2. First-line medications: isoniazid (INH), rifampin (RIF), streptomycin (SM), ethambutol (EMB), and pyrazinamide (PZA) for 4 months, with INH and RIF continuing for an additional 2 months.
3. Second-line medications: capreomycin, kanamycin, ethionamide, para-aminosalicylate sodium, amikacin, cyclizine.
4. Person is considered noninfectious after 2–3 weeks of continuous therapy.

Preventive Treatment

Identify persons at risk: INH for preventive therapy is given in a single daily dose for 6–12 months.

NURSING PROCESS

Assessment

1. Perform complete history and physical examination.
2. Perform respiratory assessment exploring presence of fever, anorexia, weight loss, night sweats, fatigue, cough, and sputum production.
3. Assess change in temperature, respiratory rate, amount and color of secretions, frequency and severity of cough, and chest pain.
4. Evaluate breath sounds for consolidation (diminished, bronchial, or bronchovesicular sounds, crackles), fremitus, egophony, and percussion (dullness).
5. Assess for enlarged, painful lymph nodes.
6. Assess emotional readiness to learn, perceptions and understanding of TB.

T

7. Review results of physical and laboratory evaluations.

Major Nursing Diagnosis

1. Ineffective airway clearance related to copious tracheobronchial secretions.
2. Nonadherence to treatment regimens.
3. Knowledge deficit about preventive health measures.

Collaborative Problems

1. Malnutrition.
2. Side effects of medication therapy, i.e., hepatitis, neurological changes (deafness or neuritis), skin rash.
3. Multidrug resistance.
4. Spread of TB infection (miliary TB).

Planning and Implementation

The major goals include maintenance of a patent airway, knowledge about the disease and treatment regimen, adherence to the medication regimen, increased activity tolerance, and absence of complications.

Interventions

PROMOTING AIRWAY CLEARANCE

1. Instruct about best position to facilitate drainage.
2. Encourage increased fluid intake.
3. Provide a high-humidity face mask/humidifier.

ADVOCATING ADHERENCE AND PREVENTION

1. Instruct that TB is a communicable disease and taking medications is the most effective way of preventing transmission.
2. Instruct patient about hygienic measures, including mouth care, covering mouth and nose when coughing and sneezing, proper disposal of tissues, and handwashing.
3. Clarify medications, schedule, and side effects.

MONITORING AND MANAGING POTENTIAL COMPLICATIONS

1. Collaborate with health care team to identify strategies to assure adequate nutritional intake and availability of nutritious foods.
2. Assess for side effects of medication therapy.
3. Encourage liver and kidney function follow-up.
4. Monitor sputum culture results to evaluate effectiveness of therapy.
5. Teach to take medications on empty stomach or 1 hour before meals because food interferes with drug absorption.
6. Teach patients on INH to avoid foods containing tyramine and histamine.
7. Inform that rifampin may discolor contact lenses; wear eye glasses.
8. Instruct about risk of drug resistance if regimen not followed continuously; failure to comply will result in multidrug resistance.
9. Caution about the spread of TB infection to nonpulmonary sites of the body (miliary TB), a consequence of late reactivation of dormant infection.

✎ PATIENT EDUCATION AND HEALTH MAINTENANCE: CARE IN THE HOME AND COMMUNITY

1. Assess the ability of the patient to continue therapy at home.
2. Arrange follow-up screening for potentially infected contacts.
3. Instruct patient and family about infection control procedures.
4. Teach and use universal precautions for body fluids, including sputum.
5. Demonstrate and stress good handwashing technique.
6. Instruct to cover mouth when coughing; use disposable tissues if available, place in paper bag, and discard.

T

Gerontologic Considerations

May have atypical manifestations in elderly, i.e., unusual behavior and altered mental status, fever, anorexia, and weight loss. Increasingly encountered in the nursing home population.

For more information see Chapter 24 in Smeltzer and Bare: *Brunner and Suddarth's Textbook of Medical–Surgical Nursing,* 8th Edition. Philadelphia: Lippincott–Raven, 1996.

TUMORS, BLADDER

See Cancer of the Bladder

TUMORS, BONE

See Bone Tumors

TUMORS, BRAIN

See Brain Tumors

TUMORS, BREAST

See Cancer of the Breast

TUMORS, CERVICAL

See Cancer of the Cervix

TUMORS, COLON

See Cancer of the Large Intestine (Colon and Rectum)

TUMORS, ENDOMETRIAL

See Cancer of the Endometrium

TUMORS, ESOPHAGUS

See Cancer of the Esophagus

TUMORS, KIDNEY

See Cancer of the Kidney

TUMORS, LARYNX

See Cancer of the Larynx

TUMORS, LIVER

See Cancer of the Liver

TUMORS, LUNG

See Cancer of the Lung

TUMORS, ORAL CAVITY

See Cancer of the Oral Cavity

TUMORS, OVARIAN

See Cancer of the Ovary

TUMORS, PANCREAS

See Cancer of the Pancreas

TUMORS, PITUITARY

See Pituitary Tumors

TUMORS, PROSTATE

See Cancer of the Prostate

TUMORS, RECTUM

See Cancer of the Large Intestine (Colon and Rectum)

TUMORS, STOMACH

See Cancer of the Stomach

TUMORS, TESTIS

See Cancer of the Testis

TUMORS, VAGINA

See Cancer of the Vagina

TUMORS, VULVA

See Cancer of the Vulva

ULCER

See Peptic Ulcer

ULCER, STRESS

See Stess Ulcer

ULCERATIVE COLITIS

Ulcerative colitis is a recurrent ulcerative and inflammatory disease of the mucosal layer of the colon and rectum. It is a serious disease, accompanied by systemic complications and a high mortality rate. Eventually 10–15% of the patients develop carcinoma of the colon. It is characterized by multiple ulcerations, diffuse inflammations, and desquamation of the colonic epithelium, with alternating periods of exacerbation and remission.

CLINICAL MANIFESTATIONS

1. Predominant symptoms: diarrhea, abdominal pain, intermittent tenesmus, ineffective straining at stool, and rectal bleeding.
2. Anorexia, weight loss, fever, vomiting, dehydration, as well as cramping and feeling an urgent need to defecate (may report passing 10–20 liquid stools daily).
3. Hypocalcemia and anemia frequently develop.
4. Rebound tenderness may occur in right lower quadrant.
5. Other symptoms include skin lesions, eye lesions (uveitis), joint abnormalities, and liver disease.

U

DIAGNOSTIC EVALUATION

1. Stool examination to rule out dysentery and test for blood.
2. Sigmoidoscopy and barium enema.
3. Blood studies.

MEDICAL MANAGEMENT

Medical treatment for both regional enteritis and ulcerative colitis is aimed at reducing inflammation, suppressing inappropriate immune responses, and providing rest for a diseased bowel, so healing may take place.

Diet and Fluid Intake

1. Oral fluids, low-residue, high-protein, high-calorie diets with supplemental vitamin therapy and iron replacement.
2. Correct fluid and electrolyte imbalance by intravenous therapy.
3. Avoid foods that exacerbate diarrhea; avoid milk, cold foods, and also smoking; total parenteral nutrition as indicated.

Drug Therapy

1. Sedative and antidiarrheal/antiperistaltic medications.
2. Sulfonamides, i.e., sulfasalazine (Azulfidine) or sulfisoxazole (Gantrisin) effective for mild or moderate inflammation.
3. Antibiotics for secondary infections.
4. Adrenocorticotropic hormone (ACTH) and corticosteroids.
5. Aminosalicylates (topical and oral).

Psychotherapy

Aimed at determining the factors that distress the patient, coping with these factors, and attempting to resolve conflicts.

Surgical Management

When conservative measures fail to relieve the severe symptoms of inflammatory bowel disease, surgery may be recommended.

NURSING PROCESS

Assessment

OBTAINING HEALTH HISTORY

1. Onset and duration of abdominal pain; presence of diarrhea, tenesmus, nausea, anorexia, weight loss.
2. Dietary pattern, including amounts of alcohol, caffeine, and nicotine used daily/weekly.
3. Family history of inflammatory bowel disease.
4. Allergies, especially to milk/lactose.
5. Assess bowel elimination patterns including character, frequency, and presence of blood, pus, fat, or mucus.

Objective Assessment

1. Auscultate for bowel sounds and their characteristics.
2. Palpate for distention, tenderness, or pain.
3. Inspect the skin for evidence of fistula tracts or symptoms of dehydration; inspect stool for blood.

Regional Enteritis

1. Most prominent symptom is intermittent pain associated with diarrhea that does not decrease with defecation.
2. Pain usually localized in the right lower quadrant.
3. Abdominal tenderness on palpation.
4. Periumbilical regional pain usually indicates involvement of terminal ileum.

Ulcerative Colitis

1. Dominant sign is rectal bleeding.
2. Distended abdomen with rebound tenderness present.

U

Major Nursing Diagnosis

1. Diarrhea related to the inflammatory process.
2. Abdominal pain related to increased peristalsis and inflammation.
3. Fluid volume and electrolyte deficits related to anorexia, nausea, and diarrhea.
4. Anxiety related to impending surgery.
5. Ineffective individual coping related to repeated episodes of diarrhea.
6. Risk for impaired skin integrity related to malnutrition and diarrhea.
7. Knowledge deficit concerning the process and management of the disease.

Collaborative Problems

1. Cardiac dysrhythmias.
2. Gastrointestinal bleeding with fluid volume loss.
3. Perforation of the bowel.

Planning and Implementation

The major goals may include attainment of normal bowel elimination, relief of abdominal pain and cramping, prevention of fluid volume deficit, maintenance of optimal nutrition and weight, avoidance of fatigue, reduction of anxiety, effective coping, prevention of skin breakdown, acquisition of knowledge and understanding of the disease process and therapeutic regimen, and absence of potential complications.

Interventions

MAINTAINING NORMAL ELIMINATION PATTERNS

1. Determine if there is a relationship between diarrhea and certain foods, activity, or emotional stress.
2. Identify any precipitating factors, as well as stool frequency, consistency, and amount.
3. Provide ready access to bathroom or bedpan; keep environment clean and odor free.

4. Administer antidiarrheal agents as prescribed and record frequency and consistency of stools after therapy has started.
5. Encourage bed rest to decrease peristalsis.

RELIEVING PAIN

1. Describe character of pain (dull, burning, or cramp-like), onset, pattern, and medication relief.
2. Administer anticholinergic medications 30 minutes before a meal to decrease intestinal motility.
3. Give analgesics as prescribed; reduce pain by position changes, local application of heat (as prescribed), diversional activities, and prevention of fatigue.

MAINTAINING FLUID BALANCE

1. Keep accurate record of intake and output (I&O) including wound or fistula drainage.
2. Monitor weights daily.
3. Assess for signs of fluid volume deficit: dry skin and mucous membranes, decreased skin turgor, oliguria, exhaustion, decreased temperature, increased hematocrit.
4. Evaluate urine specific gravity and hypotension.
5. Encourage oral intake; monitor IV flow rate.
6. Initiate measures to decrease diarrhea: dietary restrictions, stress reduction, and antidiarrheal agents.

PROMOTING NUTRITIONAL MEASURES

1. Use total parenteral nutrition (TPN) when symptoms are severe.
2. Maintain an accurate record of fluid I&O and daily weight during TPN therapy; test for glucose daily.
3. Give feedings high in protein, low in fat and residue after TPN therapy; note intolerance (e.g., vomiting, diarrhea, distention).

U

PROMOTING REST

Recommend intermittent rest periods during day; schedule or restrict activities to conserve energy and reduce metabolic rate.

REDUCING ANXIETY

1. Establish rapport by being attentive and displaying a calm, confident manner.
2. Provide time for patient to ask questions and express feelings.
3. Listen carefully and sensitively to nonverbal indicators of anxiety (restlessness, tense facial expressions).
4. Tailor information about impending surgery to patient's level of understanding and desire.

COPING MEASURES

1. Give essential understanding and emotional support for isolated, helpless, and out-of-control feelings.
2. Recognize that behavior may be affected by innumerable factors unrelated to inherent emotional characteristics.
3. Support patient's attempts to deal with stresses.
4. Communicate that the patient's feelings are understood: encourage to talk and ventilate; discuss any disturbing matters.
5. Use stress-reduction measures: relaxation techniques, breathing exercises, and biofeedback.

PREVENTING SKIN BREAKDOWN

1. Examine patient's skin, especially perianal skin.
2. Provide perianal care after each bowel movement.
3. Give care to reddened or irritated areas over bony prominences.
4. Use pressure-relieving devices to avoid possible skin breakdown.

MONITORING AND MANAGING POTENTIAL COMPLICATIONS

1. Monitor serum electrolyte levels; administer replacements.

2. Report dysrhythmias or change in level of consciousness.

3. Monitor rectal bleeding and give blood and volume expanders.

4. Monitor blood pressure; provide laboratory blood studies often.

5. Monitor for indications of perforation (acute increase in abdominal pain, rigid abdomen, vomiting, or hypotension).

✎ Patient Education and Health Maintenance: Care in the Home and Community

1. Assess for additional information about medical management (medications, diet) and surgical interventions.

2. Provide information about nutritional management (bland, low-residue, high-protein, high-calorie, and high-vitamin diet).

3. Give rationale for using steroids, anti-inflammatory agents, antibacterial, antidiarrheal medications, and antispasmodics.

4. Emphasize importance of taking medications as prescribed and not abruptly discontinuing (especially the steroids, as serious medical problems may result).

5. Explain procedure and preoperative and postoperative care if surgery is required; review ileostomy care as necessary.

6. Explain that disease can be controlled and patient can lead a healthy life between exacerbations.

7. Encourage to rest as needed and modify activities according to energy levels during a flare-up; advise to limit tasks that impose strain on the lower abdominal muscles.

8. Give information about medications and the need to take them on schedule while in home setting, i.e., medication reminders (containers that separate pills according to day and time).

U

9. Recommend low-residue, high-protein, high-calorie diet during an acute phase; encourage to keep a record of foods that irritate bowel and to eliminate them from diet.
10. Provide support for prolonged nature of disease as it is a strain on family life and financial resources.
11. Provide time for patient to express fears and frustrations.

For more information see Chapter 37 in Smeltzer and Bare: *Brunner and Suddarth's Textbook of Medical–Surgical Nursing*, 8th Edition. Philadelphia: Lippincott–Raven, 1996.

UNCONSCIOUS PATIENT

Unconsciousness is a condition in which cerebral function is depressed, ranging from stupor to coma. In stupor, the patient shows symptoms of annoyance when stimulated by something unpleasant, i.e., pinprick or loud slapping of hands; may draw back or make facial grimaces or unintelligible sounds. Coma is a clinical state of unconsciousness in which the patient is unaware of self and environment. Akinetic mutism is a state of unresponsiveness to the environment in which the patient makes no movement or sound but sometimes has eyes open. A persistent vegetative state is one in which the patient is described as wakeful, without cognitive or effective mental function. The causes of unconsciousness may be neurologic (head injury, stroke), toxicologic (drug overdose, alcohol intoxication), or metabolic (hepatic or renal failure, diabetic ketoacidosis).

DIAGNOSTIC EVALUATION

1. Neurologic examination.
2. Laboratory tests: major chemical profile, serum ammonia, osmolality, prothrombin time, serum ketones, alcohol, drug and arterial blood gases (ABGs).

MANAGEMENT

1. The first priority is to obtain a patent and secure airway.
2. Assess circulatory status (carotid pulse, heart rate and impulse, blood pressure).
3. Maintain adequate oxygenation.
4. Establish IV line to maintain fluid balance status.

NURSING PROCESS

Assessment

Assess for level of responsiveness (consciousness) by using the Glasgow Coma Scale.

1. Evaluate pupil size, equality, and reaction to light; note movement of eyes.
2. Assess facial symmetry, swallowing reflexes, and elicit deep tendon reflexes.
3. Assess for purposeful or nonpurposeful responses: decorticate posturing (arms flexed, adducted, and internally rotated, and legs in extension); decerebrate posturing (extremities extended and reflexes exaggerated).
4. Rule out paralysis or stroke as cause of flaccidity.
5. Examine body functions (circulation, respiration, elimination, fluid and electrolyte balance) in a systemic manner.
6. Suspect a toxic or metabolic disorder if patient is comatose and pupillary light reflex is preserved.
7. Assume neurologic disease present if comatose and localized signs are severe.

Major Nursing Diagnosis

U

1. Ineffective airway clearance related to inability to clear respiratory secretions.
2. Risk for fluid volume deficit related to inability to ingest fluids.
3. Altered oral mucous membranes related to mouth breathing, absence of pharyngeal reflex, and inability to ingest fluids.

4. Risk for impaired skin integrity related to immobility or restlessness.
5. Impaired tissue integrity of cornea related to diminished or absent corneal reflex.
6. Ineffective thermoregulation related to damage to hypothalamic center.
7. Altered family process related to sudden crisis of unconsciousness.

Collaborative Problems

1. Respiratory distress or failure.
2. Pneumonia.
3. Pressure ulcer.

Planning and Implementation

The goals of care during the unconscious period may include maintenance of a clear airway, attainment of fluid volume balance, achievement of intact oral mucous membranes, maintenance of normal skin integrity, absence of corneal irritation or keratitis, attainment of thermoregulation, absence of urinary retention and infection, absence of diarrhea or fecal impaction, maintenance of intact family or support system, and absence of complications.

Interventions

MAINTAINING THE AIRWAY

1. Establish an adequate airway and assure ventilation.
2. Position in a lateral or semiprone position; do not allow to remain on back.
3. Remove secretions to reduce danger of aspiration; elevate head of bed to a 30° angle to prevent aspiration; provide frequent suctioning and oral hygiene.
4. Auscultate chest every 8 hours for crackles, wheezes, or absence of breath sounds.
5. Maintain patency of endotracheal tube or tracheostomy; monitor ABGs; maintain ventilator settings.
6. Promote pulmonary hygiene with chest physiotherapy and postural drainage.

PROVIDING SAFETY

1. Provide padded side rails for protection.
2. Carry out every measure available and appropriate for calming and quieting a disturbed patient; avoid physical restraints if possible to prevent rise in intracranial pressure (ICP).

ATTAINING FLUID AND NUTRITIONAL BALANCE

1. Assess for hydration status: examine mucous membranes; assess skin for tissue turgor.
2. Meet fluid needs by giving required fluids IV and then nasogastric or gastrostomy feedings.
3. Give IV fluids and blood transfusions slowly for patient with intracranial conditions.
4. Never give oral fluids to a patient who cannot swallow; insert feeding tube for administration of enteral feedings.

MAINTAINING HEALTHY ORAL MUCOUS MEMBRANES

1. Inspect mouth for dryness, inflammation, and presence of crusting; cleanse and rinse carefully to remove secretions and crust and keep membranes moist; apply petrolatum on lips.
2. Assess sides of mouth and lips for ulceration if patient has an endotracheal tube.

MAINTAINING SKIN INTEGRITY

1. Give special attention to a regular schedule of turning and repositioning to prevent ischemic necrosis over pressure areas.
2. Give passive exercise of extremities to prevent contractures; use a splint or foam boots to prevent footdrop and eliminate pressure on toes.
3. Keep hip joints and legs in proper alignment with supporting trochanter rolls.
4. Position arms in abduction, fingers lightly flexed, and hands in slight supination.

U

MAINTAINING CORNEAL INTEGRITY

1. Cleanse eyes with cotton balls moistened with sterile normal saline to remove debris and discharge.
2. Instill artificial tears every 2 hours, as necessary.
3. Use cold compresses as prescribed for periocular edema after cranial surgery and avoid contact with cornea.
4. Use eye patches cautiously because of potential for further corneal abrasions.

ATTAINING THERMOREGULATION

1. Determine temperature of environment by patient's condition, e.g., fever.
2. Use prescribed measures to treat hyperthermia; avoid shivering.

PREVENTING URINARY RETENTION

1. Palpate bladder at intervals to determine whether urinary retention is present.
2. Insert indwelling catheter if there are signs of urinary retention; observe for fever and cloudy urine; inspect urethral orifice for drainage.
3. Use external penile catheter (condom catheter) for male patients and absorbent pads for female patients if they can urinate spontaneously.
4. Initiate bladder training program as soon as conscious.
5. Monitor frequently for skin irritation and breakdown; implement appropriate skin care.

PROMOTING BOWEL FUNCTION

1. Evaluate abdominal distention by listening for bowel sounds and measuring girth of the abdomen.
2. Monitor number and consistency of bowel movements; perform a rectal exam for signs of fecal impaction; may require enema every other day to empty lower colon.
3. Enemas may be contraindicated if Valsalva maneuver increases a compromised ICP.

4. Administer stool softeners with tube feedings.

SUPPORTING THE FAMILY

1. Reinforce and clarify information about patient's condition, to permit family members to mobilize their own adaptive capacities.
2. Listen and encourage ventilation of feelings and concerns.
3. Support them in their decision-making process concerning posthospital management and placement.

PROMOTING SENSORY STIMULATION

1. Provide continuing sensory stimulation to help overcome profound sensory deprivation.
2. Make efforts to maintain usual day and night patterns of activity and sleep; orient to time and place every 8 hours.
3. Touch and talk to patient; encourage family and friends to do the same; avoid making any negative comments about status in patient's presence.
4. Introduce sounds from patient's home and workplace by means of a tape recorder.
5. Read favorite books and provide familiar radio and television programs to enrich environment.

ATTAINING SELF-CARE

Begin to teach, support, encourage, and supervise activities of daily living (ADL) as soon as consciousness returns.

MONITORING AND MANAGING POTENTIAL COMPLICATIONS: PNEUMONIA

1. Monitor vital signs and respiratory function for signs of respiratory failure or distress.
2. Assess for adequate red blood cells to carry oxygen, i.e., total blood count and ABGs.
3. Obtain cultures to identify organism for appropriate antibiotics if pneumonia develops.

For more information see Chapter 59 in Smeltzer and Bare: *Brunner and Suddarth's Textbook of Medical–Surgical Nursing*, 8th Edition. Philadelphia: Lippincott–Raven, 1996.

UPPER URINARY TRACT INFECTION

See Pyelonephritis

URINARY BLADDER DISEASE

See Cancer of the Bladder

URINARY TRACT INFECTION, LOWER

See Cystitis

URINARY TRACT INFECTION, UPPER

See Pyelonephritis

UROLITHIASIS

Urolithiasis refers to the presence of stones (calculi) in the urinary system. Stones are formed in the urinary tract when urinary concentrations of substances, i.e., calcium oxalate, calcium phosphate, uric acid, increase. The majority of stones contain calcium or magnesium in combination with phosphorus or oxalate. Calculi may be found anywhere from the kidney to the bladder and vary in size from minute granular deposits, called sand or gravel, to bladder stones the size of an orange. Certain factors favor formation of stones, including infection, urinary stasis, periods of immobility, and altered calcium metabolism (hypercalcemia and hypercalciuria). In many patients no cause may be found. The problem occurs predominantly in the third to fifth decades and affects men more than women. Most stones are radiopaque and can be detected by x-ray.

CLINICAL MANIFESTATIONS

Manifestations depend on presence of obstruction, infection, and edema. Symptoms range from mild to excruciating pain and discomfort.

Stones in Renal Pelvis

1. Intense, deep ache in the costovertebral region.
2. Hematuria and pyuria.
3. Pain radiates anteriorly and downward toward bladder in female and toward testes in male.

Renal Colic

1. Pain acute, costovertebral area exquisitely tender.
2. Nausea, vomiting, diarrhea.
3. Abdominal discomfort may occur.

Ureteral Colic (Stones Lodged in the Ureter)

1. Acute, excruciating, colicky, wavelike pain, radiating down the thigh to the genitalia
2. Frequent desire to void, but very little urine passed; usually contains blood.

Stones Lodged in Bladder

1. Symptoms of irritation associated with urinary tract infection and hematuria.
2. Urinary retention, if stone obstructs bladder neck.
3. Possible sepsis if infection is present with stone.

U

DIAGNOSTIC EVALUATION

Confirmed by kidneys, ureter, bladder (KUB) studies, intravenous urography or retrograde pyelography.

MANAGEMENT

The basic goals are to eradicate the stone, to determine the stone type, prevent nephron destruction, control infection, and relieve any obstruction that may be present.

Pain Relief

1. Administer morphine or meperidine to prevent shock and syncope.
2. Give hot baths or apply moist heat to flank areas.
3. Encourage fluids unless vomiting to assist in passage.
4. Encourage high round-the-clock fluid intake to reduce urine concentration, dilute the urine, and ensure high urinary output.

Stone Removal

1. Cystoscopic examination and passage of small ureteral catheter.
2. Chemical analysis on stones for determination of composition.

Nutrition and Medication Therapy

1. Calcium stones: reduce dietary calcium and phosphorus; medications to acidify urine, i.e., ammonium chloride, Lithostat.
2. Phosphate stones: diet low in phosphorus; aluminum hydroxide gel.
3. Uric stones: low-purine diet; allopurinol (Zyloprim).
3. Cystine stones: low-protein diet; penicillamine.
4. Oxalate stones: maintain dilute urine and limit oxalate intake, e.g., green, leafy vegetables, beans, chocolate, tea, coffee.

Methods of Stone Removal

1. Extracorporeal shock wave lithotripsy (ESWL)
2. Percutaneous nephrostomy.

3. Electrohydraulic lithotripsy.
4. Ureteroscopy: Stones can be fragmented with use of laser, electrohydraulic lithotripsy, or ultrasound, and then removed.
5. Stone dissolution: Alternative for those who are poor risk for other therapy, refuse other methods, or have easily dissolved stones (struvite).
6. Surgical removal: Performed on only 1–2% of patients.

NURSING PROCESS

Assessment

1. Assess for pain and discomfort; severity and location along with any radiation of the pain.
2. Assess for presence of associated symptoms, i.e., nausea, vomiting, diarrhea, and abdominal distention.
3. Observe for signs of urinary tract infection (chills, fever, dysuria, frequency, and hesitancy) and obstruction (frequent urination of small amounts, oliguria, or anuria).
4. Observe urine for presence of blood; strain for stones or gravel.
5. Focus history on factors that predispose to urinary tract stones or may have precipitated current episode of renal or ureteral colic.
6. Assess patient's knowledge about renal stones and measures to prevent their occurrence or recurrence.

Major Nursing Diagnosis

1. Pain related to inflammation, obstruction, and abrasion of the urinary tract.
2. Knowledge deficit regarding prevention of recurrence of renal stones.

U

Collaborative Problems

1. Infection and sepsis (from UTI and pyelonephritis).
2. Obstruction of the urinary tract by a stone or edema with subsequent acute renal failure.

Planning and Implementation

The major goals may include relief of pain and discomfort, prevention of recurrence of renal stones, and prevention of complications.

Interventions

RELIEVING PAIN

1. Use narcotic analgesics as prescribed.
2. Encourage and assist to assume a position of comfort.
3. Assist patient by ambulating to obtain some pain relief.
4. Monitor pain closely and report promptly increases in severity.
5. Prepare for treatment, e.g., lithotripsy, if pain unrelieved.

MONITORING AND MANAGING COMPLICATIONS (INFECTION AND OBSTRUCTION)

1. Instruct to report decreased urine volume and bloody or cloudy urine.
2. Monitor total urine output and patterns of voiding.
3. Encourage increased fluid intake.
4. Begin IV fluids if unable to take adequate oral fluids.
5. Observe constantly to detect the spontaneous passage of a stone.
6. Strain urine through gauze.
7. Crush any blood clots passed in urine and inspect sides of urinal and bedpan for clinging stones.
8. Instruct to report any increases in pain; administer analgesics.
9. Monitor patient's vital signs for early signs of infection.

10. Treat infections with antimicrobials prior to stone dissolution.

✎ Patient Education and Health Maintenance: Care in the Home and Community

Provide instructions for home care and follow-up after ESWL.

1. Increase fluid intake to assist passage of stone fragments (may take 6 weeks to several months after procedure).
2. Instruct about signs and symptoms of complications, i.e., fever, decreasing urinary output, and pain).
3. Instruct that hematuria is anticipated but should disappear in 24 hours.
4. Give appropriate dietary instruction according to composition of stones.
5. Encourage to follow a regimen to avoid further stone formation.
6. Maintain a high fluid intake; drink enough to excrete 3000–4000 ml of urine every 24 hours.
7. Adhere to prescribed diet.
8. Avoid sudden increases in environmental temperatures; may cause a fall in urinary volume.
9. Teach to take sufficient fluids in the evening to prevent urine from becoming too concentrated at night.
10. Perform urine cultures every 1–2 months the first year and periodically thereafter.
11. Treat recurrent urinary infection vigorously.
12. Encourage increased mobility whenever possible and discourage ingestion of vitamins (especially vitamin D) and minerals.
13. Instruct about signs and symptoms of complications following surgical procedures that warrant physician notification.

U

14. Emphasize to family and patient the importance of follow-up to assess kidney function and to ensure removal of all kidney stones.
15. Explain prescribed medications, actions, and importance.
16. Give detailed verbal/written information about specific foods.
17. Instruct to monitor and interpret urinary pH.
18. Teach signs and symptoms of stone formation, obstruction, and infection; report these to physician promptly.

For more information see Chapter 43 in Smeltzer and Bare: *Brunner and Suddarth's Textbook of Medical–Surgical Nursing,* 8th Edition. Philadelphia: Lippincott–Raven, 1996.

UTI

See Cystitis

VAGINAL CANCER

See Cancer of the Vagina

VARICIES, ESOPHAGEAL

See Esophageal Varicies

VARICOSE VEINS

See Vein Disorders

VEIN DISORDERS (VENOUS THROMBOSIS, THROMBOPHLEBITIS, PHLEBOTHROMBOSIS, AND DEEP VEIN THROMBOSIS [DVT])

Although the above terms do not necessarily present an identical pathology, for clinical purposes they are often used interchangeably. The exact cause of venous thrombosis remains unclear, although three factors are believed to play a significant role in its development: stasis of blood, injury to the vessel wall, and altered blood coagulation. Thrombophlebitis is an inflammation of the walls of the veins, often accompanied by the formation of a clot. When a clot develops initially in the veins as a result of stasis or hypercoagulability, but without inflammation, the process is referred to as phlebothrombosis. Venous thrombosis can occur in any vein but is most frequent in the veins of the lower extremities. Both superficial and

V

deep veins of the legs may be affected. The danger associated with venous thrombosis is that parts of a clot can become detached and produce an embolic occlusion of the pulmonary blood vessels.

CLINICAL MANIFESTATIONS

1. 50% of all patients have no symptoms.
2. Obstruction of the deep veins of the legs produces edema and swelling of the extremity.
3. Skin over affected leg may become warmer; superficial veins may become more prominent.
4. Bilateral swelling may be difficult to detect.
5. Tenderness occurs later; detected by gently palpating the leg.
6. Homans' sign, (pain in the calf after sharp dorsiflexion of the foot), not specific for deep venous thrombosis because it can be elicited in any painful condition of the calf.
7. In some cases, signs of a pulmonary embolus are the first indication of a deep venous thrombus.
8. Thrombus of superficial veins produces pain or tenderness, redness, and warmth in the involved area.

DIAGNOSTIC EVALUATION

Noninvasive Techniques

Doppler ultrasonography, impedance plethysmography, duplex imaging.

Invasive Techniques

^{251}I-labeled fibrinogen scanning, contrast phlebography (venography).

MANAGEMENT

The goal of management is to resolve the current thrombus and prevent a recurrence.

Therapeutic Anticoagulation

1. Heparin: administered for 10–12 days by intermittent or continuous IV infusion; dosage is regulated by partial thromboplastin time (PTT).
2. Thrombolytic (fibrinolytic) therapy: given within the first 3 days after acute occlusion. Streptokinase, urokinase, and tissue-type plasminogen activator are used.
3. Monitor PTT, prothrombin time, hemoglobin, hematocrit, platelet count, and fibrinogen level frequently.
4. Discontinue drug if bleeding occurs and cannot be stopped.

SURGICAL MANAGEMENT

Thrombectomy is the treatment of choice.

NURSING MANAGEMENT

1. Bed rest, elevation of the affected extremity, elastic stockings, and analgesics for pain.
2. Bed rest for 5–7 days after deep venous thrombosis.
3. Use elastic stocking when patient begins to ambulate.
4. Encourage walking (better than standing or sitting for long periods).
5. Recommend bed exercises, such as dorsiflexion of the foot against a footboard.
6. Apply warm, moist packs to affected extremity to reduce discomfort.
7. Provide additional relief for pain control with mild analgesics as prescribed.

Assessment

1. Assess carefully for early signs of venous disorders in lower extremities.
2. Take history of varicose veins, hypercoagulation, neoplastic disease, cardiovascular disease, or recent major surgery or injury. The obese, the elderly, and women taking oral contraceptives are at risk.

3. Question patient about presence of leg pain, heaviness, any functional impairment, or edema.
4. Inspect legs from groin to feet, noting asymmetry and measuring and recording calf circumference (one early indication of edema is engorgement of the space behind the ankle).
5. Note any increase in temperature in the affected leg.
6. Identify areas of tenderness and any thromboses.

PREVENTIVE MEASURES

Prevention is dependent on identifying risk factors for the development of thrombus and educating the patient on appropriate interventions.

1. Remove elastic stockings for a brief interval at least twice daily; inspect skin for signs of irritation and examine calves for possible tenderness; report any skin changes or signs of tenderness.
2. Intermittent pneumatic compression (IPC) devices can be used with elastic stockings for prevention of DVT; ensure prescribed pressures are not exceeded and assess for comfort.
3. Use of subcutaneous heparin in surgical patients.

❂ GERONTOLOGIC CONSIDERATIONS

Elderly patients may be unable to apply elastic stockings properly. Teach family member who is to assist the patient to apply the stockings so that they do not cause undue pressure on any part of the feet or legs.

Elevate feet and lower legs periodically above heart level when on bed rest. Perform active and passive leg exercises, particularly those involving calf muscles, to increase venous flow preoperatively and postoperatively.

Provide early ambulation in preventing venous stasis. Encourage deep-breathing exercises because they produce increased negative pressure in the thorax, which assists in emptying the large veins.

For more information see Chapter 31 in Smeltzer and Bare: *Brunner and Suddarth's Textbook of Medical–Surgical Nursing,* 8th Edition. Philadelphia: Lippincott–Raven, 1996.

VENOUS THROMBUS

See Pulmonary Embolism

VIRAL HEPATITIS

See Hepatitis, Viral

VITAMIN B$_{12}$ DEFICIENCY

See Anemia, Megaloblastic

VULVAR CANCER

See Cancer of the Vulva

V

ZOLLINGER-ELLISON SYNDROME (GASTRINOMA)

Zollinger-Ellison syndrome is suspected when a patient presents with several peptic ulcers or ulcers that are resistant to standard medical therapy. It is identified by hypersecretion of gastric juice, duodenal ulcers, and gastrinomas (islet cell tumors) in the pancreas. Approximately one-third of gastrinomas are malignant. Diarrhea and steatorrhea (unabsorbed fat in the stool) may be evident. These patients may have coexistent parathyroid adenomas or hyperplasia and exhibit signs of hypercalcemia. The patient's most frequent complaint is epigastric pain.

For more information see Chapter 40 in Smeltzer and Bare: *Brunner and Suddarth's Textbook of Medical–Surgical Nursing*, 8th Edition. Philadelphia: Lippincott–Raven, 1996.

INDEX